ESSENTIAL
PUBLIC HEALTH
MEDICINE

ESSENTIAL PUBLIC HEALTH MEDICINE

R J DONALDSON
OBE, CStJ, DPH, FFPHM
Consultant in Public Health Medicine
Lately Director of the South Eastern Consortium for Training in
Public Health Medicine, St George's Hospital Medical School,
London

L J DONALDSON
MSc(Anatomy), MD, FRCS(Ed), FFPHM
Regional General Manager and Director of Public Health,
Northern Regional Health Authority
Professor of Applied Epidemiology,
University of Newcastle upon Tyne

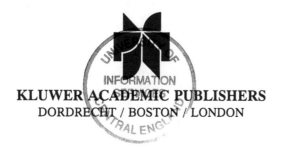

KLUWER ACADEMIC PUBLISHERS
DORDRECHT / BOSTON / LONDON

Distributors

for the United States and Canada: Kluwer Academic Publishers, PO Box 358, Accord Station,
Hingham, MA 02018-0358, USA
for all other countries: Kluwer Academic Publishers Group, Distribution
Center, PO Box 322, 3300 AH Dordrecht, The Netherlands

A catalogue record for this book is available from the British Library.

ISBN 0-7923-8826-7

Copyright

Published in the United Kingdom by Kluwer Academic Publishers,
PO Box 55, Lancaster, UK.

Kluwer Academic Publishers BV incorporates the publishing programmes of
D. Reidel, Martinus Nijhoff, Dr W. Junk and MTP Press.

Typeset by EXPO Holdings, Malaysia.

Printed in Great Britain by Cromwell Press, Melksham, Wiltshire.

Contents

About the authors

Dr R J 'Paddy' Donaldson OBE, CStJ, DPH, FFPHM, has had a long and distinguished career in Public Health Medicine. As a Medical Officer of Health he dealt with the wide range of problems of large urban populations. Later, he held senior academic appointments in London University Medical Schools where his responsibilities included designing and running major training programmes in public health. Dr Donaldson has written extensively on health topics and spoken to health professionals in Britain and many other countries. He has served on many committees which advise government.

Professor Liam Donaldson MSc(Anatomy), MD, FRCS(Ed), FFPHM, Regional General Manager and Director of Public Health, Northern Regional Health Authority and Professor of Applied Epidemiology in the University of Newcastle upon Tyne, is a senior officer of a major health care organisation in the National Health Service. His responsibilities include health policy making, management, research and teaching. He has lectured extensively to staff and students in all health care disciplines and has published widely in medical journals on topics arising from his research and on health policy matters generally. Professor Donaldson serves on a number of national committees.

PUBLISHING ACKNOWLEDGEMENTS

We are grateful to individual publishers, institutions, editors and authors for permission to reproduce material as tables, figures or illustrations. In most cases, this is acknowledged in full through reference to the source as a footnote to the presentation. We wished to take a consistent approach to citations in such footnotes so, in some cases, we have not provided the more detailed forms of words which a number of publishers requested. For this reason, we would like to make the following additional acknowledgements and special thanks here to: the Wellcome Institute Library, London for permission to reproduce the historical illustrations, to BBC Enterprises Limited for permission to reproduce the material in Table 10.2, to the editor of the *American Journal of Epidemiology* and to the authors for permission to reproduce the material in Tables 2.5, 2.7, 3.8 and 7.5, to Cambridge University Press for permission to reproduce the data in Table 7.4, to Oxford University Press for permission to reproduce the material in Figure 8.6, to the Health Education Authority for permission to reproduce material in Table 1.5, Figures 3.1, 3.14 and 3.17, to the Office of Population Censuses and Surveys, the Department of Health, the Central Statistical Office and the World Health Organisation for permission to present various analyses of official statistics throughout the book.

A number of figures and tables are reproduced with the permission of the Controller of Her Majesty's Stationery Office and are Crown Copyright.

COVER ILLUSTRATIONS

The background illustration is of a children's nursery in the Victorian era (see page 306) and the portrait illustrations are of: (centre) Hippocrates (born 460 BC), (bottom left) Louis Pasteur (1822–1895), (bottom right) Bernardin Ramazzini (1663–1714), and (top left) James Lind (1716–1794). Descriptions of the contributions of these individuals to the history of public health are given in Chapter 3.

Introduction

Were it not for the change in the name of the specialty of community medicine to public health medicine which occurred in the late 1980s in the United Kingdom, this book would have been the second edition of *Essential Community Medicine*. The original text aimed to bring together, in one volume, the principles and applications of epidemiology, the main health problems experienced by populations and by the main groups within them, the strategies for intervention to promote health and prevent disease, the main themes underlying health policy formation and a description of the provision of health and social services.

The fact that *Essential Community Medicine* became a standard text in so many institutions of learning and training as well as the large and very positive response we have had from students and practitioners in a variety of disciplines, emboldens us to claim that we largely fulfilled these aims. Students, both undergraduate and postgraduate, in a number of disciplines have even written to us to say that they were successful in examinations through reading the book and receiving no other teaching. As experienced teachers we would not encourage nor would we condone such an approach. Nevertheless, we are heartened that the book provided the breadth and depth of knowledge required.

In building upon these foundations, why then have we seen the need so radically to revise what has become *Essential Public Health Medicine*? Firstly, the last decade has been one of major change, not just in the understanding of the epidemiology of diseases but in the concepts and philosophy of public health and in the structure and functioning of health care services. Secondly, we have benefited from the constructive comments of students and colleagues on the original text.

Each chapter has been entirely recast. Many new themes have been introduced and many subjects dealt with in the earlier book have been brought up-to-date. We have also introduced much material of direct practical relevance.

Chapter 1 of *Essential Public Health Medicine* describes the ways in which an assessment can be made of the health and health needs of a population. The main sources of information on health and health services are reviewed with examples of their uses. The common measures of morbidity and mortality are described together with illustrations about how they are used to describe health problems in populations.

In Chapter 1, we have also introduced a new section on classification systems. We describe the latest version of the International Classification of Diseases (ICD–10) as well as the increasingly important Read Clinical Classification, Diagnostic Related Groups (DRGs) and Healthcare Resource Groups (HRGs). We also cover other health status measures which have emerged, including the influential Quality Adjusted Life Years (QALYs) concept. Throughout this first chapter, we have placed special emphasis on providing simple descriptions and definitions of the concepts involved and on explaining the origins of the common types of routinely available and specially-collected data.

Chapter 2 is an entirely new chapter. It draws together the main approaches of public health investigation starting with the ways in which descriptive epidemiological data can be used to examine the frequency of diseases within and between populations and over time. The main study methods of epidemiology – cross sectional or prevalence studies, cohort studies, case–control studies and randomised controlled trials – are described much more fully than in the earlier book. Emphasis is placed not just on the conceptual basis of these important methods of investigation but on their strengths and weaknesses and their applicability in particular situations. The final section of Chapter 2 gives examples of practical investigations in public health. Each is described from our own experience so that we are able to draw attention to the reality of carrying out such investigations as well as how to interpret and act upon the findings which emerge from them. The field of study is sometimes referred to as 'quick and dirty' investigation. We do not subscribe to this philosophy and our emphasis is on the need for rigour even when a pragmatic approach needs to be taken in deciding the scope of a study and the speed with which it is carried out.

Chapter 3 is also virtually a new chapter. It discusses the concept of health and deals with the subject of health promotion encompassing health education, disease prevention and health protection. The main strategies in health promotion are described in this chapter and the main health problems amenable to intervention in this way are discussed. There are new sections on drug and alcohol abuse, infection with the Human Immune Deficiency Virus (HIV) which causes the Acquired Immune Deficiency Syndrome (AIDS), inequalities in health and nutrition. The previous sections on coronary heart disease, stroke, accidents and presymptomatic screening have been expanded and brought up-to-date.

Special emphasis is given in Chapter 3 to the promotion of health in the younger age groups where the foundations of healthy living can be laid. Many young people become involved in different types of risk-taking behaviour during their teenage years. In the case of smoking, drinking, drug or solvent misuse, such behaviour has considerable impact on current as well as future health. Unhealthy patterns of behaviour can be developed during adolescence which are carried through into maturity and adulthood. Not only must young people be informed and educated, they must be encouraged to practise and adopt a range of strategies which deal with peer and media pressure and allow them to enjoy healthy lifestyles. Chapter 3 discusses these issues and the challenges of, and strategies for, achieving behaviour change in all age groups, particularly young people.

In these first three chapters, many of the scientific foundations of public health medicine are laid down. Throughout the reader is made aware of the strengths and limitations of data, of how data are turned into information and of the challenges in changing human behaviour and designing programmes to promote health and prevent disease.

The modern welfare state is a large and complex structure with diverse origins and traditions. The 1990s sees it in a state of major flux with the introduction of fundamental reforms to the National Health Service and to local government services particularly with the advent of new arrangements for Community Care. Chapter 4 brings together in one place a description of the present structure, organisational framework and method of functioning of this wide range of services.

The implications of the NHS and Community Care Act 1990 are fully described as is the way in which the health service is managed. New sections deal with quality in health care, including total quality management, medical audit, the Patient's Charter and other aspects of health consumerism. The sections on the planning, management and funding of the health service have also been substantially expanded.

Early life is the time when the foundations of health are laid but when some of the risks are greatest. Chapter 5 deals with the health of mothers and children. The main epidemiological features of health and disease in infancy and childhood are described as are the risks to fetal and maternal health. The main measures of fertility in a population are described, so too are the main trends over time in fertility and the factors which can influence the number of completed pregnancies in a population. The causes of death at different periods of infancy are also discussed and the various mortality rates in early life are defined. The range of approaches which can be taken to promote health in pregnancy and childhood are described as are the maternity and child health services themselves.

Increasingly, more and more people in many countries of the world are living into late old age. They will have needs which must be met not just by those services which diagnose and treat illness but also those which enhance their capacity for independent living and provide appropriate support where this is not possible. There are other groups within the population with special needs: adults and children with physical disability, people with mental illness and those with mental handicap (also called learning disability). All these groups need services which are broad based and delivered by a wide range of agencies within the community which are working towards a common purpose. They also need services which are based upon a clear assessment of their needs. This means being familiar with all relevant sources of data and the ways in which they can be used to describe the needs of a group within the population. Chapters 6 (Physical Disability), 7 (Mental Health) and 8 (Elderly People) are concerned with these groups. In these chapters greater emphasis has been placed on defining needs as well as describing the framework of service provision required. The development of care in the community and the need for co-ordination of the work of different care agencies and the professional staff working within them is particularly emphasised. The importance of taking account of, and meeting, the needs of family members and other informal carers is also stressed.

Chapter 9 deals with communicable diseases. We have retained the approach of describing individual diseases which we used in the earlier book but have also introduced a new classification of these important public health problems. We have described more diseases. In *Essential Public Health Medicine* there is also a new emphasis on practical approaches to the investigation and surveillance of communicable diseases, especially the handling of outbreaks and untoward incidents.

The importance of the relationship between the quality of the physical environment and people's health has long been recognised. Moreover, there have been a number of major incidents around the world which have all too dramatically highlighted some of the contemporary threats and hazards, both to the wellbeing of individuals and to the planet itself as with, for example, the Chernobyl nuclear accident and the release of toxic chemicals in Bhopal, India. There is still an enormous amount to be learned about the influence of the environment on health.

The growth in interest and rapidly rising concerns about wider environmental issues make it certain that there will be an increasing focus on the links between environmental and health issues. In Chapter 10, we describe the impact of the environment on health as well as strategies for promoting health through the creation of healthier environments.

In introducing *Essential Public Health Medicine* to our readers both old and new, we believe we have built upon the successful formula of its predecessor. However, looking at it afresh, revising and introducing much new material, we have been able to encompass the entire scope of modern public health medicine as well as describing and discussing the range of services required to provide a comprehensive system of care. We look forward to continuing to receive the views of our readers in providing the kinds of constructive comments which we have found so valuable in the past.

We would like to acknowledge our special thanks to a number of colleagues who have so generously provided their specialist expertise in commenting on the book. They are: Raj Bhopal, Sarah O'Brien, Martin White, Keith Boddy, Jim Smith, Edmund Hey, Leonard Barron, Richard Thomson, David Flory, Angus McNay, David Kay, Deborah Richardson-Kelly, Eugene Milne, Antek Lejk, Marie O'Donnell, Barbara Howe, Mike Barnes, Ian Dalton, Frances Howie, Allan Colver, Tom Fryers, Tim van Zwanenberg, Bill Kirkup, Neil Craig, Sheila Delaney, Chris Foy, Peter Hill, John Woodhouse, Joan Shaw and Brenda Sherwin. Any omissions or errors of fact and interpretation are our own.

Finally, we owe a deep debt of gratitude to Wendy Smith, Anna Martyn and to Phil Johnstone (our publisher).

1 Assessing the health of the population: Information and its uses

INTRODUCTION

One of the great strengths of the National Health Service, and one which has endured since its inception in 1948, is the concept of responsibility for the health of geographically defined populations, not just the patients who seek help from the service.

This is in contrast to the health care systems of some other countries where the population for which health care is provided is not so readily identifiable or comprises, for example, those subscribing to a health insurance plan. In Britain, a framework of service provision helps to ensure that a comprehensive range of care, based in general practice, in hospital and in the community, is made available to local populations on the basis of their health needs.

The assessment of a population's health needs is not, however, a straightforward process. Health is not easily defined, other than in broad terms, and it certainly cannot be measured with precision. Instead, a wide range of sources of data are available, some used as proxies, to illustrate, with appropriate analysis, different aspects of the health of a population living in a particular place: its size and composition; the people's lifestyles; the illnesses and diseases which are experienced; and those of its numbers who are born or who die. By piecing together information from different sources, of different types and to which different levels of importance are attached, it is possible to begin to develop an understanding of the health of a population.

This first chapter describes the main ways of obtaining data which can contribute to the assessment of a population's health. A distinction needs to be made between 'health related' and 'health service' data. 'Health related' refers primarily to demographic data (population size for example); or data describing mortality and fertility experience. 'Health service' refers to data about the use which a population makes of the health service, such as number of episodes of inpatient hospital care; number of contacts with general practitioners or the use of community nursing services. This distinction is important because many 'health related' data are not collected by the health service but by the government under Acts of Parliament. There is a legal requirement to carry out population counts at certain times and to register a birth or a death. In contrast, much health service data are collected as part of the normal operational work of the service, though without the formal rigour of, for example, a birth or death certification process.

All sources of health data, to a varying degree, are subject to quantitative and qualitative deficiencies which limit the conclusions which can be drawn from them. These drawbacks are best appreciated by being familiar with the way in which the data are gathered.

POPULATION: SIZE AND COMPOSITION

Fundamental to any consideration of population is a periodic count of the number and characteristics of people in a given area. This is known as the population census.

The census

A census has been carried out every ten years in Great Britain since 1801, except in 1941 during the Second World War. Authority for the census is enshrined in the 1920 Census Act. Before each census there is extensive public consultation on conduct and content.

The law requires that all people alive on the night of the census are enumerated in the household or establishment where they spent that night. A household is defined as one person living alone or a small group of people, who may or may not be related, living at the same address, temporary residents being included. The country is divided into enumeration districts, commonly each being several hundred households. An enumerator for each district ensures that the head of the household completes a form giving details of every person in that household.

In the 1991 Census, data were collected about the household as well as about individuals. The former comprise postcode, type of building, number of rooms, tenure, the presence of certain amenities (bath, shower, toilet, central heating) and the number of cars or vans. The head of household then lists the names of people in the household, in each case stating their: sex; date of birth; marital status; usual address; relationship to head (for example, wife, daughter); whereabouts on the night of the Census (if absent); address one year previously; country of birth; ethnic group; the presence of long term illness, health problem or handicap which limits daily activities; whether they are working and details of occupation and employment; higher education; the address of students and school children; and usual means of transport to work. Similar information is required for members of the household absent on census night. People aged 18 years or over are asked also about higher qualifications. In Scotland and Wales, questions are asked about people's ability to speak, read or write Gaelic or Welsh.

The census is co-ordinated by the Office of Population, Censuses and Surveys (OPCS), which collates and processes all of the census data, under conditions where strict confidentiality is observed. Names are not entered into computers for processing but used only for internal checking of completeness and accuracy of forms. In analysis, great care is taken not to differentiate very small communities in which an individual person might be identified.

All data about households and individuals, other than that for persons aged 16 years and over, are processed fully. The individual questions about persons aged 16 years and over are processed only on a 10% sample basis, given the costs involved in their coding. Publication of results takes three forms. Firstly, in published reports, secondly, in analyses made available on request and thirdly, advances in computer technology have greatly improved the facility to handle census data so that relatively inexpensive packages are available to enable handling of analyses (including mapping) down to small areas, on local mainframe and micro computers.

The completeness of the census is difficult to estimate. Clearly, enumeration of 100% of the population is the aim. Problems in underestimation include the tendency to overlook very young children and the homeless. Accuracy is also difficult to assess. Statements on age and marital status are sometimes inaccurate, and particular problems arise with vague and imprecise statements of occupation, on which social class analysis is based. Nevertheless, and notwithstanding these difficulties, the decennial census represents a most valuable periodic count of the population, for use as a baseline in further analyses.

Ethnic minority populations

The 1991 census was the first to include a question on ethnic groups and therefore enabled the analysis of local populations in these terms. Ethnic minority people have special needs which are important to the provision of health services (Table 1.1). The non-white population makes up approximately five per cent of the population of Britain. The largest proportion of this population lives in London with relatively high proportions also living in the West Midlands, East Midlands, West and South Yorkshire, and the North West (Figure 1.1). The ethnic minority population is not a homogenous group. The main groups are those of Afro-Caribbean or of Asian (Indian, Pakistani or Bangladeshi) origin. Nor is the ethnic minority population evenly distributed within the population of Britain. The populations of Bradford, Birmingham, Southall, Tower Hamlets and Leicester all contain substantial numbers of 'Asians' but these same populations are very differently composed. Whether an Asian man or woman is a Hindu, a Muslim or a Sikh, whether he or she came to Britain directly from India, Pakistan, Bangladesh or had lived or been brought up in East Africa, may all be important influences on the kinds of health problems to be expected, and the appropriate approach required for the planning and provision of services.

Generally, the age structure of people belonging to ethnic groups is younger than the indigenous population but as the population ages the special problems of their elder members will pose challenges for services in the future.

Table 1.1: *Ethnic minority populations: areas where cultural differences have implications for health or the provision of services*

- Uptake of services
- Presentation of illness
- Perceptions of health and disease
- Lifestyle and cultural practices
- Encounters with services
- Patterns of disease
- Use of alternative medicine

Source: Donaldson LJ, Odell A. Planning and providing services for the Asian population: a survey of District Health Authorities. Journal of the Royal Society of Health 1984; 6:199–202.

Population estimates and projections

Whilst the population census takes place usually every ten years, there is clearly the need to produce statements of population size, and details of characteristics such as age and sex, for periods between census points. Such statements are produced annually and are called population estimates.

Population estimates are derived by taking the census as a baseline, adding births, subtracting deaths and making an allowance for migration. Since births and deaths are events which have to be registered as a legal requirement, these

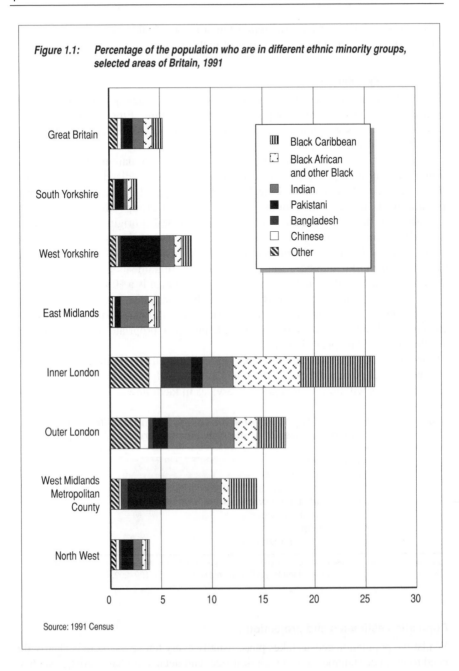

Figure 1.1:   Percentage of the population who are in different ethnic minority groups,
               selected areas of Britain, 1991

Source: 1991 Census

components of estimation are reasonably sound. The weakness in the process is the allowance made for migration. Information on external migration (that is in and out of Britain) is reasonably accurate, but an understanding of internal migration has to be based on an accumulation of local knowledge, including things such as new housing development, clearance of old housing estates and the mass movement of population to other areas.

Population estimates become less reliable as time moves away from the census baseline, but they are nevertheless valuable and, for many uses, they are quite adequate.

Population estimates deal with populations between census points. In contrast, population projections are attempts to forecast the characteristics and size of populations into the future, making assumptions about fertility, mortality and migration. Population projections can be quite accurate in the short term. For example, a projection of the number of people aged 65–74 years in 20 years time will be quite accurate, as the number of people aged 45–54 years now is known, as is the expected mortality of this age group. On the other hand, a projection of the number of school children in 30 years time will be less accurate because current fertility experience may not be maintained for the next 15 to 25 years. For this reason, population projections are often produced as a series, giving alternative figures based on whether low, intermediate or high levels of fertility are assumed.

SOME IMPORTANT CLASSIFICATION SYSTEMS

The remainder of this chapter deals with other kinds of health related data, as well as some examples of health service data. As many of these data use certain classification systems, this section provides some prior description of them. There are three main classifications: those relating to diagnoses and causes of death, those relating to operative procedures and interventions, and those associated with geographical location.

International Classification of Diseases, Tenth Revision (ICD-10)

The World Health Organisation, by international agreement, produces 'The International Statistical Classification of Diseases and Health Related Problems' or 'ICD' as it is commonly known, and this is used in many countries as the principal means of classifying and coding both mortality and morbidity experience.

The latest revision of the ICD, known as ICD-10, was published by the World Health Organisation in 1992, and replaced its predecessor, ICD-9, as the standard coding system. The existence and widespread use of such an internationally agreed disease classification is of vital importance. Without it, comparisons of statistics over time and between different places would not be possible in any valid or meaningful form. Through the years, the classification has moved from being disease orientated, and primarily a means of assigning causes of death, to include a wider framework of illness and other health problems.

The tenth revision groups diagnoses, signs and symptoms, causes and other factors into 21 chapters, starting with those relating to infectious and parasitic diseases and ending with codes for factors influencing health status and contact with health services (Table 1.2). The codes are alphanumeric, and run from A00.0

to Z99.9, excluding the letter U, which is reserved for additional codes and changes arising between revisions of the classification. The first three characters of a code define a category, with the fourth character supplying extra detail. Hence K26 is the category 'Duodenal ulcer' and K26.1 is 'Duodenal ulcer – acute with perforation'. Figure 1.2 shows a short extract from the chapter on diseases of the digestive system to illustrate the range of code numbers available for a common surgical condition. The classification thus provides a glossary which allows for greater precision and uniformity in medical diagnosis. It allows coding of varying medical terminology for essentially the same condition and brings together similar conditions in a stock classification.

Table 1.2:   *Composition of chapters in the tenth revision of the International Classification of Diseases (ICD–10)*

Chapter number & designation		Range of codes
I	Certain infectious and parasitic diseases	A00–B99
II	Neoplasms	C00–D48
III	Diseases of the blood and blood-forming organs and certain disorders involving the immune mechanism	D50–D89
IV	Endocrine, nutritional and metabolic diseases	E00–E90
V	Mental and behavioural disorders	F00–F99
VI	Diseases of the nervous system	G00–G99
VII	Diseases of the eye and adnexa	H00–H59
VIII	Diseases of the ear and mastoid process	H60–H95
IX	Diseases of the circulatory system	I00–I99
X	Diseases of the respiratory system	J00–J99
XI	Diseases of the digestive system	K00–K93
XII	Diseases of the skin and subcutaneous tissue	L00–L99
XIII	Diseases of the musculo-skeletal system and connective tissue	M00–M99
XIV	Diseases of the genito-urinary system	N00–N99
XV	Pregnancy, childbirth and the puerperium	O00–O99
XVI	Certain conditions originating in the perinatal period	P00–P95
XVII	Congenital malformations, deformations, and chromosomal abnormalities	Q00–Q99
XVIII	Symptoms, signs and abnormal clinical and laboratory findings, not elsewhere classified	R00–R99
XIX	Injury, poisoning and certain other consequences of external causes	S00–T98
XX	External causes of morbidity and mortality	V01–Y98
XXI	Factors influencing health status and contact with health services	Z00–Z99

Source: Ashley, J. The international classification of diseases: the structure and content of the 10th revision. Health Trends 1990/91; 4: 135–7.

Classification of Surgical Operations and Procedures (OPCS-4)

In Britain, the primary classification of operative procedures and other interventions is the Fourth Revision of the Office of Population, Censuses and Surveys Classification of Surgical Operations and Procedures, known as OPCS-4. The codes use a similar format to those in ICD-10 and cover procedures within anatomical systems as well as subsidiary codes for methods (laser therapy for example) and specific sites of operation (such as upper inner quadrant of the breast).

Figure 1.2:   Extract from the chapter on diseases of
the digestive system within the tenth revision of
the International Classification of Diseases (ICD-10)

K35   **Acute Appendicitis**

K35.0   **Acute appendicitis with generalized peritonitis**
Appendicitis (acute) with:
- perforation
- peritonitis (generalized)
- rupture

K35.1   **Acute appendicitis with peritoneal abscess**
Abscess of appendix

K35.9   **Acute appendicitis, unspecified**
Acute appendicitis without:
- perforation
- peritoneal abscess
- peritonitis
- rupture

K36   **Other appendicitis**
Appendicitis:
- chronic
- recurrent

K37   **Unspecified appendicitis**

Reproduced, by permission, from: ICD-10 International statistical classification of
diseases and related health problems. Tenth revision, Volume 1. Geneva, World Health
Organization, 1992, p. 569.

The Read Clinical Classification

A relatively recent development (certainly in contrast to the longstanding
diagnostic and surgical systems described above) is the Read Clinical
Classification, referred to commonly as the Read codes. This is a comprehensive,
coded, computerised, hierarchically arranged thesaurus of terms used in health care.
The 5-character alpha-numeric codes cover both diagnoses and operations, as well
as other features such as history and symptomatology, findings on examination and
signs, laboratory and radiological procedures, occupations, social information and
drugs and appliances. The Read Clinical Classification contains over 250,000 codes
including a synonym list of 150,000 terms. It is still being added to. Read codes
were endorsed by the Department of Health as the standard clinical coding system
for general practice in 1990. It is intended that they will be used in all National
Health Service information systems. Read codes are designed to be a superset of a
number of other standard coding systems, including ICD-10 and OPCS-4; they are
thus at least as detailed as these classifications and can be translated back to them.
Read codes are intended to cover most types of information in a clinical record.
Doctors can continue to use their preferred clinical terms which are then converted
automatically by computer software into a Read code.

Postcodes

Classification by geographical location of residence is of increasing importance in health care, both for epidemiological and administrative purposes. For example, locating the homes of individuals with a particular disease permits exploration of that disease's relationship with specific geographical features or it can allow calculation of disease rates for specific communities. The precision of geographical location needed will depend on the particular analysis being performed. It makes sense, therefore, to use a building block from which appropriately sized 'patches' can be assembled. Ideally, one would wish to use the precise grid reference of each home but this is not routinely collected. Postcodes, however, are readily available and are now the primary geographical unit of all mortality, fertility and health service recording in Britain. The postcode is based on a maximum of seven characters, for example, NE30 4ET. In this example, 'NE' denotes the postcode area, of which there are about 120 in the country. The '30' represents a postcode district, and the '4' the postcode sector within a district. Finally, the 'ET' identifies a small geographical area (commonly about 15 households) within a sector which is known as the unit postcode. There are 1.7 million unit postcodes in the United Kingdom. Naturally, there are problems with the use of postcodes. For example, not all people know or remember them accurately and, inevitably, there are delays in the issuing of new postcodes to cover housing development.

All birth, death and most patient-based service data are now postcoded. This fact and the availability of computer programs to assign postcodes to local or health authority areas and approximate grid references means that postcodes are a very powerful tool for geographical analysis of health data (Figure 1.3).

Diagnosis Related Groups (DRGs)

Codings of diagnoses and operations using the classification systems described in this section are essentially primary, in that they represent the finest level of detail routinely available. Increasingly, classification systems at a secondary level are being used. These take one or more of these, or other, primary classifications together with factors such as age and sex, to produce broader groupings that describe clinical activity called measures of case mix. Diagnosis Related Groups (DRGs) are probably the best known example of these, having been used by the Medicare system in the United States since 1983 for reimbursement of health service charges. The most widely used version of this system has 467 groups, each defined by one or more of: diagnosis, surgical procedure, comorbidities and complications, age, sex and discharge disposition. Such groupings have been examined in the British hospital service in an attempt to describe case mix in clinically coherent and iso-resource terms.

Healthcare Resource Groups (HRGs)

More recently, Healthcare Resource Groups (HRGs) have been developed, and continue to be refined as a specific British evolution of DRGs, both for use within hospitals, and possibly as a vehicle for contracting purposes.

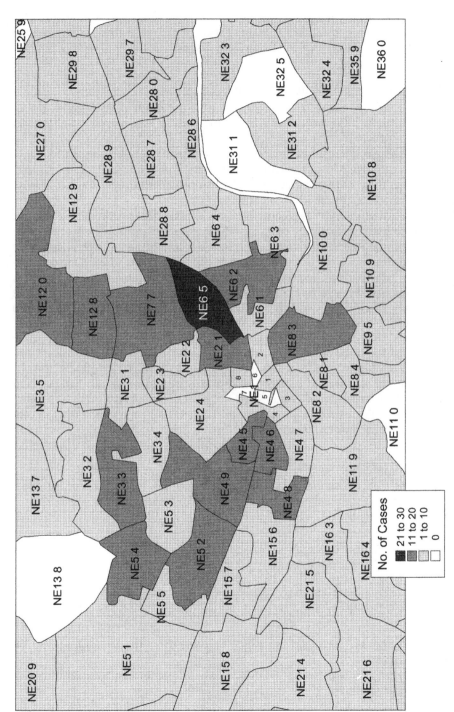

Figure 1.3: Distribution of Chlamydia cases in an urban conurbation by postcode sector, 1992

MORTALITY

Examination of a population's mortality experience is still a good starting point in assessing its health even though today many diseases are not immediately fatal.

Registration and certification of death

In Britain, and most developed countries, it is a legal requirement to record deaths. Provision for this was made in an Act of Parliament in 1836 and made compulsory in 1874.

This process is organised by the Office of Population, Censuses and Surveys (OPCS), through a local network of registration and sub-registration districts throughout the country, administered by Superintendent Registrars and Registrars who are appointed by the local authority.

When a death occurs, the registered medical practitioner concerned is required by law to issue a medical certificate of the cause of death (Figure 1.4). This statement must indicate the date the deceased was last seen alive, whether the body was seen after death, the length of time between onset of any disease and death, as well as whether the certified cause of death is based on post-mortem evidence. This certificate may be sent by post to the local Registrar of Deaths, although it is commonly given to the so called qualified informant (usually a close relative) who must attend the Registrar's office to give, orally, details of place and date of death, name, sex, date and place of birth of the deceased, and the deceased person's occupation and place of residence. Normally, the Registrar is then able to complete a local death Register and issue an order permitting disposal of the body. Returns on deaths are sent weekly to the OPCS for processing, where the 'International Statistical Classification of Diseases and Related Conditions' is used to code cause of death. Another extract is also sent to the Director of Public Health of the health district in which the dead person resided.

Certification of cause of death

The cause of death certification falls into two sections. Part I asks for the direct cause of death (Ia) together with conditions (if any) leading to the direct cause of death. For example:

Ia Uraemia
Ib Acute retention of urine
Ic Benign prostatic hypertrophy
            or
Ia Acute myocardial infarction
Ib
Ic

Part II asks for the significant condition contributing to death, if any, as for example:

II Diabetes mellitus

A common problem with medical certification is the use of mode of dying (cardiac arrest, renal failure) as cause of death. This is of no value. If no other details

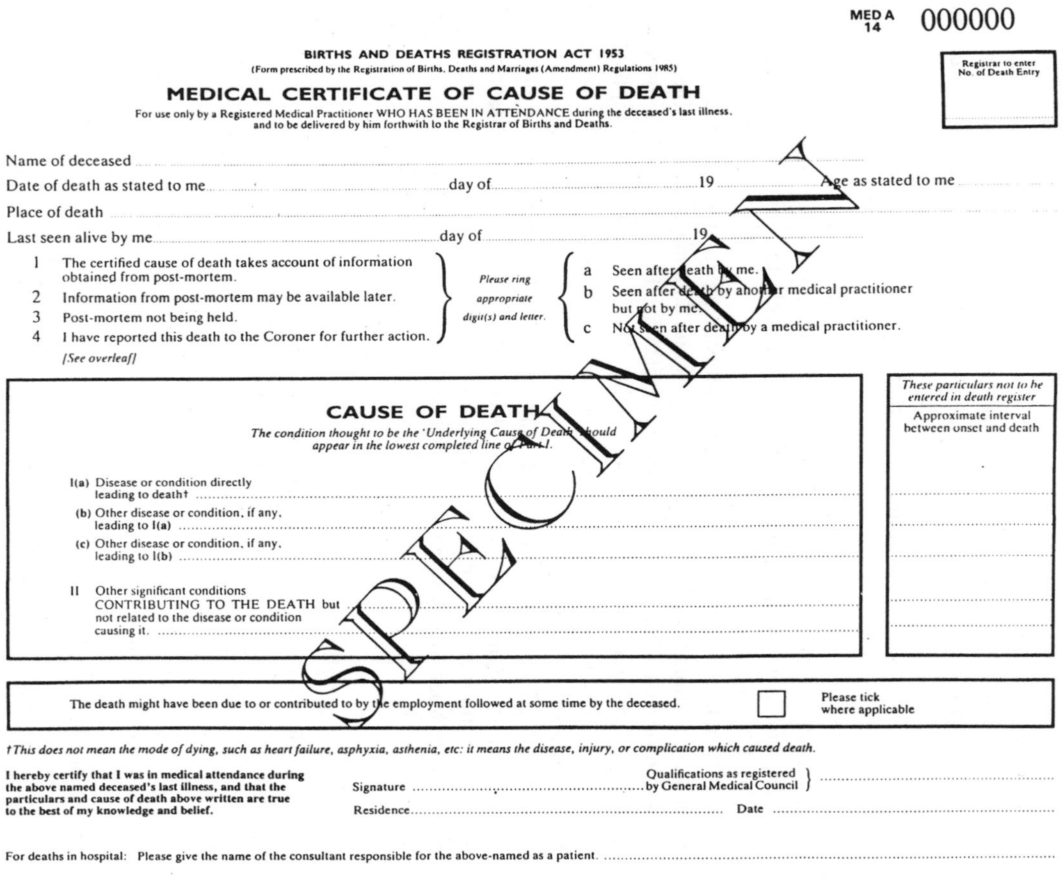

MED A 14 000000

Registrar to enter No. of Death Entry

BIRTHS AND DEATHS REGISTRATION ACT 1953
(Form prescribed by the Registration of Births, Deaths and Marriages (Amendment) Regulations 1985)

MEDICAL CERTIFICATE OF CAUSE OF DEATH

For use only by a Registered Medical Practitioner WHO HAS BEEN IN ATTENDANCE during the deceased's last illness, and to be delivered by him forthwith to the Registrar of Births and Deaths.

Name of deceased ....

Date of death as stated to me .... day of .... 19 .... Age as stated to me ....

Place of death ....

Last seen alive by me .... day of .... 19 ....

1 The certified cause of death takes account of information obtained from post-mortem.
2 Information from post-mortem may be available later.
3 Post-mortem not being held.
4 I have reported this death to the Coroner for further action.
[See overleaf]

Please ring appropriate digit(s) and letter.

a Seen after death by me.
b Seen after death by another medical practitioner but not by me.
c Not seen after death by a medical practitioner.

CAUSE OF DEATH

The condition thought to be the 'Underlying Cause of Death' should appear in the lowest completed line of Part I.

I(a) Disease or condition directly leading to death† ....
(b) Other disease or condition, if any, leading to I(a) ....
(c) Other disease or condition, if any, leading to I(b) ....

II Other significant conditions CONTRIBUTING TO THE DEATH but not related to the disease or condition causing it. ....

These particulars not to be entered in death register
Approximate interval between onset and death

SPECIMEN

The death might have been due to or contributed to by the employment followed at some time by the deceased. ☐ Please tick where applicable

†This does not mean the mode of dying, such as heart failure, asphyxia, asthenia, etc: it means the disease, injury, or complication which caused death.

I hereby certify that I was in medical attendance during the above named deceased's last illness, and that the particulars and cause of death above written are true to the best of my knowledge and belief.

Signature .... Qualifications as registered by General Medical Council ....

Residence .... Date ....

For deaths in hospital: Please give the name of the consultant responsible for the above-named as a patient ....

Figure 1.4: Medical certificate of cause of death

are obtained, such cases would normally be referred to the coroner, as would all cases where the cause is unknown or where there are suspicious circumstances. About a quarter of all deaths are certified by the coroner, usually following a post-mortem examination by a pathologist appointed by the coroner. The coroner must enquire into deaths associated with accidental, violent, unnatural and sudden causes.

The certifier must distinguish direct causes of death from other contributory causes and must show the underlying cause of death in the lowest completed line of Part I of the certificate. Coders at the Office of Population, Censuses and Surveys make the assumption that the certifier has followed this practice. In which case the so-called 'general rule' in coding underlying cause of death applies. In guidelines issued by the World Health Organisation, this general rule must be overridden in certain circumstances, most commonly when the completion of Part I of the certificate does not follow a proper clinical sequence of events. Under these or similar circumstances, coders follow rules which help them to select the underlying cause of death. These issues concerning certification of cause of death and its coding are important because they determine ultimately the content of population level mortality data.

Mortality notification has the advantage that it is legally required, and refers to an event which is unlikely to be missed. Even so, some data may be unreliable. If the qualified informant is a close relative, clearly data are likely to be more accurate than if details are given by someone more remote. However, the qualified informant may be vague about the deceased person's actual occupation, or may give the most senior occupation held during life, even if it was not that held at the time of death. Even the medical reason given for death may be subject to uncertainty, being based largely on clinical opinion in many cases. Deaths in the elderly are often ascribed to terminal conditions such as 'bronchopneumonia', when the certifier is unsure of the precise cause, whereas a death in a young person may be investigated more fully.

Measures of mortality

The basic unit of measurement used in studying mortality in populations is the rate. The rate consists of three components: a numerator, which is the number of people in the population who have died, a denominator which is the total number of people in the population and the time period during which deaths took place.

The use of a rate allows a comparison between different populations, different subgroups within the same population or populations at different times. A statement of absolute numbers, such as '100 deaths from coronary heart disease occurred last year in District A compared with 700 in District B' may be of value to the local undertakers in helping to assess their likely workload, but does not tell us whether mortality from coronary heart disease is a greater health problem amongst the inhabitants of District A compared to District B, since the relative sizes of the two populations are not given.

Crude death rate

The simplest form of mortality measure is the crude death rate, which takes the number of deaths in a period, usually a year, and expresses that number per 1000 population at risk of dying in the middle of the year, using the mid year population estimate described earlier.

Use of crude death rates has the advantage that mortality can be expressed in a single figure. This is helpful in comparing mortality within an area over a period of time, so long as the age and sex structure of the population does not change too much. The disadvantage of crude death rates is that they cannot be used to compare mortality experience between areas because of the possible different age and sex structures of the populations in those areas. A new town, for example, is likely to have a lower crude death rate than a seaside retirement resort. This is because in the former, there will be fewer people in age groups at risk of dying, compared to the latter.

Specific mortality rates

The need to look beyond crude death rates leads to the use of specific rates. A specific mortality rate refers to the number of deaths occurring in a subgroup of the population. Age and sex together with cause are the most commonly described subgroups. Occupation, social class and the ethnic group are others. Thus, the annual age-specific death rate for 15–24 year old males would be expressed as: number of deaths in the year of men aged 15–24 years divided by the number of men of that age in population. If this value is multiplied by 1000, it gives the rate per 1000.

In practice, age-specific rates are nearly always also sex-specific since important differences exist between males and females in their risk of dying from or developing certain diseases (Figure 1.5).

Death rates may be expressed for individual causes of death rather than the all cause rates that have been described thus far. Most health problems show an effect of some kind with age, as shown in Figure 1.5, so that crude death rates are inadequate to describe conditions which are heavily loaded at the extremes of life. The study of age/sex and other specific rates is by far the best way of examining how mortality or other measures vary between different populations. However, by moving away from the crude death rate in order to observe such detailed measures, an attractive feature of the crude rate is lost, namely, its ability to convey an impression in a single figure.

Standardised rates

A more useful summary measure in these circumstances, one which takes account of the different age structures of two populations so that their mortality experience can be compared directly, is provided by standardisation. In age standardisation, a single standardised death rate is calculated in which allowance has been made for the age (and usually also sex) structure of the population in question.

There are two methods of standardisation: indirect and direct. Both involve choosing a standard population (for example, the population of England and Wales in 1990), which is broken down into specific age (and usually sex) groups.

In the **indirect method** of standardisation, the death rates experienced by each age group of the standard population (for example, females aged 15–24 years in England and Wales) are applied to the population of the same age groups in the

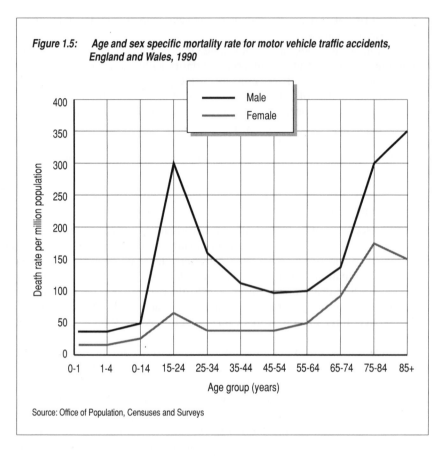

Figure 1.5:   Age and sex specific mortality rate for motor vehicle traffic accidents, England and Wales, 1990

Source: Office of Population, Censuses and Surveys

study area. This shows how many females aged 15–24 years in the study area would have died if the standard population's death rate had prevailed. After the calculation has been performed for all age groups the resulting total number of deaths is added up. These deaths did not actually occur, but are those which would have occurred if the study population had experienced the same mortality as the standard population, and hence they are referred to as *'expected'* deaths. The 'expected' number of deaths can then be compared to the actual, or *'observed'*, number of deaths. The most common means of comparison is the Standardised Mortality Ratio (SMR). This is the ratio of observed deaths to expected deaths and is usually expressed as a percentage. By definition, the standard population has an SMR of 100% (i.e. observed and expected deaths are the same). SMRs over 100 (the % sign is usually not used) represent unfavourable mortality experience, and SMRs below 100 show relatively favourable mortality experience, the effect of differences in the age and sex profile of each population having been taken into account.

Table 1.3 illustrates the process of calculating the SMR for deaths in females aged 15–64 years, in one part of the country, compared to the standard female population of England and Wales. The SMR of 106 for the area in question indicates that the mortality rate was 6% higher than that for England and Wales.

In indirect standardisation, the death rates occurring in the standard population are applied to the study population. In the **direct method** of standardisation the reverse process is used. The age specific death rates of the study population are applied in turn to the numbers in each corresponding age group of the standard population, to give the number of deaths which would have occurred in the standard population if the death rates in each study population had applied. This number of deaths is divided by the total standard population to give an age standardised death rate for the population under study.

In these examples, standardisation has been used to examine mortality in different areas. The process can be applied to any sub-groups of the population

---

Table 1.3   Indirect standardisation: worked example of the calculation of a standardised mortality ratio (SMR)

The aim is to compare the mortality experience of women (aged 15–64 years) in one part of the country (the study population) with that of all women of the same age group in England and Wales (the standard population).

Age-specific death rates for all females in England and Wales (Standard population)

	Deaths per 100,000 population
15–24 years	29.7
25–34 years	44.2
35–44 years	110.7
45–54 years	290.2
55–64 years	855.4

Population of females in the study population

	Population
15–24 years	70,100
25–34 years	72,000
35–44 years	65,000
45–54 years	57,200
55–64 years	59,400

"Expected" number of deaths of females living in the study population if their experience was the same as all females in England and Wales

		"Expected" deaths
15–24 years	29.7 x 70,100 / 100,000 =	21
25–34 years	44.2 x 72,000 / 100,000 =	32
35–44 years	110.7 x 65,000 / 100,000 =	72
45–54 years	290.2 x 57,200 / 100,000 =	166
55–64 years	855.4 x 59,400 / 100,000 =	508
Total expected deaths	=	799

"Observed" (actual) deaths of study population
females aged 20–64   =   849

SMR (as a percentage)   (England and Wales = 100)

$$\frac{\text{observed deaths}}{\text{expected deaths}} \times 100 = \frac{849}{799} \times 100 = 106 \text{ (SMR)}$$

where suitable data are available, for example, social class or occupational group. Although most commonly used to take account of age and sex, standardisation can also be used to adjust for differences in other characteristics. For example, perinatal mortality rates may be standardised for birth weight. The essence of standardisation is that it holds or eliminates the effect of the characteristic being standardised (for example, age, sex) so that the effect of other factors can be examined. Once a factor has been used in standardisation, it cannot be used to explain variation between rates. Figure 1.6 shows Standardised Mortality Ratios for cervical cancer in parts of England. The differences cannot be explained by the fact that different regions had different age structures, since it is age which has been standardised.

Avoidable deaths

Avoidable death is a concept which addresses deaths from those causes and in age groups where preventive measures or better clinical management might have avoided deaths (Figure 1.7). There are difficulties with this approach when comparing different parts of the country, particularly in taking account of different disease severity, which may account for the variation observed. Nevertheless, the avoidable deaths concept has proved valuable in providing a focus for further investigation.

Another approach is to examine deaths according to years of life lost prematurely. In a typical calculation, number of deaths under 75 years are multiplied by the number of years of life lost (at zero age, an average of 74.5 years; at 74 years, an average of 0.5 years) to give total years of life lost. This total figure can then be expressed both absolutely, and as a rate relative to the population at risk (Figure 1.8).

DESCRIBING MORBIDITY

The lessening reliability of mortality data as a window on illness and disease makes it important to establish and maintain systems of information which describe, more directly, the size of the pool of such morbidity in the population. Yet, no single source of routinely collected health data will provide a comprehensive picture of the range of illnesses and diseases from which people suffer. Moreover, much of the information which is available is incomplete, largely because a substantial number of cases may not be counted.

It is difficult to imagine a service industry in the non-health sector functioning without a clear idea of the size of various groups of customers within the population who will require, or benefit from its services. Yet, this is just the position the health service is in.

Mortality more or less defines itself, death being so clear cut, whereas morbidity does not always do so. Whilst there may be a relatively common understanding of what represents a strangulated hernia, there may be less of such an understanding, even amongst doctors, about what threshold of blood pressure represents hypertension. Self reporting of illness is also enormously variable. Patients do not have common thresholds in presenting illness to a general practitioner. One person's problem may not be perceived as such if experienced by another.

A wide diversity of data about illness or disease (morbidity data) are collected,

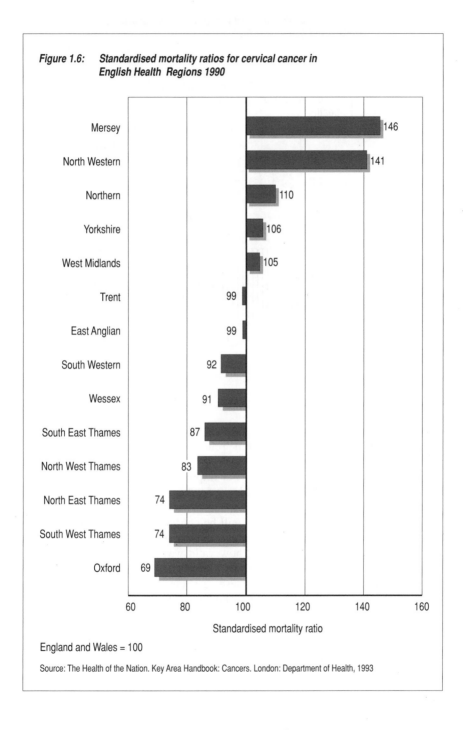

Figure 1.6:   Standardised mortality ratios for cervical cancer in
English Health Regions 1990

Standardised mortality ratio

England and Wales = 100

Source: The Health of the Nation. Key Area Handbook: Cancers. London: Department of Health, 1993

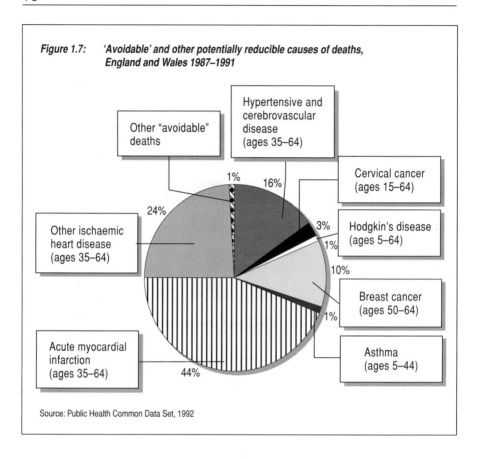

Figure 1.7:   'Avoidable' and other potentially reducible causes of deaths, England and Wales 1987–1991

Hypertensive and cerebrovascular disease (ages 35–64)

Other "avoidable" deaths

Cervical cancer (ages 15–64)

Other ischaemic heart disease (ages 35–64)

Hodgkin's disease (ages 5–64)

Breast cancer (ages 50–64)

Acute myocardial infarction (ages 35–64)

Asthma (ages 5–44)

1%   16%   3%   1%   10%   1%   24%   44%

Source: Public Health Common Data Set, 1992

some nationally, others only locally, some routinely, others on an ad hoc basis for a specific purpose, some as a statutory requirement, others on a voluntary basis. In considering the value of such data, it is important to be fully aware of their limitations. These are best appreciated by understanding the source and method of collection of the data.

Mostly, those using morbidity data, will be concerned with two issues. Firstly, they will want to understand how complete a coverage of the disease problem the data provide, and secondly, to decide how valid was the method of ascertaining whether disease was present or absent. Many routinely available sources of morbidity data are deficient in both these respects. If they are based upon the collection of information about patients who have made contact with services (and many are) they will not comprehensively give information about all cases of the disease which exist in the population.

In considering how completely a particular source of morbidity data describes the disease problem in the population, it is helpful to bear in mind the 'iceberg' concept depicted in Figure 1.9. The phenomenon whereby only a proportion of patients make contact with health services and, in particular with the hospital services, is often referred to as the tip of the iceberg. The process which leads people into the tip of this iceberg is complex and depends on many factors such as:

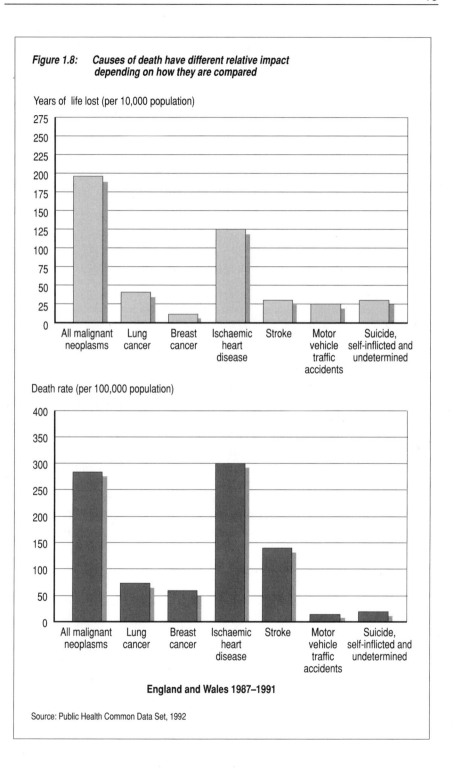

Figure 1.8: *Causes of death have different relative impact depending on how they are compared*

Years of life lost (per 10,000 population)

Death rate (per 100,000 population)

England and Wales 1987–1991

Source: Public Health Common Data Set, 1992

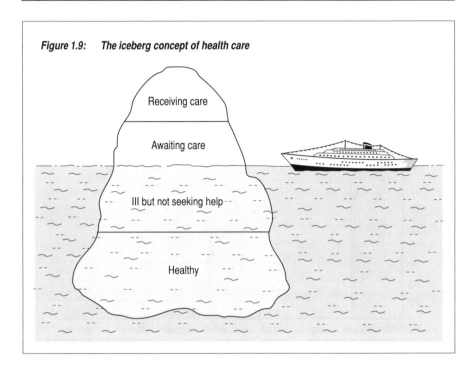

Figure 1.9:   *The iceberg concept of health care*

Receiving care

Awaiting care

Ill but not seeking help

Healthy

the patient's perceptions of his ill health; his own attitude and that of his family and friends, and society in general, to illness; and the availability of medical services.

A number of types of morbidity data are collected, analysed and presented on a routine basis. Examples include notifications of communicable diseases (described in detail in Chapter 9), data on hospital inpatients, notifications of congenital malformations (described in detail in Chapter 6), abortion statistics and cancer registration. Many other types of morbidity data are available routinely or on an *ad hoc* basis but are less useful in assessing the health of a population on a day-to-day basis.

In this section, four examples of morbidity recording systems are described. Those based upon hospital patients, general practice patients, people in the general population and disease registers.

Hospital morbidity systems

Traditionally, many countries have used hospital inpatient data as an indicator of morbidity. However, such data can only take account of those conditions for which inpatient care is required. Diseases for which the patients do not require hospitalization will not be revealed by examining hospital inpatient statistics only. Many 'important' health problems (for example, the common cold, migraine, backache), at least as judged by the proportion of the population affected by them and the economic impact of working days lost, will seldom lead their sufferers to require hospital inpatient care.

For relatively serious conditions, such as asthma, hernia or arthritis, a proportion of people afflicted will not make the decision to seek health care (even though they may recognize themselves as ill). A further proportion will visit their general practitioners only. Others will come to the attention of hospital services as outpatients or inpatients. Only the very last group will be recorded in a system of morbidity data based on hospital inpatients. In some disorders where hospitalisation is virtually mandatory, such as fractured neck of femur or perforated duodenal ulcer, hospital rates may approximate to the total size of the disease problem in the population. These situations are so few, that conclusions about incidence of disease based on hospital inpatient data should be interpreted with great caution.

Hospital Episode Statistics (HES)

The Hospital Episode Statistics (HES) system of data recording seeks to capture every episode of inpatient care which takes place within a National Health Service hospital in England. An 'episode' is defined as a period of treatment under the care of a particular hospital consultant. Patient-based inpatient and day case events are recorded daily in every hospital on a computerised Patient Administration System (PAS) or on forms in those hospitals where such a computerised system is not yet in place. The data are transferred to district and regional level and then to the Office of Population, Censuses and Surveys (OPCS).

The range of data collected cover: contract details (for example, hospital of treatment, health authority of residence), patient administrative details (for example, birthdate, sex, usual address), admission details (for example, referring general practitioner, dates of admission and discharge, mode of admission), consultant episode details (for example, consultant, specialty), clinical details (primary and subsidiary diagnoses, operations and procedures undertaken). For maternity admissions, details of the delivery record are entered as are details about the baby itself. For psychiatry cases, additional information is collected annually on longstay patients (those over one year) and on patients detained under one of the sections of the Mental Health Act.

Whilst Hospital Episode Statistics provide a useful potential source of information on illnesses treated in hospital, in the authors' experience their value is limited for this purpose by the quality of clinical information recorded as well as the completeness of returns made by some hospitals.

Morbidity recording in general practice

At present, the general practitioner records the details of each consultation on a medical record. There is no standardised way of recording clinical information and very often, because of pressure of time and because they carry many details in their memories and do not wish to add bulk to the medical record, the general practitioners' records of a consultation will comprise a few words or at most a few sentences. This contrasts with most hospital records of an episode of care which comprise several pages of text.

National morbidity study of general practice

No details of general practice consultations, whether clinical or administrative, are routinely collected either locally or nationally. The richness of general practice as a potential source of data on morbidity in the population led, in the period 1970–1972, to the setting up of a National Morbidity Study of General Practice, organised jointly by the Royal College of General Practitioners (RCGP), the Office of Population Censuses and Surveys and the Department of Health. This was a more elaborate version of an earlier study which had been carried out in the early 1950s. The study has been continued at approximately ten year intervals since and uses a sample of volunteer general practices in England and Wales.

General practice as a source of morbidity data for the community has many attractions. A high proportion of the population is registered with a general practitioner. General practitioners deal with the wide range of less serious disorders which do not present to hospital. The general practice population allows greater insight into the early stages of the natural history of illnesses and, in the majority of cases, it is the point of entry into the health-care system. It does not, of course, tell us anything about illnesses which are unrecognised by the patient or for which the patient undertakes self-medication. A more serious drawback, however, is that there is no system operating routinely to collect such data from general practice. The National Morbidity Study is not a random sample of general practitioners (although they are chosen to represent different regions of the country). An enthusiastic general practitioner who wishes to participate in such a study is unlikely to be representative of all general practitioners, so the results are unlikely to be typical of the country as a whole. Nor can geographical analysis be taken down to local level.

Despite its limitations, the National Morbidity Study of General Practice is the best guide to patterns of less-serious illness, both within subgroups of the population and for different parts of the country. Moreover, it can be used as a starting point for a more detailed look at an individual problem. Some individual general practices have established their own morbidity recording system and where these are available and properly organised they can yield important information for local health needs assessment.

Age-sex registers

Most general practices file records alphabetically by the surname of the patient. This is essential to allow the receptionist to retrieve the correct case notes when a particular patient attends for consultation. It does not, however, enable the general practitioner to identify particular groups (for example, all schoolchildren) within the practice population. The general practice age-sex register is a file of the practice population arranged by age and sex. Such registers began as systems using small index cards bearing the name, sex, date of birth and address of each patient, possibly together with other details (for example, National Health Service number). These cards were then filed in age bands for males and females separately. With the growing availability of relatively cheap computers, many practices now have computerised age-sex registers. This enables other data to be added on each patient (for example, the need for repeat prescriptions or the presence of chronic illness such as diabetes).

The age-sex register is a relatively simple device. It can give the modern general practitioner invaluable assistance in a number of ways. It can provide a list of the names of patients in particular age-sex groups for which special preventive or surveillance measures can then be organised. For example: the very elderly (who may be visited regularly at home); pre-school children (who are given a full course of immunisation and vaccination); middle-aged men (who may be offered blood pressure checks).

In addition, the register can serve as a denominator for the calculation of age-sex specific rates or be used as a sampling frame for research studies.

General household survey

One way of obtaining information on illness which does not present to the health service at all, is to choose people from the general population and obtain information about their health directly. The General Household Survey (GHS) includes the collection of such information.

The General Household Survey began in 1971 and has been running ever since. It is a continuous survey based upon a representative sample of around 12,000 private households in Britain. Interviews are conducted throughout the year with the adult members of these households and, in addition, parents are asked for details of each child in the household under 16 years of age. The information collected is not restricted to health. Indeed, the survey serves many government departments and includes questions on housing, economic activity, pensions, leisure activities, education and the family. The questions on health relate to acute illness, health during the previous year, presence of chronic illness, consultations with a doctor, visits to hospital (as an inpatient or outpatient), wearing of glasses or contact lenses, as well as smoking and drinking habits.

The General Household Survey gathers data on self-reported morbidity and disability. Questions are asked about both acute and long-standing illness and, if present, whether they limit or restrict activity in any way. Figure 1.10 illustrates the use of such data and shows a steadily increasing trend for long-standing illness. However, such changes should be interpreted with caution in view of the subjective nature of the reported information.

The main limitation of the General Household Survey is that, since it relies on the evidence of the individual, errors may be introduced due to forgetfulness, differing perceptions of illness, or withholding certain information. Moreover, diagnostic labels are attached to the illness by the patient. Although the interviewers, who are not medically qualified, are trained to probe for as much clarifying detail as possible, they are unlikely to conform with the terminology or accuracy of a medical practitioner's diagnosis.

Despite these disadvantages, the General Household Survey enables major and minor illness to be described in the population as a whole. It avoids the disadvantages of data systems which monitor contact with health services in that it seeks to count both declared and undeclared illness. Data are collected along with information on a wide range of other subjects, thus allowing associations between such variables and health indices to be explored in a preliminary fashion.

Registration of disease

A register has four main characteristics:

(a) it identifies individuals;
(b) these individuals each have the same particular feature in common, which is the focus of interest for the register;

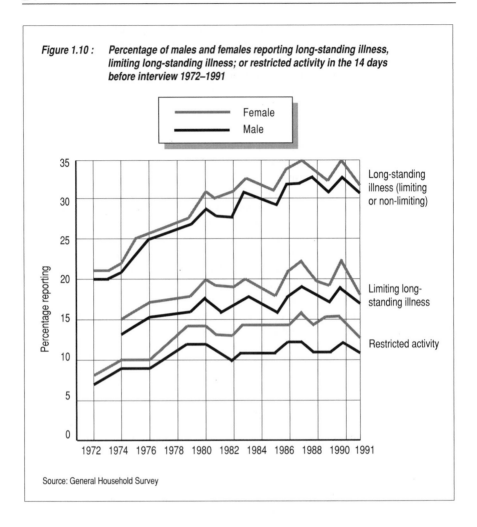

Figure 1.10 :   Percentage of males and females reporting long-standing illness,
                limiting long-standing illness; or restricted activity in the 14 days
                before interview 1972–1991

Source: General Household Survey

(c) it is longitudinal in that the information held about individuals is updated in a
     defined systematic manner;
(d) it is based on a geographically-defined population.

A number of registers are currently maintained in the health field and serve a
range of different purposes.

Cancer registration

The National Cancer Registration scheme has been operating since the end of
World War II, although a system was in operation in some parts of the country in
the 1920s when radium treatment commenced. It is organised on the basis of health
regions and information is also processed nationally by the Office of Population,
Censuses and Surveys which maintains a National Cancer Registry. Each Regional
Cancer Registry holds details of the identity and of the type of neoplasm for each

person in the region who has been diagnosed as having cancer (certain premalignant tumours are also included).

The National Cancer Registry at the Office of Population, Censuses and Surveys, through notification by each region, assembles a minimum data set. This includes: patient identification details (name, previous surname, address, postcode, sex, date of birth, marital status, NHS number, date of first diagnosis, date of death); details of the tumour (site of primary growth, type of growth, grade, stage, basis upon which the diagnosis was made) and certain other details relating to the tumour and its treatment. Regional Cancer Registries may also collect as optional other data (for example, ethnic origin, occupation, industry of the patient and head of household) which can also be notified nationally. Such data enable the incidence of cancer to be examined geographically, within sub-groups of the population and over time. They also enable survival to be compared for cancer at different sites. Such analyses can reveal the improving survival for cancer at some sites due to more effective treatment (Figure 1.11).

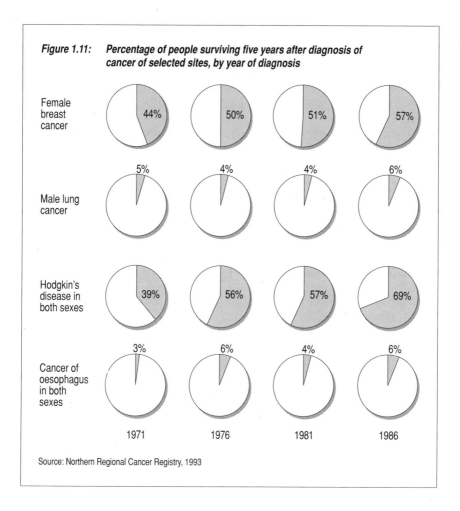

Figure 1.11:   Percentage of people surviving five years after diagnosis of cancer of selected sites, by year of diagnosis

Female breast cancer: 44%, 50%, 51%, 57%

Male lung cancer: 5%, 4%, 4%, 6%

Hodgkin's disease in both sexes: 39%, 56%, 57%, 69%

Cancer of oesophagus in both sexes: 3%, 6%, 4%, 6%

1971   1976   1981   1986

Source: Northern Regional Cancer Registry, 1993

Other case registers

Registers have been established to study other conditions such as psychiatric illness, child abuse, ischaemic heart disease, stroke and trauma. It has been argued that the proliferation of such registers, accumulating large amounts of data, must incorporate checks to ensure high quality or their cost will not be justified. The availability of cheap, small computers and the growing interest of clinicians in automating records increases the risk of unplanned growth of registers.

Establishing and running a register

Before a register is established, consideration must be given to why the register is required, what disease is being registered, how cases are to be identified and reported, what information will be recorded on each case, how information will be stored and communicated, who will be responsible for producing analyses and servicing requests, who will produce reports, and what the financial implications will be. To be of any real value, a disease register, once established, must be maintained to a high quality. This means addressing at least two fundamental issues: completeness of case ascertainment and validity. Unfortunately, this is not always recognised and the resources set aside to run the register may be insufficient to allow quality control issues to be tackled. The day-to-day problems of running a case register are formidable and include searching for missing records, making good incomplete or inaccurate records, the elimination of duplicate entries, resolving coding queries, ironing out computing difficulties and responding to requests for analyses.

One of the main problems of any registration system is achieving comparability of diagnosis. Wherever possible, strict rules should be laid down, so that there are well-defined criteria which must be present before a particular diagnosis is made. Variations in diagnostic and classification practices can give rise to problems when comparing data for different countries, different parts of the same country, or the same population over time. Duplication sometimes occurs, but with proper organisation it is usually possible to identify whether an incoming record belongs to an existing registration or not. However, undercoverage (cases eluding registration) is an almost intractable problem with all registers. Most registers rely on some agreed procedure of notification of cases by health workers, with varying degrees of success.

The decision to establish a register should not be undertaken lightly. It requires proper justification, skilled organisation, adequate resources and, above all, dedicated and imaginative leadership.

Uses of registers

Whilst in practice, many disease registers have a single disease focus, they also have the potential for multiple uses. In addition to measuring the amount of disease in the population, they can monitor temporal trends, they can be used in patient follow-up, they can enable comparisons of treatment outcomes, they can facilitate service evaluation, they can be used as the basis for studies of disease causation, they can be used for research and medical audit, they can be used to organise services for patients.

Measures of morbidity

There are two types of measure of illness or morbidity. They are incidence and prevalence. It is important to be able to distinguish between them (Table 1.4).

Incidence and prevalence

The incidence rate measures the number of new cases of a particular disease arising in a population at risk in a certain time period. In contrast, prevalence measures all cases of the disease existing at a point in time (point prevalence) or over a period in time (period prevalence). Although one often speaks of the prevalence rate of a particular disease, strictly speaking it is not correct to refer to prevalence as a rate. More correctly it is a ratio, since it is a static measure and does not incorporate the idea of cases arising through time. The point prevalence measure is often compared to a snapshot of the population. It states the position at a single point in time. In measuring a particular disease, prevalence counts individuals within the whole spectrum of that disease from people who have newly developed the disease to those in its terminal phases; whereas incidence just counts new cases. Thus, prevalence results from two factors: the size of the previous incidence (occurrence of new cases of the disease) and the duration of the condition from its onset to its conclusion (either as recovery or death).

In most chronic diseases complete recovery does not occur. Many people develop diseases (for example, chronic bronchitis, peripheral vascular disease, stroke) in middle age which they may carry until their death. The incidence of a condition is an estimate of the risk of developing the disease and hence is of value mainly to those concerned with searching for the causes or determinants of the disease. Knowledge of the prevalence of a condition is of particular value in planning health services or workload, since it indicates the amount of illness requiring care. Relatively uncommon conditions (i.e. those with a low incidence) may become important health problems if people with the disease are kept alive for a long period of time (producing a relatively high prevalence figure). An example of such a condition is chronic renal failure which is rare, yet because dialysis and transplantation can keep sufferers alive, it becomes an important health problem which consumes considerable resources.

Table 1.4:   *Measures of morbidity*

- Incidence: The number of new cases of a disease occurring per unit of population per unit time.
- Point prevalence: The number of people with a disease in a defined population at a point in time.
- Period prevalence: The number of people with a disease in a defined population over a period of time.

DATA ON LIFESTYLE AND RISK FACTORS

Determining the extent of particular lifestyles or risk factors within a population is an important aspect of assessing its health need. As with morbidity data, the sources of data on lifestyle are very disparate. In many cases, such data are collected for purposes not directly connected with health. For example, the National Food Survey, conducted on behalf of the Ministry of Agriculture, Fisheries and Food, began in 1940 and is based on a random sample of private households in Great Britain. It provides information on food consumption and expenditure. Information on smoking and alcohol consumption, collected through the General Household Survey, also has wider applications.

From time to time, major surveys are carried out on behalf of Government to establish lifestyle or risk factor prevalence. For example, a national survey of physical activity patterns and fitness levels was carried out jointly by the Sports Council and the Health Education Authority and reported in 1992 (Table 1.5).

Table 1.5:   Proportion of men and women undertaking 20 minute periods of physical activity to different levels within the previous four weeks

Frequency and intensity activity level	Description	Men %	Women %
Level 5	Twelve or more occasions of vigorous activity	14	4
Level 4	Twelve or more occasions mixed between moderate and vigorous activity	12	10
Level 3	Twelve or more occasions of moderate activity (not vigorous)	23	27
Level 2	Five to eleven occasions mixed between moderate and vigorous activity	18	25
Level 1	One to four occasions mixed between moderate and vigorous activity	16	18
Level 0	None	17	16
Total		100	100

Source: Allied Dunbar National Fitness Survey. London: Health Education Authority/Sports Council, 1992

National health survey

A health survey for England is run annually. The survey is based on a random sample of adults aged 16 years and over living in private households in England (covering approximately 17,000 people). The survey has three main components: a health and socio-economic questionnaire, physical measurements (height, weight, demi-span, waist/hip ratio and blood pressure) and a blood sample (tested for haemoglobin, ferritin and cholesterol). Most major topics are repeated each year to enable comparison over time.

Local health surveys

Although information from sources like these provides valuable insights into health related lifestyles and risk factors on a national basis, it cannot readily be extrapolated to populations at local level. Increasingly, local health programmes are seeking to promote health, prevent illness and premature death. Information on the prevalence of risk factors and health-related behaviours is required for this purpose. The gap in public health information at local level can be addressed by commissioning or conducting lifestyle assessments involving postal or face-to-face interview questionnaire surveys of the population. It is essential that such local surveys seek to adopt valid survey instruments and survey methods. Comparisons over time and with other populations are then possible. It is also important that local surveys are properly resourced so that there can be comprehensive data capture, control of quality as well as effective analysis and communication of the findings.

OTHER HEALTH STATUS MEASURES

A separate set of measures seek to go beyond the more clear cut health events which have been described so far. Such measures have been developed because many existing indicators do not measure fully the effects that disease has on people's physical, social and emotional well-being. There is a need to address issues such as quality of life and the concept of health itself.

Health and disease rating scales

Measures which attempt to do this fall into two main categories. Disease-specific measures focus on the aspects of health which are considered to be especially important in determining the quality of life for patients suffering from particular conditions. For example, some rating scales have been developed for arthritic patients which provide summary measures of symptoms including pain, function, range of motion of joints and the absence of deformity.

In contrast, general health scales attempt to measure the aspects of quality of life which are important to everybody, irrespective of their health status. Very few such measures are in regular use but they have been widely developed in a research context. One example is the Nottingham Health Profile[1] which asks people a series of questions and assigns a score for each of six categories (physical mobility, pain, sleep, energy, social isolation, emotional reactions). Each category is scored 0 to 100, and rather than combining the scores to derive a summary health status measure, the score in each category is presented separately.

Quality Adjusted Life Years (QALYs)

A general health status measure which takes a different approach is the quality adjusted life year (QALY). Rather than painting a picture of the population's health from which the need for health services can be inferred, QALYs assess need in terms of the capacity of health services to improve the population's health.

Health improvements are measured in terms of life expectancy, adjusted according to changes in quality of life resulting from the use of health services. Quality of life is usually measured by assessing two or more aspects of people's health, such as pain, disability, mood or capacity to perform self-care, social activities or main activities like housework or paid employment. These assessments are then reduced to a single measure of changes in quality of life. Combining this measure with information on life expectancy gives an estimate of health improvement in terms of QALYs gained.

Because the capacity to improve the population's health is inevitably constrained by the resources available to health care, the increase in QALYs arising from the use of health services is usually compared to the cost of treatment.

QALYs are an appropriate measure to focus on the predominant modern health problem, chronic disease. Table 1.6 shows how QALYs can be used to compare all kinds of health care, from preventive services to acute and rehabilitative care. However, whilst QALYs continue to be developed in a research context, their routine use in the health service is limited by the practical and theoretical difficulties of deriving valid single indices of quality of life, and by reservations regarding the fairness and appropriateness of QALYs as a basis for assessing the need for different health services.

Table 1.6: Cost per quality adjusted life year (QALY) league table

Treatment	Service cost per QALY gained (£)
Special chiropody at home, 75 years and over	229
GP's advice to give up smoking	274
Chiropody in a clinic for ages 60–75 years	694
Pacemaker implantation	957
Hip replacement	1025
Valve replacement for aortic stenosis	1260
CABG*: severe angina, left main disease	1416
CABG: severe angina, triple disease	1731
CABG: moderate angina, left main disease	1822
Kidney transplantation	4099
Heart transplantation	6983
Haemodialysis at home	15029
Haemodialysis in hospital	19129

Source: Bryan S, Parkin D, Donaldson C. Chiropody and the QALY: a case study in assigning categories of disability and distress to patients. Health Policy 1991; 18: 169–185
(*CABG = coronary artery by-pass graft)

HEALTH SERVICE ACTIVITY DATA

Almost all activity in the health service is covered by some form of aggregated data collection. Such data are principally used operationally to judge service usage or performance.

Körner data

The main system for recording health service activity is the Körner aggregate returns (named after the Chairman of a Steering Group which reviewed health information requirements in the early 1980s). Information is collected on patient activity in the hospital and community health services in England and includes the following categories:

- accident and emergency attendances
- ambulatory care attendances
- hospital inpatient and day case admissions

- activity in radiological, laboratory and other diagnostic departments
- clinic activity
- activity associated with paramedical services
- activity associated with health visiting and community nursing.

Information dealing with other aspects of the health service (for example, the estate, transport, manpower, finance) are also routinely gathered and analysed.

Körner returns are made at different intervals. Some are made quarterly, some annually. They provide aggregated returns which enable patient activity data to be compared between localities or over time and which allow such data to be linked to manpower and finance data. They are usually presented for broad clinical specialty groupings and do not enable clinical or demographic variables to be analysed.

Returns are classified by a particular code number. For example, KH07 is a quarterly return recording the number of people waiting for hospital inpatient admission. An illustration of its use to compare service performance is shown in Figure 1.12 where the variation in the number of people waiting for inpatient treatment in English health regions is shown. Return KH08 collects data on National Health Service operating theatre use and availability and allows, for example, the efficient use of such theatres to be reviewed (Figure 1.13).

Resource management systems

Possibly of potentially great value are the systems now being established to examine case mix within hospitals. In principle, operational systems are established in individual departments – X-Ray, Pharmacy, Pathology for example and used also to feed data into a central computer, where it is linked to an individual patient, the ultimate aim being to identify the total resource consumed by that patient during an episode of care. Patient Administration Systems (PAS) may be one of the feeder systems. The philosophy of resource management however goes much deeper than mere data collection, and is intended to influence the management culture within a hospital, to encourage professional staff to be more aware of the resource implications of their clinical decisions. It is largely under the aegis of resource management that attempts have been made to apply the Diagnosis Related and Health Care Resource Groups (described in an earlier section) analysis to workload, to try to describe activity in clinically meaningful and iso-resource use terms.

Record linkage and data networks

Medical record linkage is the process whereby health records from two or more different sources and containing different types of information are brought together to provide a single file for an individual. Such a process greatly enhances the usefulness of the information collected. For example, the linkage of cancer registration statistics with mortality data enables survival rates to be compared between different groups of people with different types of cancer.

The advent of advanced computer technology makes linkage easier. Even so it is a complex matter with the need to ensure compatibility of computer systems, accurate linkage information and procedures for resolving anomalies. In addition to linkage of records, data communication networks help the flow of information to users. It is becoming increasingly common to see electronic transfer of information

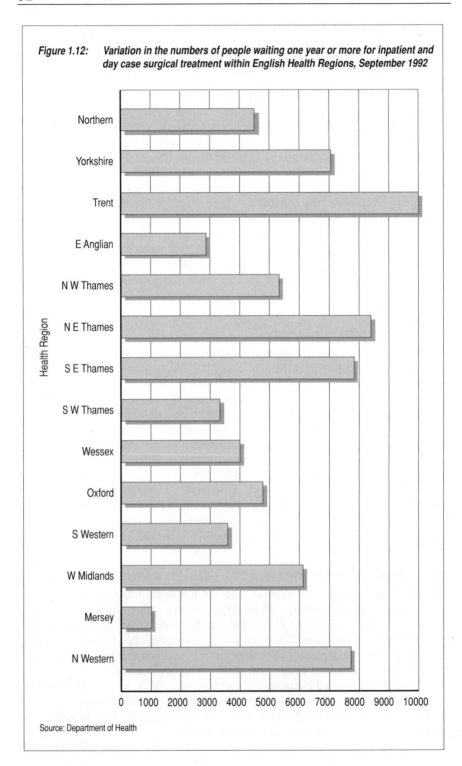

Figure 1.12: Variation in the numbers of people waiting one year or more for inpatient and day case surgical treatment within English Health Regions, September 1992

Source: Department of Health

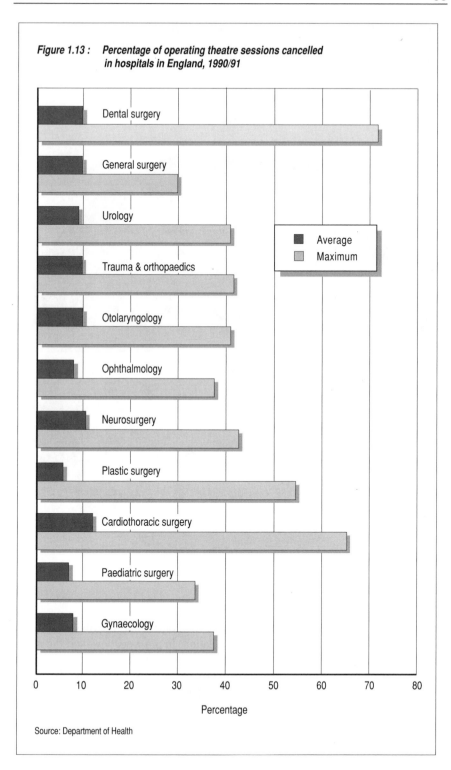

Figure 1.13 :   Percentage of operating theatre sessions cancelled
                in hospitals in England, 1990/91

Source: Department of Health

from large data bases to users with microcomputers. In the case of both record linkage and data networks, it is essential to ensure data protection and confidentiality.

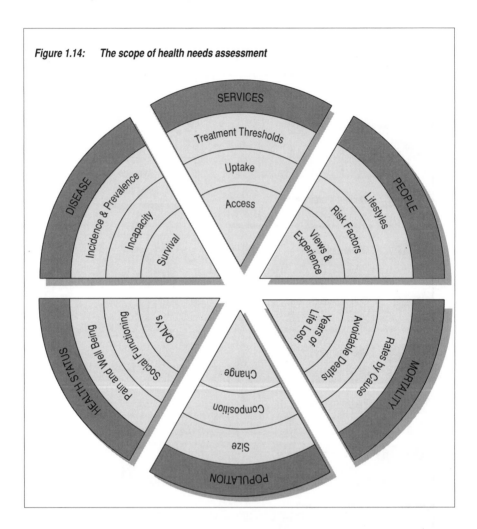

Figure 1.14: The scope of health needs assessment

CONCLUSIONS

All the sources of data covered in this chapter (and others not described) can be of value in assessing the health needs of a population. In practice, however, the needs assessment process involves a variety of approaches, including the use of routinely available data to provide continuous surveillance of health patterns or trends; *ad hoc* analysis of routinely available data to answer a particular question or throw light on a particular problem and the gathering of data which are not available routinely. The form of the needs assessment will differ according to the purpose for which the information is required. Figure 1.14 shows the main categories of information which are required to make an assessment of a population's health needs.

2 Approaches to investigation: Examining health and health service problems in the population

INTRODUCTION

The investigation of health problems in populations, and of the health services which provide care to them, is a key function of public health.

Anyone leading, or participating in, such investigative work should have a good knowledge of the range of routinely available data about health and health services, some of which are described in Chapter 1. On the other hand, as is made clear in Chapter 1, it is equally important to have an understanding of their strengths and weaknesses because there are enormous dangers in the uncritical use of routinely available health data. Indeed, it is all too common to see analytical reports written for bodies responsible for taking major policy, or resource-allocation decisions which contain conclusions far more sweeping than should be drawn given the limitations of the data.

Those involved in public health investigative work must also be familiar with, and skilled in, the methods and techniques of epidemiology.

Epidemiology is one of the population sciences basic to public health. The techniques and methods of epidemiology and its general approach in terms of a population perspective on health, disease, and health services leads it to have a very widespread application throughout the field of public health. The epidemiological perspective is a key component in identifying health needs; examining the pattern of disease problems within and between populations; searching for the causes of disease; formulating health promotion and disease prevention strategies; studying the natural history of disease; and planning and evaluating health services.

This chapter deals with the way in which epidemiological techniques and methods can be used to investigate the health problems of, and the health services provided for a population.

COMPARING DISEASE PATTERNS BETWEEN AND WITHIN POPULATIONS: DESCRIPTIVE EPIDEMIOLOGY

Chapter 1 described the range of information which could be used to describe the health of a population. Having assembled the necessary information to be able to examine a particular indicator (for example, mortality under the age of 65 years from coronary heart disease or the incidence of fractured neck of femur), the next questions which inevitably will occur to the investigator will involve comparisons. How does the population under study compare with other populations? How does the occurrence of the problem in the population currently, compare with earlier time periods? Are different sub-groups within the population affected by the health problem to a greater or lesser degree? Comparisons of this kind are the basis of hypothesis formulation and problem solving.

The use of health information in this way, whether derived from routinely available data or assembled by special surveys, is usually referred to as *descriptive epidemiology*.

When using the technique of descriptive epidemiology, it is particularly important to take a cautious and stepwise approach to interpreting the findings and before drawing conclusions, no matter how tentative. This is not just good scientific practice, it is the duty of the responsible investigator to the population which he or she is studying.

For example, to present information showing that the incidence of childhood leukaemia in one part of a city is higher than another without first checking the cancer register (and other data sources) for comprehensiveness of ascertainment of cases, for the validity of the recorded diagnoses on individual children, and for the accuracy of the places of residence attributed to the cases, could not only be highly misleading but it could also cause great public disquiet and anxiety (perhaps needlessly).

It is essential that before conclusions are drawn about differences in the occurrence of health problems between different populations, or over time, consideration is given to whether the differences may not be real.

Are differences real? Three important questions

In determining whether differences between populations or over time truly reflect different levels of a particular disease, it is helpful to address three questions.

What are the criteria for defining the disease?

It is well known that there are variations in medical practice (between different time periods, different places and even individual doctors on different occasions) which influence the way in which a particular diagnostic label is applied to a particular condition.

An illustration of apparent variations in the occurrence of psychiatric illness which can be explained partly by variations in the diagnostic process, is provided by considering a cross-national study carried out in the mid-1960s. It had long been recognised that there were apparent differences in the frequency of certain psychiatric illnesses in the United States of America compared with the United Kingdom. If such differences were real, then valuable clues as to the causes of certain psychiatric illnesses might be available. These considerations gave rise to an investigation into the differences.

Table 2.1 shows the results of an analysis of two samples of patients in psychiatric hospitals in London and in New York. There appeared to be a much higher percentage of schizophrenics and alcoholics in the New York sample than in the London sample. In contrast, patients with depression and mania were much more common in the London sample. Using a standardised interviewing technique each patient in the sample was examined by a member of a team of project psychiatrists as soon as possible after admission, and independently of the hospital staff. Table 2.2 shows the results of comparing the original hospital diagnoses with the subsequent project diagnoses in the two samples. Once alcoholics and drug addicts had been excluded, the comparison of the two sets of project diagnoses

Table 2.1: **The hospital diagnoses of the London and the New York samples**

	New York Percentage (n =192)	London Percentage (n =174)
Schizophrenia	61.5	33.9**
Depressive psychoses	4.7	24.1**
Mania	0.5	6.9**
Depressive neuroses	1.6	8.0**
Other neuroses	2.6	5:7
Personality disorders	1.0	4.6*
Alcoholic disorders	19.8	3.4**
Drug dependence	0.0	0.6
Organic psychoses	5.2	1.7
Other diagnoses	3.1	10.9**

* difference significant at 5% level
** difference significant at 1% level
Source: Cooper JE et al. Psychiatric Diagnosis in New York and London: a comparative study of mental hospital admissions. London: Oxford University Press, 1972.

showed no significant difference for schizophrenia, personality disorders, neurosis (other than depressive) and organic psychosis. This suggests that the original differences – in terms of hospital diagnoses – between two centres were largely the result of variation in the diagnostic criteria used by the psychiatrists.

The report concluded that the most important of these differences was that the New York concept of schizophrenia was much broader than that used in London, and included cases which many British psychiatrists would have called depressive illnesses, neurotic illnesses or personality disorders (see Figure 2.1).

Variation amongst doctors in the choice of labels for particular clinical problems or causes of death is quite commonplace. Whilst it may not be of paramount importance as far as the individual doctor and patient are concerned, it becomes central when data are aggregated for the purpose of producing a population count

Table 2.2: **The project diagnoses of the London and New York samples after the exclusion of alcoholics and drug addicts**

	New York Percentage (n =192)	London Percentage (n =174)
Schizophrenia	39.4	37.0
Depressive psychoses	26.8	24.2
Mania	7.7	6.7
Depressive neuroses	9.2	15.2
Other neuroses	2.1	4.2
Personality disorders	5.6	3.6
Organic disorders	3.5	3.6
Other diagnoses	5.6	5.5

Source: Cooper JE et al. Psychiatric Diagnosis in New York and London: a comparative study of mental hospital admissions. London: Oxford University Press, 1972.

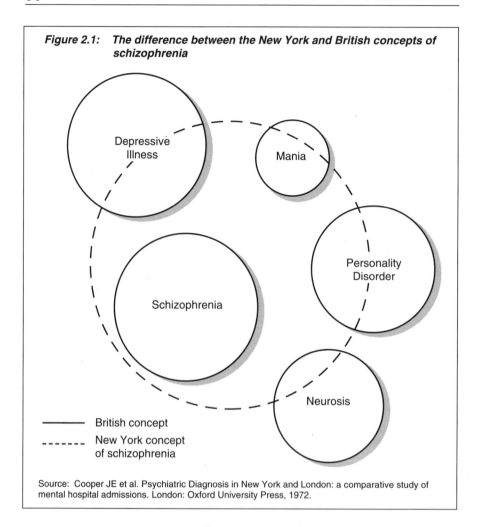

Figure 2.1:   The difference between the New York and British concepts of schizophrenia

────── British concept

- - - - - New York concept
of schizophrenia

Source: Cooper JE et al. Psychiatric Diagnosis in New York and London: a comparative study of mental hospital admissions. London: Oxford University Press, 1972.

of the number of cases of a disease or the number of deaths from a particular cause. It is even more important to establish the diagnostic criteria which have been used to count cases of the disease when comparisons are made between different populations or when a disease trend over time is observed. Otherwise, spurious conclusions about apparently major differences may be made (just as in the psychiatry example described above). This potential problem is applicable to all diseases, no matter how objectively the diagnosis is made.

Have all cases of the disease been identified?

False impressions about the amount of disease in one population compared to another may also be gained through a failure to take account of differences in the efficiency of case detection.

For example, the observation that the frequency of a particular cancer is commoner in a Western country compared to a developing country, using cancer registration data, may lead to speculation about risk factors in the two countries. Such a line of thought would be unwise without first examining the efficiency of the two cancer registration systems. The apparently higher occurrence of the cancer in the Western country may simply reflect the fact that it has an efficient, well-maintained cancer registry which detects and records most cases of cancer which occur. The cancer registry of a developing country, perhaps covering a rural population which does not readily have access to medical services, may not be so efficient at detecting cases of the cancer. But this does not necessarily mean that they are not occurring as often as in the Western country, merely that they are not being recorded.

This is a rather obvious example to illustrate the importance of being aware of possible differences in disease detection rates when making comparisons. It should be remembered that this pitfall can be encountered when comparing disease frequency from region to region, city to city, and hospital to hospital and not just between developing and developed countries.

A particularly common source of fallacious reasoning about disease differences between populations stems from descriptive studies based upon hospital inpatient data. This is also an issue of differential case ascertainment. Because the true incidence of the condition in the population is seldom known, it must be remembered that hospital cases of the disease can only approximate incidence in diseases where a high proportion of people who develop them are hospitalised. Since there are relatively few diseases which fall into this category, it follows that differences between populations in the occurrence of a particular disease based upon studies of hospital admission rates should be treated with great caution because they are likely to reflect differential admission rates for the condition rather than differences in the true incidence of the disease in the population.

Is the population at risk accurately defined?

In any measure of disease frequency, it will be necessary to express the number of cases of the disease in relation to the population from which they arose. A difference between two populations in the incidence of a disease or in mortality from a particular cause may be related to differences in the characteristics of the populations (such as age and sex) which affect the rate of disease. Once such characteristics are corrected for, an example being through standardisation (see Chapter 1), the differences in disease experience are no longer apparent. It is important to recognise this possibility at an early stage before too much interest is shown in apparent major variations in disease frequency.

It is also important to be sure that all cases of the disease or deaths are related to an identifiable, (ideally) geographically defined population upon which accurate estimates are available of its size and structure. Hospital catchment populations which can change rapidly over time, and may vary according to the type of diseases being examined, are notoriously unreliable in this respect.

THE APPROACH OF DESCRIPTIVE EPIDEMIOLOGY

Provided these limitations are always borne in mind when comparisons of disease frequency are being made, important observations may result from examining the pattern of diseases within populations.

Beyond simply the interest which is engendered by studying any population health problem, the process of descriptive epidemiology has three specific purposes. Firstly, to identify the scope for research into the causation of diseases or other health problems which might lead ultimately to their prevention; secondly, to help plan services for the whole population; and, thirdly, to highlight populations or groups within the population which are in special need of health service initiatives.

Example of a descriptive epidemiological approach yielding clues to causation

Figure 2.2 shows the findings of a study which used routinely available data to describe the trend over time in mortality from asthma.

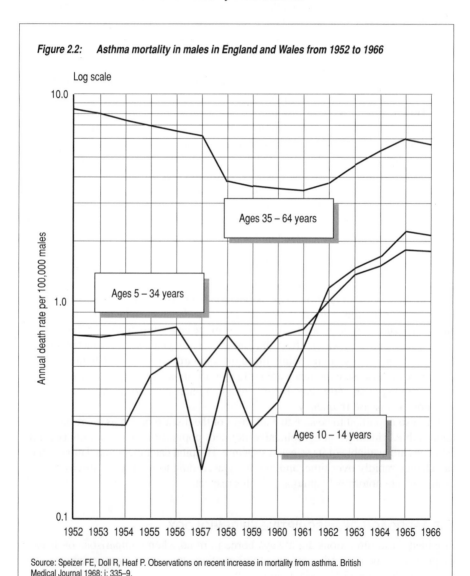

Figure 2.2:   Asthma mortality in males in England and Wales from 1952 to 1966

Source: Speizer FE, Doll R, Heaf P. Observations on recent increase in mortality from asthma. British Medical Journal 1968; i: 335–9.

The most striking observation from this trend was the rapid increase in the mortality rate from the disease which occurred in boys aged 10 to 14 years over the period from the mid-1950s to the mid-1960s.

This led the investigators to seek an explanation for this tragic apparent increase in loss of life and to discover whether the trend might be reversible. However, before going further it was important for them to bear in mind that such a change may be artefactual rather than real.

For example, was it possible that asthma was being more frequently used as an underlying cause of death by doctors completing death certificates in circumstances where previously some other terminology had been used? This was excluded by the investigators who found no downward trend in deaths from other respiratory disease diagnoses to coincide with the apparent increase in asthma deaths.

Having excluded this and other artefactual possibilities for the increase in asthma mortality, two other explanations were considered. Firstly, that the disease (asthma) had become more common (the incidence had increased) but that the proportion of asthmatic children who died from their disease remained static (i.e. that the case fatality rate remained stable) or, alternatively, that the disease had not become more common (the incidence was stable) but that the children who developed the disease died more often from it (the case fatality rate had risen).

The investigators in this study could find no evidence from other data sources to suggest an increase in the incidence of asthma and therefore concluded that the rise in mortality shown in Figure 2.2 was due to an increase in case fatality. There was a strong suspicion that the change was due to medications used to treat childhood asthma at that time and the next phase of the study was to seek information from the general practitioners of the children who had died of asthma about the drugs which had been used to treat them prior to death.

At the time, corticosteroids had been recently introduced into clinical practice and one of the known side-effects was suppression of the adrenal gland and therefore there was a suspicion on the part of the investigators that this group of drugs may be implicated in causing the deaths of asthmatic children. However, the survey of general practitioners revealed that this was not the case but that bronchodilators in the form of pressurised inhalers had been used in a high proportion of cases. Isoprenaline, administered in the form of an inhaler, was the drug most commonly involved. This drug can, amongst other side-effects, produce abnormal heart rhythms when taken to excess and there was clearly a possibility that children self-administering the drug to relieve acute bronchospasm might have used it indiscriminately and excessively when symptoms were severe.

At the time this drug had been available without prescription. As a result of the findings of the study it was subsequently made available only on prescription. Warnings were circulated to all doctors about these side-effects and printed warnings were also included in the instructional material for patients using these pressurised inhalers. As a result of these measures, mortality from asthma declined.

This is a classic example of descriptive epidemiological investigation leading to successful preventive action. Usually, however, it would first be necessary to move from the suggestion of causation created by the descriptive approach to investigate the presumed causal factors using more specialised epidemiological methods before drawing firm conclusions and taking definitive action. In this case, however, the findings were of sufficient importance and the public health problem was of such great concern, that immediate action was justified.

The subject of preventable deaths in asthma has continued to be controversial. Whilst the trend in Britain, and in some other Western countries, declined following the 1960s, a further increase has occurred in New Zealand whose cause has not been fully elucidated. The discussion of this later trend has led some observers to question the explanation for asthma deaths put forward in the earlier work.

Patterns of disease; time, place, person

The technique of descriptive epidemiology traditionally examines disease patterns across three main dimensions: in relation to *time*, in relation to *place* and in relation to *person*.

Describing disease in relation to time

When describing the way in which the occurrence of a disease varies with time there are three common methods of examining the relationship: seasonal variation; epidemic curves; and long-term (secular) trends. However, any temporal cyclicity may be studied (for example, diurnal rhythms or patterns).

Seasonal variation. Many diseases exhibit seasonal variations in their occurrence: peaks in the frequency of these diseases occur regularly at particular times of the year. Respiratory infections, for example, are more common in the colder months. In some non-infectious conditions seasonal variations have been clearly demonstrated, but no satisfactory explanation has, as yet, indicated why they should occur. For example, Figure 2.3 shows apparent seasonal variation in the onset of insulin-dependent diabetes mellitus in children. It can be seen that there is a higher occurrence in the winter months (January, February and December). Data of these kinds have led to suggestions that insulin-dependent diabetes in children may be caused or precipitated, in a small number of susceptible individuals, by an infectious agent, possibly a virus.

Such findings must be interpreted cautiously because they raise questions about the extent of detection of cases and the way in which the onset of the disease is determined. Even if such a seasonal pattern is established, this is not proof of a causal link between any particular infectious agent and the disease. However, it is a further example of how examination of the pattern of disease can provide a clue which may prompt further investigation, which in turn may lead to a greater understanding of its causal mechanism.

Epidemic curves. The increase in the frequency of a disease over a relatively short period of time above its baseline level of occurrence is termed an epidemic.

Sometimes the term is also used to describe increase in frequency, over a period of years, of diseases which have had a stable (and lower) level of occurrence for decades. Coronary heart disease and lung cancer are often referred to as the modern epidemics. Trends over years, or decades and longer, however, are usually described as secular trends.

Secular trends. The study of the pattern of diseases over long periods of time, years, decades, or even centuries, highlights many changes. Major diseases of the past have faded from importance, whilst others have become increasingly prominent.

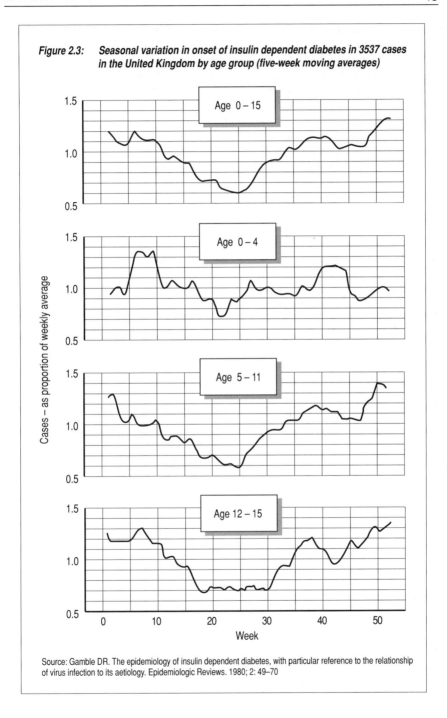

Figure 2.3: Seasonal variation in onset of insulin dependent diabetes in 3537 cases in the United Kingdom by age group (five-week moving averages)

Source: Gamble DR. The epidemiology of insulin dependent diabetes, with particular reference to the relationship of virus infection to its aetiology. Epidemiologic Reviews. 1980; 2: 49–70

As will be clear from the discussion earlier in the chapter, there are many pitfalls in interpreting secular trends in the frequency of a disease. Its true frequency may not have changed over time but improvements in methods of detection and diagnosis, fashions in diagnosis, changes in the criteria used to define or classify it, may suggest that it has.

Some of the most spectacular secular changes in the pattern of disease in Western industrialised countries have involved the decline in the importance of the infectious diseases as major health problems and causes of death. The decline in infant and childhood mortality, largely as a result of general measures (sanitary reforms, improvements in living standards and nutrition) which reduced the impact of the infectious diseases, improved life expectation for modern Britons compared to their Victorian counterparts. This secular change in mortality from infectious diseases in turn, therefore, had wider implications beyond its immediate impact for the size and structure of the population.

Tuberculosis was one of the great scourges of the recent past, often referred to as the 'white man's plague'. Bunyan, in his writings, gave it the chilling and evocative title 'Captain of the men of death'. In 1855, for example, 13% of deaths from all causes were attributed to tuberculosis. By the beginning of the 1990s the figure had fallen to 0.1%. Although the disease is now a much less common cause of mortality and morbidity, it is still important as a health problem world wide, particularly in immigrant groups in the United Kingdom.

The decline in mortality from tuberculosis (Figure 2.4) had begun before the advent of specific medical measures. This highlights another principle in interpreting secular trends. If the frequency of a disease is already declining it must not be assumed automatically that the introduction of a specific measure has brought it about.

The decline in importance of infectious diseases in Britain, particularly since the beginning of the century, has coincided with an upsurge in the importance of so-called 'chronic diseases'. The dramatic increase in coronary heart disease and lung

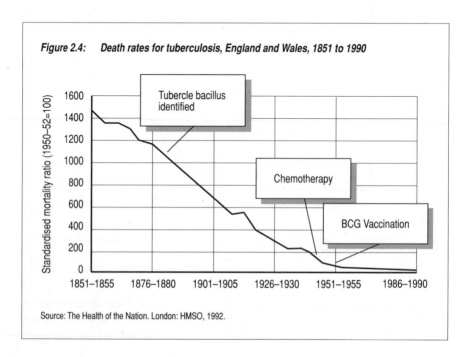

Figure 2.4:   Death rates for tuberculosis, England and Wales, 1851 to 1990

Standardised mortality ratio (1950–52=100)

Tubercle bacillus identified

Chemotherapy

BCG Vaccination

1851–1855   1876–1880   1901–1905   1926–1930   1951–1955   1986–1990

Source: The Health of the Nation. London: HMSO, 1992.

cancer must in part reflect an awareness of them amongst clinicians and pathologists as disease entities, so that although they occurred in the past, deaths from them were attributed to other causes.

Describing disease in relation to place

Description of the pattern of disease in geographical terms can be undertaken in a number of ways, although there are three main aspects: national variation (within a country); international variation (between countries); smaller area variation (for example, urban/rural).

National variation

For many diseases in the United Kingdom, there is variation in morbidity and mortality rates between different geographical areas. Chronic bronchitis, for example, is more common in the urban industrial areas of northern England than in the rural areas of the south. Other diseases are also distributed in a similar way. The overall result is that general mortality within Britain is lower for the population of southern England and East Anglia and higher for parts of northern and north-western England, Wales and Scotland (Figure 2.5). The reasons for this are multifactorial and complex.

International variation

Many diseases vary in frequency between different countries and on occasions this may give clues to causation. Table 2.3 shows the variation in the prevalence of neural tube defects (spina bifida, anencephaly and encephalocele) between 14 populations in European countries. Registers of congenital malformations had been established to monitor the occurrence of such birth defects and enable comparisons to be made.

Table 2.3: *Total reported prevalence (number and rate per 10,000 births) of neural tube defects (including livebirths, stillbirths, and induced abortions) in 14 European Registries 1980–1986*

Registry	All neural tube defects	
	Number	Rate per 10 000
Dublin	565	34.5
Galway	47	24.4
Glasgow	342	37.4
Liverpool	366	25.6
Northern Ireland	670	34.4
South Glamorgan	119	31.3
Hainaut	64	11.2
Groningen	72	14.3
Odense	41	12.6
Paris	229	10.7
Strasbourg	79	12.1
Marseille	79	11.1
Florence	71	11.2
Malta	25	11.2

Source: EUROCAT Working Group. Prevalence of neural tube defect in 20 Regions of Europe and the impact of prenatal diagnosis 1980–1986. Journal of Epidemiology and Community Health 1991; 45: 52–58.

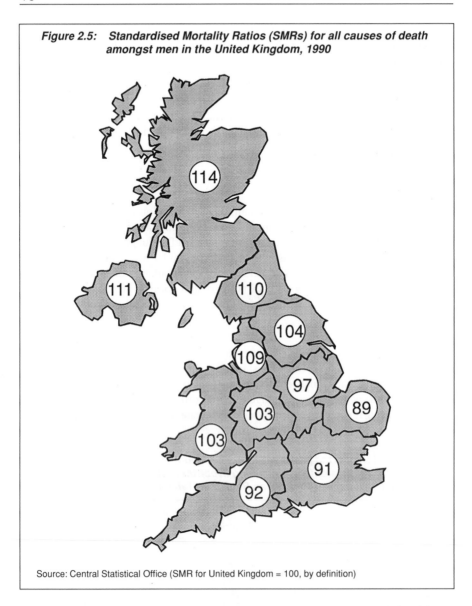

Figure 2.5: *Standardised Mortality Ratios (SMRs) for all causes of death amongst men in the United Kingdom, 1990*

Source: Central Statistical Office (SMR for United Kingdom = 100, by definition)

As Table 2.3 shows, considerable variation was seen between the different populations. Moreover, rates were generally higher amongst births occurring in the British and Irish centres than those in other European countries.

The reasons why some countries show a higher prevalence of neural tube defects than others is not known but the observation emphasises the need for studies to elucidate causation. Until it becomes possible to prevent all cases of neural tube defect, reducing its impact requires folate supplementation preconceptually and successful antenatal detection programmes coupled with termination of affected pregnancies (see also chapter 6).

Small areas

An example of the analysis of health data in relation to smaller geographical areas is illustrated by the work carried out in Teesside County Borough which was formed in 1968 and disbanded in 1974 with the reorganisation of local government. The Borough covered 49,000 acres and had a population of almost 400,000. Lying close to an industrial belt of large chemical and steel complexes on the banks of the estuary of the River Tees was a collection of old urban centres with a high proportion of poor housing. Moving away from the river, pollution lessened and the countryside opened up. The objective of the work was to identify the deprived sections of the population and to bring services to support them.

From census data three housing characteristics were used for all the separate small enumeration districts in Teesside. These were: (a) proportion of houses lacking one or more basic amenities (w.c., bath, hot and cold water); (b) proportion of houses with more than 1.5 people per room; (c) proportion of houses which were privately rented. Using predetermined criteria, the enumeration districts with poor housing characteristics were categorised as 'downtown'. The population was approximately a fifth of the total. The remainder of Teesside was referred to as 'the rest'.

A number of health indices were then compared in order to examine differences between these two types of area. When compared for standardised mortality ratios (SMRs) for various causes of death, infant mortality or illegitimacy rates, the 'downtown' areas persistently fared worse than the rest of Teesside. The cause of death analysis is shown in Figure 2.6 and demonstrates the unfavourable mortality experience of people living in the 'downtown' areas, particularly with respect to respiratory disease and suicides, accidents and violence. This study thus identified the multiple deprivation of the inner urban area: poor housing, high unemployment, poor health, and low uptake of services. Through these findings action was taken to deploy services to meet these problems, although it must be appreciated that such problems, rooted in social, economic, cultural and environmental factors, will not be resolved by action within the health service alone. Indeed, at the beginning of the 1990s active research programmes were still underway in the Teesside area to try and explain the reasons for the poor health of people living in some small communities and to assess the respective contributions of deprivation, environment and lifestyle to poor health and premature death.

Describing disease in relation to person

There are many more ways of examining the pattern of disease in relation to the characteristics of people than by either time or place.

Most diseases show a distinct pattern when looked at in terms of age, sex, occupation and social class. In addition, there are diseases which vary with ethnic origin and with marital status. Some examples of patterns of disease in relation to some of these variables are described in this section, though there are many others.

Age and sex

Almost all diseases show a marked variation with age. Indeed, mortality rates from all causes show a distinctive pattern (Figure 2.7). Once the first few years of life have been passed, there are relatively few deaths per unit of population until the

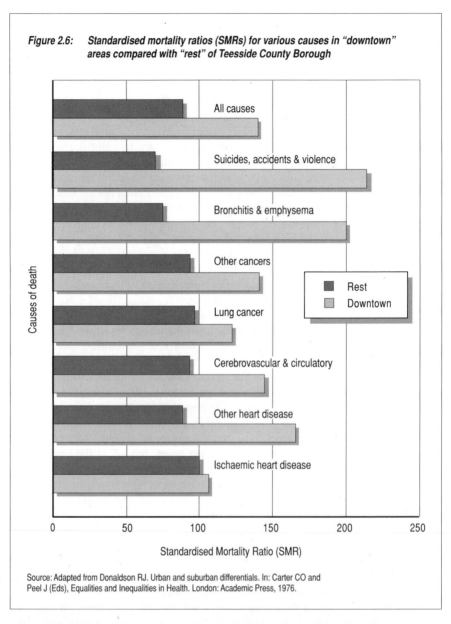

Figure 2.6:   Standardised mortality ratios (SMRs) for various causes in "downtown" areas compared with "rest" of Teesside County Borough

Source: Adapted from Donaldson RJ. Urban and suburban differentials. In: Carter CO and Peel J (Eds), Equalities and Inequalities in Health. London: Academic Press, 1976.

age of about 35 years, when death rates begin to increase sharply with each successively higher age group.

There are differences, too, in the importance of various causes of death at each age. Figure 2.8 shows that in the younger age groups, accidents and violence are a more important cause of death than diseases, whilst in the older age group, diseases of the respiratory and circulatory systems and cancer come to the fore.

Not all disease shows a straightforward increase in occurrence with age. Figure 2.9 shows that even within a disease category, for example, fractures, there can be

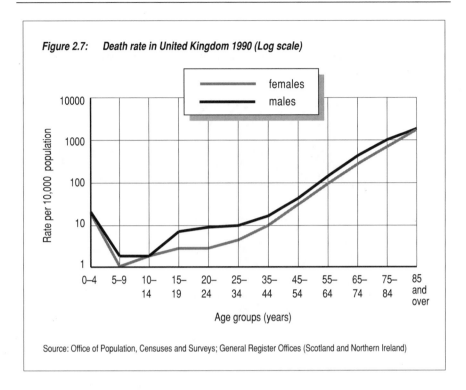

Figure 2.7: *Death rate in United Kingdom 1990 (Log scale)*

Source: Office of Population, Censuses and Surveys; General Register Offices (Scotland and Northern Ireland)

very different age patterns according to the fracture site. Fractures of the neck of the femur (Graph A, Figure 2.9) show a very low incidence in childhood and early adult life, with a steadily increasing rate for both sexes from middle age upwards. Apart from a small peak in childhood, fractures of the upper end of the humerus (Graph B, Figure 2.9) show a similar pattern. The tibial and fibular fractures (Graph C, Figure 2.9), show a peak occurrence in young men, largely as a result of sporting and road traffic accidents whilst fractures of the lower end of the radius and ulna (Graph D, Figure 2.9), where a common mechanism is a fall on the outstretched hand, show a peak in both sexes in the younger age group as well as in older women.

Figure 2.10 is derived from the same study of fracture incidence in a geographically-defined population but this time compares the size of the male and the female incidence rate at each site in two broad age groups, people over 55 years of age and people under 55 years of age. The incidence rate for males and females in each age group is compared by means of their ratio. The purpose of analysing these data in this way was to try to throw light on the possible influence of menopausal changes on fracture incidence.

There were interesting differences between the sexes at different ages according to the site of fracture. These fell into two broad patterns. In the first pattern of fracture sites (Graph A, Figure 2.10), there was a male excess in both younger and older age groups. In the second pattern (Graph B, Figure 2.10) female incidence began to predominate over male after the age of 55 years.

This sex pattern in fracture incidence at different sites points to a number of possible explanations: osteoporotic fall in bone mass around the time of the menopause, a

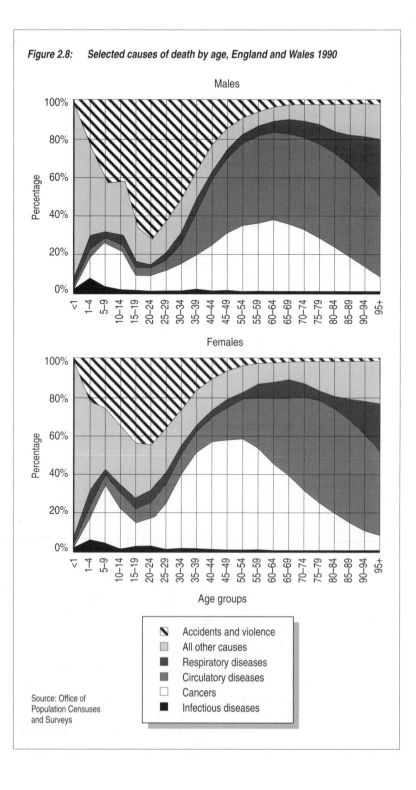

Figure 2.8:   Selected causes of death by age, England and Wales 1990

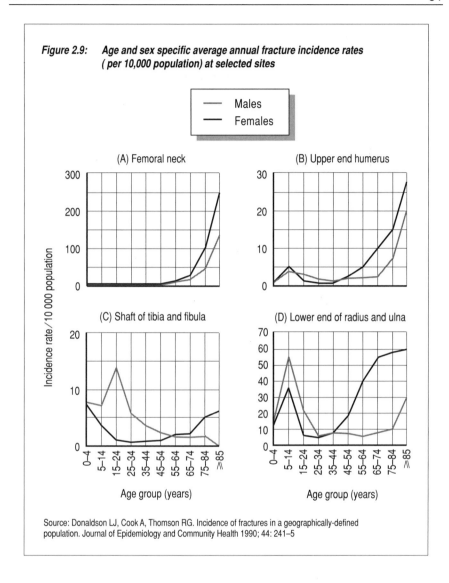

Figure 2.9:   Age and sex specific average annual fracture incidence rates
(per 10,000 population) at selected sites

—— Males
—— Females

(A) Femoral neck

(B) Upper end humerus

(C) Shaft of tibia and fibula

(D) Lower end of radius and ulna

Incidence rate/10 000 population

Age group (years)

Age group (years)

Source: Donaldson LJ, Cook A, Thomson RG. Incidence of fractures in a geographically-defined
population. Journal of Epidemiology and Community Health 1990; 44: 241–5

greater propensity to falls amongst older women and neuromuscular deterioration
with age which may reduce the degree of skeletal protection when trauma occurs.

As with any descriptive epidemiological data, these interesting sex differences in
the incidence of a disease do not provide direct evidence of causal association but
do point the way for further epidemiological studies aimed at elucidating causation
and possibly scope for prevention of an important public health problem.

Occupation and social class

The study of mortality in groups of workers in particular occupations or industries
has a long tradition, and through the years, has uncovered particular risk factors for
particular diseases which have arisen in the working environment.

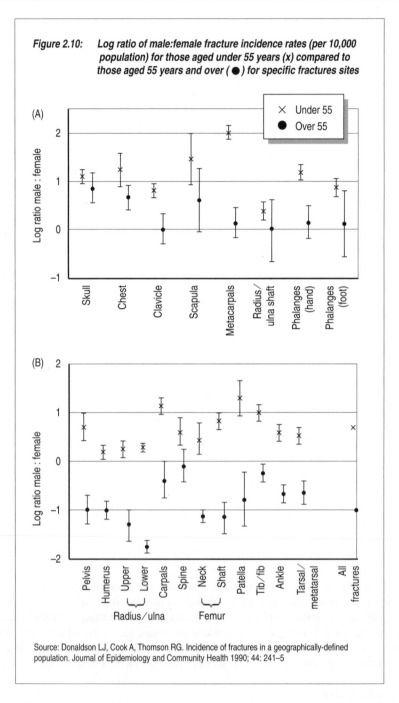

Figure 2.10: *Log ratio of male:female fracture incidence rates (per 10,000 population) for those aged under 55 years (x) compared to those aged 55 years and over (●) for specific fractures sites*

Source: Donaldson LJ, Cook A, Thomson RG. Incidence of fractures in a geographically-defined population. Journal of Epidemiology and Community Health 1990; 44: 241–5

In 1911, the Registrar General in Britain first used a hierarchical classification of social class based on occupation. The move to collect and present data in this way was prompted by the concern expressed by many of the social reformers of the time such as Charles Booth (1840-1916) and Seebohm Rowntree (1871-1954), about the high rates of mortality amongst the poor, in particular infant mortality. The classification grouped people according to the skill required for, and the social standing carried by, their particular occupation.

Data on occupation continue to be used to produce various methods of social and economic classification. Broadly, the assumption underlying this approach is that someone's occupation is a good guide to his or her position within society.

A very wide range of approaches to defining social class have been used by Governmental agencies in different countries or by research workers. Most measures take, either singly or as a composite measure, three aspects about the person: occupation, education and income.

In Britain, occupation remains the main basis for such social and economic classifications and detailed data about occupation are collected at birth, marriage, death, at the time of the census, and in responses given to Government social surveys.

Classification of occupation. Two widely used classifications are derived from such occupational data by grouping of occupations. Social class based on occupation (also called the Registrar General's social class or simply social class) and socio-economic groups.

The basis of the collection of occupational data for these official purposes (and hence their aggregation to produce social class and socio-economic group measures) is the Standard Occupational Classification. This classification is intended to be applicable to all paid jobs. On the basis of the typical work activities associated with the job, occupational groups have been created. The grouping is on the basis of occupations which are similar in terms of the level of skills (experience or qualifications) needed to carry them out and the nature of the work activities.

At the first level, the Standard Occupational Classification comprises approximately 3,800 detailed occupational titles (for example, bank-note engraver, mussel gatherer, member of the Stock Exchange). These are aggregated into 374 unit occupational groups (for example, caretakers, nursery nurses, glass product and ceramics makers) which in turn are further aggregated into 77 minor occupational groups (for example, woodworking trades, filing and records clerks, catering occupations). Finally, there are 22 sub-major groups and the highest level of aggregation which is called major occupational groups (for example, clerical and secretarial occupations, managers and administrators, plant and machine operators) of which there are nine.

Social class based on occupation. Strict rules are in existence to ensure that occupational groups are correctly assigned to their social class.

In addition, there are a number of more complex issues surrounding the usage of the system generally and in specific circumstances. For example, when considering the position of an unemployed or retired person, should their last occupation be chosen as representative or the main occupation followed during their work career? In practice, for people in work, the current occupation is used and for those not in work, it is their last main paid occupation which is used.

Another example of the potential complexity of assigning a social class to someone relates to the position of women and children. Traditionally the occupation of the (usually male) head of household has been used to assign a social class to other household members viewed as dependent. This is still the case for many purposes. However, as the position of women in society, at work and in the home has changed and as household structures have become more varied, the appropriateness of assigning social class to household members using the head of household's occupation has increasingly been debated. There is no easy way round the difficulty when trying to characterise a household. However, for some statistical purposes, married women who are employed are classified by their own occupations.

In general, each occupational group is given a basic social class, although certain groups (for example, managers or foremen) are allocated to a higher social class than others in their occupational group on the basis of their level of responsibility.

The present social class categories are as follows:

I		Professional occupations
II		Managerial and technical occupations
III	N	Non-manual skilled occupations
III	M	Manual skilled occupations
IV		Partly skilled occupations
V		Unskilled occupations

Table 2.4 shows data comparing mortality in men by social class living in three different parts of England. Whichever of the three regions the men lived in, the familiar gradient of increasing mortality with lower social class is evident. Also apparent, however, is a geographical difference within social classes so that, for example, Social Class I men living in the North have a much worse mortality experience than their counterparts in East Anglia. The geographical difference is even more striking when mortality amongst men in Social Classes IV and V in the North are compared with the same social class groups in East Anglia.

This is one example of a well established North-South gradient in Britain which is apparent for many causes of death. It is not fully explained but differences in lifestyle and environment undoubtedly contribute to producing these discrepancies.

The familiar pattern of increasing mortality on moving down the social-class scale is a feature of all age groups from birth, through childhood into adult life.

Table 2.4: **Mortality experience of men aged 20 to 64 years belonging to different social classes living in certain parts of England**

Social Class	North	South East	East Anglia
		(Standardised Mortality Ratios)	
I	72	61	65
II	83	69	65
IIIN	106	87	80
IIIM	115	97	80
IV and V	152	112	93
ALL	114	89	79

Source: Adapted from The Nation's Health (Edited by Smith and Jacobson) London: King's Fund, 1988, which used data for 1979/80 and 1982/3.

Socio-economic groups. This is an alternative way of classifying the population on the basis of employment status and occupation. It was introduced in 1951 and has been extensively amended since then. There are 20 categories, for example, 'agricultural workers' or 'professional workers, self-employed'. Unlike social class the numbering of the groups is not hierarchical. The groups are sometimes combined into six 'collapsed categories', as used in Figure 2.11. This analysis shows the proportion of cigarette smokers in each socio-economic group and allows the factors which might contribute to differential smoking rates to be explored.

Ethnic origin

The study of disease and mortality in populations of different ethnic origin can provide important clues to disease causation. There is a particular tradition in descriptive epidemiology of studying the disease and mortality experience of immigrant populations, to see whether their disease experience remains as in their country of origin or changes to their new country of residence.

The study of an ethnic minority population which retains distinct cultural traditions and practices in comparison to a longstanding indigenous population can also yield clues to disease causation. Figure 2.12 compares the occurrence of cancer at different sites for Asians (defined as people not of United Kingdom descent who originate from India, Pakistan or Bangladesh or people of Indian or Pakistani descent who originate from East Africa) and non-Asians living in Leicestershire, England.

A relatively complex statistical approach was necessary to compare the incidence of cancer in the two populations because, at the time of the study, concurrent denominator data on the Asian population were not available (the study was before the time of the 1991 census when ethnic origin questions enabled much more reliable information on the size and structure of the ethnic minority populations to be made available).

It is not necessary to understand the details of the methodology for the purpose of this illustration, merely to note (as is shown in Figure 2.12) the apparent excess (over the 'expected' occurrence) amongst Asians of cancers of the tongue, oral cavity, pharynx, oesophagus, and of some other sites.

It is, of course, important to exclude spurious explanations of the kind discussed earlier and particularly to consider the possibility that the findings might be due to selective immigration. In this case could Asian people have come to Britain because they were already suffering from cancer (for example, to obtain treatment)? This is always an important potential explanation to consider in studies of immigrant populations. However, it was considered implausible in this particular example.

Of particular relevance to the excess of Asian cancer cases at the particular sites found in the study shown in Figure 2.12 is the habit of betel chewing. In countries where betel is chewed, its common accompaniment in the chew, tobacco, has been implicated in the causation of cancerous and precancerous lesions of the oral cavity. It has further been suggested that elements in the betel chewing habit other than tobacco – that is, the areca nut, the betel leaf, or the lime additive – may be causally linked to oral cancer as well as pharyngeal and oesophageal cancer.

The Asian population, one of the main ethnic minority populations of present day Britain is still relatively young in its age structure. Chronic diseases such as

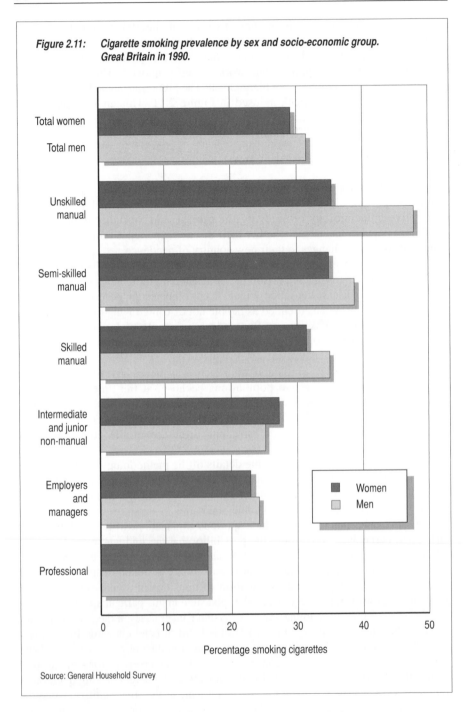

Figure 2.11:   *Cigarette smoking prevalence by sex and socio-economic group.*
                 Great Britain in 1990.

Source: General Household Survey

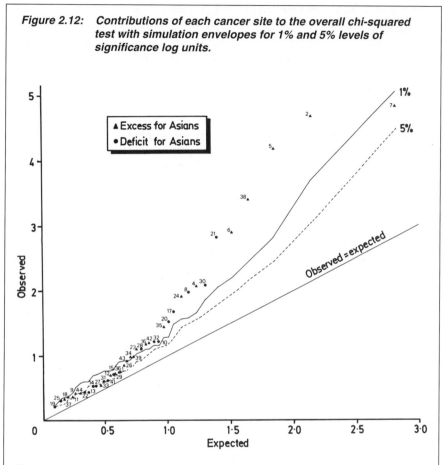

Figure 2.12: *Contributions of each cancer site to the overall chi-squared test with simulation envelopes for 1% and 5% levels of significance log units.*

Site of cancer: 1 Lip, 2 tongue, 3 salivary glands, 4 gum, floor of mouth, other mouth, 5 oro-, naso-, hypopharynx, 6 other oral cavity, 7 oesophagus, 8 stomach, 9 small intestine, 10 colon, rectum, 11 liver, bile ducts, gallbladder, extrahepatic bile ducts, 12 pancreas, 13 peritoneum, 14 other and ill-defined (digestive organs, and peritoneum), 15 nasal cavities, etc, 16 larynx, 17 trachea, bronchus, lung, 18 pleura, thymus, heart, 19 bone and cartilage, connective tissue, 20 malignant melanoma, 21 other skin, 22 breast, 23 uterus unspecified, 24 cervix, 25 placenta, 26 body of uterus, 27 ovary and tubes, 28 other female genital, 29 prostate, 30 testis, 31 penis and other male genital, 32 bladder, kidney, ureter, 33 eye, 34 brain, other nervous system, 35 thyroid, 36 other endocrine, 37 other ill defined sites, 38 lymph nodes, other and unspecified, 39 secondary of respiratory and digestive system and other site, unspecified, 40 lymphosarcoma and reticulosarcoma, 41 Hodgkin's disease, 42 other lymphoid, 43 multiple myeloma, and 44 leukaemia

Source: Donaldson LJ, Clayton DG. Occurrence of Cancer in Asians and non-Asians. Journal of Epidemiology and Community Health 1984; 38: 203–207.

cancer are uncommon. This will not always be so. As the population ages, there will be a need to be able to anticipate the main health problems of this community. Observational studies, such as the one illustrated here, can never prove cause and effect but do provide important pointers to areas where further epidemiological inquiry is indicated. They also indicate a need to establish the prevalence within the ethnic minority population of traditional practices and behaviours which may be of public health importance.

CROSS SECTIONAL OR PREVALENCE STUDIES

The previous section has dealt with the techniques of descriptive epidemiology in which comparisons are made, in mortality or the occurrence of disease between populations, within groups of the same population, and over time. Most of the examples given derived the information for making such comparisons from routinely available health data.

Quite often, it will be important to describe the size of a health problem within a population but it will be found that routinely available data are not adequate to fulfil this task. For example, a health authority wishing to establish the prevalence of dementia within its population would not readily be able to do so from available sources of data. Leaving aside problems with the quality of death certification in the elderly, mortality statistics would completely under-estimate the problem because only a relatively small proportion of people with the disease at any one time are dying from it. Similarly, statistics derived from hospital admissions (whether to psychiatric or general wards) would also underestimate the problem because a high proportion of people with dementia might be expected to reside within the community and not be in contact with hospital services.

It is in such circumstances that consideration may be given to carrying out a survey to gather data directly about members of the population to gain a more accurate estimate of the prevalence of the disease in question.

If such a special study is to be carried out, it will also usually be widened to include the gathering of other relevant information on the population under study, other than purely the disease of interest. Thus, a prevalence study of the extent of dementia in the population would be unlikely to limit itself to assessing elderly people for the presence or absence of dementia but would also gather data on factors such as their domestic circumstances, their capacity for self-care and their physical status.

Surveys in which information is gathered directly from members of a population can be carried out for reasons other than to establish the prevalence of a disease and this section describes the general approach to such surveys and why they may be carried out. Notwithstanding the precise purpose of a particular population survey, two general terms are often used to describe them: prevalence studies and cross sectional studies. Both terms emphasise a key feature of such surveys, that they describe the population at a point in time, like a snapshot.

Aims of cross-sectional surveys

As has already been described, one purpose in carrying out a cross-sectional survey is to establish the prevalence of a disease in the population. Another purpose is to describe the characteristics of the population when there are no routinely available data to do this. This may be to establish a particular aspect of the population's need for health or social services or to establish the prevalence of risk factors (for example, intravenous drug abuse, cigarette smoking, obesity) which can be the basis of health promotion programmes. A population may also be surveyed to establish people's views on health or health services, thereby yielding information not otherwise available and which may also be of major importance in planning and developing services. Whatever the aims of a cross-sectional study, many of the aspects of the methodology will be broadly similar.

Outline of methodology

The cross-sectional study is a type of epidemiological investigation which seeks to gather data on one or more aspects or characteristics of individuals resident in that population at a particular point in time. Because it will seldom be feasible or necessary to gather such data about every member of the population, usually a sample is chosen to be studied. On the basis of the findings within the sample, general conclusions are drawn about the population.

Choosing the study population

Assembling the population for this kind of study involves gaining access to a representative list of members of the population and then applying the technique of sampling to this list.

Sampling

A number of important considerations should be borne in mind when choosing a sample. Uppermost is the need to appreciate that, in taking a sample, the underlying objective is to make true statements about the population itself.

The technique of drawing a sample has an important bearing on this process. There are two main ways of obtaining a sample of people; firstly, by the quota method and secondly, randomly.

Quota sampling. The quota sample is often employed by market research organisations. This method involves the interviewer seeking a specified number of people to fit into a pre-agreed sample configuration. Men or women of particular ages or social backgrounds may be sought out, for example, by approaching people in the street. This type of sampling is generally unsatisfactory because it is unlikely to result in a sample which is representative of the whole population. For instance, a sample of middle-aged men, drawn by quota sampling in a shopping centre in mid-morning, would be unlikely to be truly representative of all middle-aged men in the particular town. Groups such as the unemployed or shift workers would tend to be over-represented.

Random sampling. The basic and most commonly used sampling method in survey research is the random sample. There are a number of different ways of obtaining a random sample, but all have the following in common: the results can be generalised to the total population from which the random sample was drawn and the precision of the estimate derived from the sample can be calculated statistically.

Choice of a sampling frame

The first step in drawing a random sample is to construct a suitable sampling frame. A sampling frame is merely a list (actual or notional) of the population. The nature of the sampling frame will vary according to the purposes of the survey. A sample for a survey of infant feeding practices might be drawn from all birth registrations in a particular area. In a survey of occupational diseases, the sampling frame might be the employment records of particular firms.

Many population surveys in public health medicine will aim to conduct an investigation in a sample of the population of a geographically defined area: say a health authority. Obtaining a suitable sampling frame, (i.e. a list of the residents of that authority), from which to draw a suitably sized sample survey is not a straightforward proposition. A traditional approach is to use the electoral roll, which supplies a list of people qualified to vote listed by the street within the different electoral wards of a town or city. As a sampling frame representative of the general population, however, this has serious limitations. The most obvious is that people below voting age are excluded. In addition, the rolls are often out of date as people move into or out of the area.

As more general practitioners have combined into large group practices, the potential for the use of age-sex registers as representative sampling frames has increased. The computerised central registers of Family Health Services Authorities (FHSAs) also have extremely important potential in this respect. It is important here, too, to realise that the register may be inflated by people who have died or left the area but whose names have not yet been removed from it.

Having obtained a suitable sampling frame, there are a number of different approaches to obtaining the random sample. The most direct is to choose people at random from the sampling frame until the required sample size is achieved (simple random sample).

A simple 10% random sample of a population of 1000 people would involve picking at random 100 names from amongst the 1000 listed. It is absolutely essential however that each time a name is chosen, every individual has an equal chance of being picked. One technique for ensuring that this is the case is through the use of a table of random numbers. In the example above, the people in the population are numbered from 000 to 999. Using a special table of random numbers, 100 numbers are then picked and the people corresponding to the numbers listed become the sample. Modern computer technology can be used to generate a random sample if the sampling frame is held on a computer data base.

Another approach is to draw a systematic random sample in which individuals are picked from the sampling frame in sequence. A 10% random sample drawn in this way would involve choosing every 10th name on the list (a 1 in 10 sample), only the first selection being made from the table of random numbers.

This is often a much more convenient way of drawing a sample. Systematic sampling is usually a perfectly satisfactory method, but it depends on people or items listed on a sampling frame being arranged in a way that does not introduce bias. For example, a 1 in 10 systematic sample drawn from a list of married people in which the husband's name always came first would result in either every person chosen being female or every person being male.

Stratification. This may be used to ensure adequate representation of different sections of the population. The population is divided into sections or strata, for example social classes, age groups, or places of residence. A random sample is then drawn from within each stratum. Stratified sampling has the additional advantage that it allows a different size of sample to be taken from each stratum.

Multistage sampling. This is often a convenient technique in large surveys. For example, a survey of lung disease in steel workers might take as its first-stage sampling frame a list of all towns with steel works. Having chosen an appropriate number of towns randomly, a second stage sampling frame consisting of the names of employees could be drawn from the towns which had initially been chosen. The workers for examination would then be drawn at random from the second frame. The advantage of having adopted a two-stage sampling technique is clearly that the need to draw up a named list of steel workers in the country was by-passed, thus saving time and avoiding difficulty and cost to the investigators.

Gathering data on the sample

The information to be gathered on members of the sample, once it has been drawn, will depend on the aims of the population survey. However, a number of general principles apply.

Definition of what to collect

At the outset, decisions need to be taken about the information which is required to address the aims of the study and how it is to be collected. There will be some types of information which address the central research question (for example, a person's blood pressure in a population survey of hypertension) whilst other information will be gathered because it provides important background on the characteristics of the sample or because it may be relevant to the analysis of the main factors under study.

Consideration must next be given as to how best to obtain the data in order to provide the required information. This may sound like a simple matter but it seldom is. Consider a seemingly straightforward variable such as social class which might be collected as an important piece of information in a population survey of mothers' infant feeding practice. Interviewers questioning members of the sample could not simply ask the mothers: 'what is your social class?'. The responses to such a general question by a population, with varying perceptions of what was meant by the concept of social class, would yield data from which no valid conclusions could be drawn about the social class of the respondents in relation to the Registrar General's definitions. A proper approach would involve the construction of a question which would provide the elements necessary to categorise the respondent by social class. Ideally, such a question should be derived from established survey work in the field and of proven validity.

There are two general ground rules which are helpful to bear in mind when addressing these issues about information gathering. The first is always to take a pedantic approach to considering the way in which each piece of information, even the simplest, is to be derived. For example, to derive age, should respondents be asked their precise age, to place their age in a banding or age group, or should they be asked their precise date of birth? This needs to be discussed in the planning stage of the survey and a decision taken on what seems appropriate, bearing in mind the aims of the study and the method of data collection. The second ground rule is to use, wherever possible, established and validated measures or questions. For example, in a questionnaire survey of lifestyle which seeks to establish levels of alcohol intake in the population, rather than the investigators thinking up their own question to elicit information they should make use of the format of questions used in well-respected previous studies in this field.

Special and more difficult judgements have to be made when gathering data to provide information about the prevalence of a disease. The first step is to agree on an operational definition of the disease under study and the method by which it is to be measured or detected. Even a formally stated definition of a disease may be of little practical value in conducting a survey to determine its prevalence. It is necessary to agree and lay down strict criteria which must be fulfilled in order that a person is counted as having the disease. Table 2.5 shows an approach which has been used in obtaining a list of criteria to define a chronic disease. It illustrates the contrast with the clinical situation, where the features of an illness which are taken as the basis for attaching a particular diagnostic label, may vary markedly between different doctors. The reasons underlying those decisions may not always be apparent. In planning a population study to determine the prevalence of a disease it is essential to resolve and adhere to a working definition or the results collected will have no meaning outside the context in which they are collected.

Table 2.5:   1987 Revised American College of Rheumatology criteria for rheumatoid arthritis

Criterion no.	Criterion description
1	Morning stiffness of at least one hour's duration
2	Arthritis of at least three joint groups with soft-tissue swelling or fluid observed by a physician
3	Arthritis involving at least one of the following joint groups: proximal interphalangeal, metacarpophalangeal, and wrists
4	Symmetrical arthritis
5	Subcutaneous nodules
6	Positive rheumatoid factor test
7	Radiographic changes typical of rheumatoid arthritis

Source: Hochberg MC, Spector TD. Epidemiology of Rheumatoid Arthritis: update. Epidemiologic Reviews 1990; 12: 247–51.

Method of data collection: the survey instrument

The choice of the method through which the data necessary to address the aims of the study will be derived is another important decision in planning a population survey. To a certain extent, this will also depend on the aims of the investigation.

The term used to describe the method of data collection is the *survey instrument* and sometimes it can literally be an 'instrument' (for example, a sphygmomanometer used to measure blood pressure in a population survey of hypertension). More often, however, the survey instrument is the document in which survey data are recorded: for example, a questionnaire to be administered by trained interviewers or a pro-forma used to extract data in a standardised format from various clinical records.

A detailed consideration of questionnaire design is beyond the scope of this book but there are a number of important aspects to be considered, for example: the structuring of questions (including the relative merits of closed versus open); the order in which questions should be asked; the avoidance of questions likely to lead to ambiguous or biased answers; the layout of the questionnaire; the coding of responses to facilitate analysis.

Questionnaires are of two broad kinds: those which will be administered face-to-face by an interviewer and postal questionnaires. Although postal questionnaires have the advantage that they allow a much larger sample size, they can have serious disadvantages in terms of the restricted range of topics which can be covered and in the generally higher levels of non-response which tend to occur with this method of questionnaire administration.

Whatever survey instrument is chosen, it is important that before the full-scale survey is undertaken, a *pilot study* is carried out on a small number of people within the sample. This allows difficulties with the questionnaire or other aspects of the survey to be ironed out or corrected before the survey proper is commenced.

Standardisation of measurement and interview technique

Variation between measurements is another important consideration in a population survey and as the example of the measurement of blood pressure shows (Figure 2.13), it can have a wide variety of sources. The main concern is with systematic variation or bias.

Some variation can be reduced by standardising the procedures in the study as, for example, when physical examinations are being carried out. This will best be ensured by training examiners and checking their technique (for departure from the standard) at intervals during the conduct of the study.

If interviewers are being used to elicit information from members of the study population by questionnaire, they must be trained. This can be done by recording pilot interviews on videotape. Thus the interviewers and the study organisers can assess the results together and correct any faults in technique.

These are only some aspects of the process of preparing and monitoring interviewers who are responsible for gathering the survey data. There are many others including: agreeing rules to be adopted when the respondents are reluctant to answer the questions posed, what to do when other family members seek to

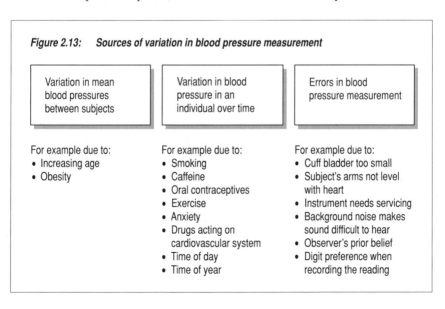

Figure 2.13: **Sources of variation in blood pressure measurement**

Variation in mean blood pressures between subjects	Variation in blood pressure in an individual over time	Errors in blood pressure measurement
For example due to: • Increasing age • Obesity	For example due to: • Smoking • Caffeine • Oral contraceptives • Exercise • Anxiety • Drugs acting on cardiovascular system • Time of day • Time of year	For example due to: • Cuff bladder too small • Subject's arms not level with heart • Instrument needs servicing • Background noise makes sound difficult to hear • Observer's prior belief • Digit preference when recording the reading

participate in answering questions on the respondents behalf, and the extent to which interviewers should react to or make observations on responses made to the questions.

A lack of clarity on these and many other aspects of interviewing can risk the results obtained being invalid or biased in ways which may be impossible to detect or eliminate from the analysis. This is why the choice of interviewers is particularly important, as is their training and experience in both the general techniques of interviewing and the issues which are specific to the particular investigation.

Variation arising from scientific instruments used in surveys can be reduced by introducing strict quality control. In studies using laboratory measurements, test solutions or reagents can be employed to ensure standardisation.

The problem of non-response

A major difficulty when gathering data in population surveys is the problem of non-response or non-cooperation.

The planning and organisation of the study should be geared to obtaining the highest possible recruitment of the sample under investigation. Key factors for success in minimising non-response will include: the nature of the initial approach made to members of the sample; the wording of a letter of introduction; the institution on the notepaper heading and, who the signatory is. These are factors which can make the difference between a very high rate of participation in the subsequent interview and a disastrous level of refusals or non-response.

It is inevitable, however, that some degree of non-response will remain, even after the most careful planning and the most strenuous efforts to reduce it. The main concern with non-response is that the non-responders are unlikely to be typical of the remainder of the sample. Depending on the circumstances, they may be more (or less) likely to suffer the disease or other subject of the investigation and hence their omission is likely to lead to bias when drawing conclusions from the results of the sample. Aside from initial attempts to keep non-response to a minimum, when it does occur the first approach is to make extra efforts on this group to gain their co-operation. Where this fails, a second strategy is to obtain as much indirect evidence as possible about the non-responders so as to make an estimate of the kind of bias which may be introduced by their omission.

Sometimes it is asked what level of response rate is acceptable? This question is almost impossible to answer in general terms because it depends on the nature and aims of the study. The concept to be borne in mind, however, is a simple one. Unless data on the sample (originally chosen) are fully captured, then the findings will not be truly representative of the whole population from which the sample was drawn. This is after all the purpose of the prevalence survey.

Some degree of non-response is, however, a feature of nearly all population surveys. The aim should be to achieve a response rate in the 95 to 100 per cent range. Some surveys do manage to do this although it would seldom be expected in postal surveys. However, it is more common to see reports of surveys with response rates in the mid to upper 70 per cent range. This is far less satisfactory but can still yield valuable findings, particularly if some data are available on the non-responders and if conclusions are drawn more cautiously than would be the case with higher response rates.

A further problem in interpreting data from population surveys to establish disease prevalence is the need to be fully aware that the population being dealt with is a survivor population. If the disease has an appreciable mortality the most severe cases will have died and any cross-sectional study will not include the entire spectrum of disease.

STUDIES TO INVESTIGATE DISEASE CAUSATION

One of the most important areas of investigation in public health is the exploration of hypotheses involving factors which may be responsible for causing disease. It is of particular importance because, if such links can be established, then there may be scope for prevention by intervening against causal agents.

A causal hypothesis may spring from clinical impression, from laboratory observations or from examining descriptive data in populations in relation to time, place or person as was described in the first section of this chapter.

Thereafter, the testing of the hypothesis that the factor, or factors under examination may be responsible for causing the disease is a matter for carefully designed studies using epidemiological methods, each of which has its own special characteristics governing its use.

The previous section of this chapter has demonstrated that the techniques of descriptive epidemiology require a clear understanding of the sources of available data, the ways in which they can be used to make comparisons and, particularly, the limits which must be placed on any conclusions which can be drawn. This is even more important when using the more specialised study methods of epidemiology, two of which (cohort and case-control studies) are described in detail in this section.

One of the principal reasons for the existence of such study methods, and their complexity, is the fact that the investigator of causal relationships in human populations is denied the experimental approach.

If the laboratory scientist wishes to investigate whether or not a suspected cause results in a particular outcome or effect, he frequently does have at his disposal the experimental approach. Suppose, for example, that a particular chemical is suspected of causing breast cancer in white mice. The investigator could take a strain of white mice and allocate them at random into two groups. One group would receive the presumed causal chemical, the other group would be treated identically in all ways, except that the mice would not receive the chemical. The investigator would then observe the occurrence of breast cancer in the two groups of animals and draw conclusions. In the laboratory experiment, the investigator is in control of the events and as a result has an extremely powerful and direct method at his disposal. Similar experiments to test the effect of a suspected causal factor in groups of humans are usually quite unacceptable. Thus, if the same chemical which caused breast cancer in the white mice was suspected of causing breast cancer in human females, an experiment could not be carried out in which one group of women was given the chemical and the other was not. Experiments may, sometimes, be performed on groups of people where removal of a suspected causal factor or addition of a supposed beneficial factor could result in an improvement in health, although the ethical aspects of such studies needs the most careful consideration. The most usual experiment carried out in human subjects is the controlled clinical trial in which new therapies are tested out on people with particular diseases.

Sometimes, fortuitously for the investigator but often to the great misfortune of the population concerned, natural experiments take place which allow conclusions to be drawn about causation. Much of the knowledge on the role of atomic radiation in the cause of cancer has stemmed from observing the development of the disease in the survivors of Hiroshima and their progeny.

Usually, however, the experimental approach is ruled out for ethical reasons when investigating the effects of causes in human populations. Instead the search concentrates on associations between the factor, or set of factors, and a disease. This 'observational' approach (to distinguish it from the 'experimental') involves comparing the disease experience of two or more groups of people in relation to their possession of certain characteristics or exposure to a suspected factor or factors.

There are two main approaches to investigating causal hypotheses: cohort and case-control studies (Figure 2.14). Each has its own specific design features. Both involve comparisons being made between different groups of people but the basis of this comparison is entirely different in the two types of study.

In the cohort study, the comparison is being made between people who have been exposed to the hypothesised risk factor and people who have not been exposed to it; each group is then studied to see whether they develop the disease. In the case-control study, the disease is already present in one group (the 'cases') and absent in another (the 'controls'); the two groups' previous exposure to the hypothesised risk factor is then compared.

Before each of these methods is described in more detail, two important points should be borne in mind. Firstly, most health professionals, managers and students, even those specialising in the public health field, will never themselves carry out a cohort study or a case-control study (except when investigating outbreaks of communicable disease). However, some of the decisions which they take will be based upon the evidence of such studies undertaken by others. This is why it is important to have a good understanding of each methodology, when it is appropriate to apply it, what its potential limitations are, and where the possible sources of bias lie. Whole texts have been written on these study methods, particularly dealing with the statistical analysis of the data which are produced, but it is not essential to have an understanding of these matters to an advanced level. It is much more important to grasp the basic principles of both cohort studies and case-control studies.

The second point to be borne in mind is that the decision to make use of these specialised methods cannot be undertaken lightly. Their use is a matter for careful deliberation and would usually only be undertaken by a team of researchers or investigators, including (or with the advice of) a statistician skilled in the design and analysis of such studies. The next sections describe the main features of the two methods.

Cohort studies

Outline of methodology

The cohort study is a type of epidemiological investigation in which a population apparently free of the disease under study (or sample of such a population) is assembled and each individual is categorised according to whether they have been exposed to the risk factor(s) of interest. The cohort is then followed up to see whether individual members of it develop the disease under study (or other

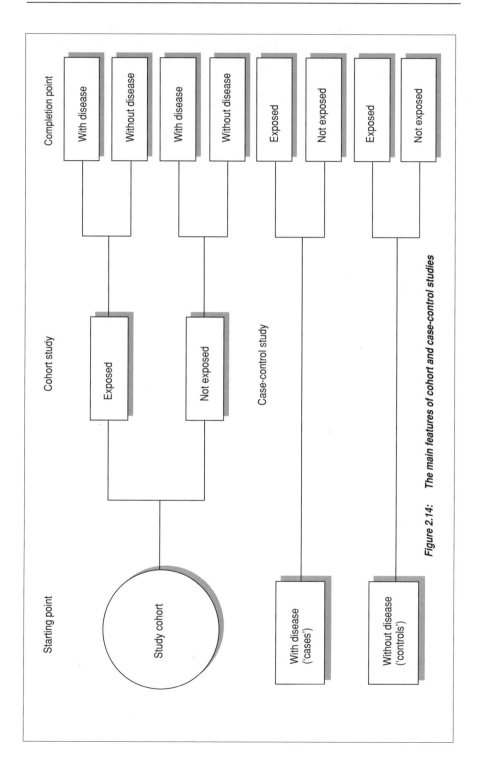

Figure 2.14: The main features of cohort and case-control studies

diseases). Comparisons are then made between the occurrence of the disease in the 'exposed' compared to the 'non-exposed' groups within the cohort. If the intention is to test the hypothesis that smoking causes lung cancer, the initial step is to classify the study cohort into smokers and non-smokers. The cohort is then followed up over time and cases of lung cancer are detected as they occur. The results would then be analysed to show what proportion of the smokers developed lung cancer compared to the proportion of non-smokers.

A cohort study may be conducted prospectively or retrospectively. In a prospectively conducted cohort study, the initial exposure data are collected on the members of the cohort and the investigators then wait for cases of the disease to crop up over time. This is the commonest type of cohort study, so much so that the terms 'cohort study' and 'prospective study' are sometimes used synonymously.

It is possible however, to conduct a retrospective cohort study, where data on the cohort's exposure as well as its disease experience, are already available. This can only really be contemplated where good past records exist to define a historical cohort. For example, suppose that a very large general practice had maintained very comprehensive records on medications prescribed to the practice population over a long period of time. If in the present day, a particular drug became suspected of causing a type of cancer, the records of such a practice may allow a retrospective cohort study to be carried out. In such a study, a cohort would be assembled at some notional past date from the old practice population records and the people within it would be classified according to whether they had been prescribed the drug of interest or not. Their past and present medical records would then also be examined to record their disease history and particularly whether they developed the cancer which was under study.

This is a simplified description of a complex methodology but in the relatively unusual situation where past data are available comprehensively on a large population, the retrospective cohort study has advantages of speed and lower cost compared to the more common prospective approach.

Choice of a study population

A cohort is a group of people who share a similar experience at a point in time. A birth cohort is people born on a particular day or in a particular year and a marriage cohort, those married in a given year. People residing in a particular geographical area or workers in an industry at a certain time also constitute a cohort.

In a cohort study investigating a causal hypothesis, the precise choice of cohort will depend on the nature of the disease under investigation. The cohort might be a group of people who have been exposed to a particular hazard (for example, a serious water pollution incident), a large workforce in a particular industry (for example, asbestos workers) or the population of a geographically defined area (for example, a small town).

Characterising the cohort

The way in which data are assembled to characterise the initial cohort of people to be followed up will very much depend on the aims of the study. In a cohort study examining the risk of cancer arising from an industrial hazard, it is likely that quite detailed information would be gathered on the employment history of the workers concerned, their likely exposure in the workplace to quantified levels of the presumed risk factor, as well as whether they had other habits or characteristics which might influence the possibility of them developing the disease (for example, cigarette smoking). In a cohort study examining the risk of development of heart disease in a population, a sample of the population might form the study cohort and each member might be assessed by questionnaire, as well as by clinical and biochemical examination to determine their baseline status in terms of the risk factors under investigation.

The follow-up phase

The follow-up phase of a cohort study, conducted prospectively, requires very careful planning and preparation. Particularly in studies where a long follow-up period is required, the difficulties in keeping track of members of the cohort who move away from the area can be very great and the process can be expensive. Considerable stability is also required in the investigative team, particularly amongst its leaders, if the study is to be brought to a successful conclusion.

A number of decisions need to be made when this phase of the cohort study is being designed. One important decision is how, and at what intervals, re-assessments of the original members of the cohort will be made. This decision is somewhat easier when the outcome under study is a clear end point such as death. In such circumstances sources of mortality data can be kept under constant review and the records of members of the original cohort can be flagged as the deaths occur to denote the outcome. Where the study is examining less dramatic outcomes, such as the progress of children whose mothers were exposed (and not exposed) to a particular hazard in pregnancy, it would be necessary (in this example) to decide on the time periods at which the children in the original cohort would be given further developmental assessments. Clearly, it would be quite impractical to undertake this with great regularity on the very large numbers of children who would be involved.

Case-control studies

The main attraction of a case-control study, especially when compared to a cohort study, is that it is relatively quick and cheap to undertake. Gathering data does not involve a long period of follow-up of the study population. That is not to say that the methodology is free of problems and these along with its main features are described in this section.

Outline of methodology

The case-control study is a type of epidemiological investigation in which an assessment is made of the extent to which people with an established disease ('cases') and a comparable group who do not have the disease ('controls') have been exposed to a risk factor believed to be responsible for causing the disease.

For example, if it is the intention to investigate the hypothesis that smoking causes lung cancer, the investigation begins by taking people with lung cancer and suitable controls who do not have lung cancer. Enquiries are then made to discover how many of the lung cancer patients were smokers and how many of the control patients were smokers.

The method of investigation in a case-control study is, almost without exception, retrospective. The investigator looks back in time on the past exposure history of present day cases of the disease and of the controls.

Choice of a study population

In practice, the design of a case-control study is much more difficult than this broad outline of the methodology implies. One of the key initial decisions for the investigator is to decide on the way in which the cases and controls which make up the study population will be chosen. If wrong decisions are made at this stage of the investigation, then the sources of bias which are introduced could render the results of the study invalid and useless.

Selection of 'cases'. The choice of 'cases' should start with the formulation of a clear operational definition of what constitutes a 'case' of the disease under study. Decisions will need to be taken on whether to study a broad diagnostic category (for example, adult acute leukaemia) or a more homogenous diagnostic grouping (adult acute myeloid leukaemia). This decision depends on the nature of the investigation but, in general, the more heterogeneity in the diagnostic group, the less likelihood of being able to link a specific risk factor to the disease causation. On the other hand, the narrower the category of disease for inclusion of 'cases' in the study, the less general applicability will the findings have. For example, a case-control study to investigate possible risk factors in osteoarthrosis which took as 'cases' people with disease of the metacarpal joints and which yielded a finding of an apparently new risk factor for the disease would have thrown light on the causation of osteoarthrosis. However, general conclusions could not necessarily be drawn about osteoarthrosis of other joints in the body because the 'cases' were limited to people with disease at one particular site.

Having established a 'case' definition, it is most important to identify a source of all cases so that all eligible cases can be recruited into the study.

Selection of controls. The choice of an appropriate 'control' group is the issue which will usually cause the greatest discussion amongst investigators planning a 'case-control' study. Whilst the issues involved in selecting 'controls' are complex, and often particular to the circumstances of the study, it is important to keep in mind the central purpose of the 'control' group. This is to provide an indication of the level of exposure to the risk factor in a 'healthy' population to which the exposure experienced by the people who have developed the disease can then be compared. Put in the simplest terms, suppose that a 'case-control' study was carried out to test the hypothesis that regular consumption of a particular kind of herbal tea led to the occurrence of pancreatic cancer. Say that 40% of 'cases' were found to be drinkers of the herbal tea, such a finding would be of much less interest if 40% of the general population were regular herbal tea drinkers than if only 2% were. In this example, the 'controls' are there to represent the same types of people as the 'cases' and allow an estimate to be made of the 'normal' pattern of herbal tea drinking.

In practice, to find 'controls' which are representative of a general population from which the 'cases' are presumed to have arisen, can be extremely difficult. For example, some 'case-control' studies using hospital 'cases' take as their 'control' group, patients who attended the hospital for the treatment of diseases other than the one which is the subject of the study. This approach has advantages in that access to controls is usually relatively easy and information can be gathered in a similar fashion to the 'cases'. It is also open to a number of potential sources of bias. For example, the hospital may have different catchment populations for the disease which is the subject of the study (the 'cases') and for the disease from which the 'control' group patients were suffering. In such circumstances, the 'controls' may not be representative of the general population from which the 'cases' were drawn, so the degree of their exposure to the risk factor may be an unreliable basis for comparison with the 'cases'.

'Controls' which are drawn from the general population do not suffer from this drawback but are less easy to identify and to gain cooperation from. The way in which they provide information may also be different to the 'cases' in ways which may introduce bias.

The relative advantages and disadvantages of different types of controls has led to many investigators using two sets of 'controls' in 'case-control' studies, one drawn from hospital and the other from the community.

Matching cases and controls

A great deal of emphasis is often placed on the question of 'matching' in 'case-control' studies. This is the process whereby 'controls' are matched to 'cases' on the basis of certain characteristics which are also known to be present in the 'cases'. The purpose of 'matching' is to eliminate the effect of so-called 'confounding' variables. Confounding can occur in other types of epidemiological investigation and is a term used to describe circumstances where there are factors, in addition to the risk factor under study, which may influence whether the disease occurs. If such confounding factors are unevenly distributed between study groups then they can distort the comparisons which are being made (and hence the conclusions which are drawn). One of the commonest confounding variables is age. The occurrence of many diseases is strongly associated with age. If in a case-control study, there are major differences in the age structure of 'cases' and 'controls', this may distort other more important comparisons between the two groups. In descriptive epidemiological studies, standardisation (described in Chapter 1) is the method through which the confounding effect of age is reduced.

The technique of matching should be used very sparingly because there are serious problems which can result from overmatching. With modern statistical analytical techniques the matching of characteristics of cases and controls can also be undertaken during the analysis stage. The tendency in 'case-control' studies now is to take account of confounding variables (except age and sex) in the analysis of results rather than eliminate them at the study design stage of matching.

Assembling data on the exposure

Data on the exposure to the hypothesised risk factor(s) amongst 'cases' and 'controls' is usually obtained retrospectively by one, or both, of two main methods. Firstly, it is obtained by abstracting information from medical or other records pertaining to the 'cases' and the 'controls' and secondly, from the 'cases' and 'controls' (or where there have been deaths, their relatives) by interview.

Inherent in these approaches are further potential sources of bias. Records may not provide either comprehensive or detailed information to satisfy fully the requirements of the investigation. This is hardly surprising because such records seldom will have been created in the knowledge that they would be needed for a study. For example, retrospectively obtaining data on exposure from medical records of lung cancer patients and hospital patients with other diseases (used as controls), it would be more likely that a smoking history would be recorded in the lung cancer patients because of the known association between that disease and cigarette smoking than in those with other diseases.

A further potential source of bias arises when exposure data are obtained retrospectively by interview. A person with the disease may be more likely to remember or report an exposure (perhaps because he is trying to rationalise the presence of the disease) than a person serving as a control who is disease free. For example, a surgeon notices that many female patients presenting at his outpatient clinic with breast lumps give a past history of localised trauma. To investigate this further, he takes two groups of women: one group comprises those who have presented to the outpatient clinic with a breast lump; the other comprises a sample of healthy women of similar ages. Each group of women is asked if they can recall having any bang, knock or bruise of the breast during the previous 12 months. A much higher occurrence of such trauma is found in the group with breast lumps than amongst the control group of healthy women. Should it then be concluded that localised trauma predisposes to the formation of breast lumps? This is possible but unlikely. Women who have developed a breast lump are often in a very anxious state and their principal fear is that the lump is malignant. They will often cling to any alternative explanation of the origin of the lump. Hence, when such women are questioned about a history of trauma they are far more likely to remember and volunteer some trivial occurrence, than will those women without breast lumps.

Since data are obtained retrospectively on the exposure, whether by abstraction of case notes or by interview survey, the serious problems arise when there are differences in the completeness of information or selectivity between the two groups ('cases' and 'controls'). The investigator may not be aware of it and may draw misleading conclusions, such as in the examples given above. It is not possible fully to guard against this but, an additional measure which may help, is to ensure that the person gathering the data (whether abstracting it from records or questioning patients) relies on a structured format and is 'blind' to whether the individuals are 'cases' or 'controls'.

ANALYSIS OF DATA FROM COHORT AND CASE CONTROL STUDIES: MEASURES OF RISK

A common measure of association derived from epidemiological studies of causation is the *relative risk*. This measure expresses how many more times the disease occurred in the group which were exposed to the risk factor than the group which was not.

Relative risk

In a cohort study, the relative risk is calculated from the ratio of incidence rates in the exposed group and the non-exposed group:

Incidence of the disease in the exposed group = I_e
Incidence of the disease in the non-exposed group = I_n

Relative risk $=$ $\dfrac{I_e}{I_n}$

If no association, relative risk $= 1$

Odds ratio

In a case-control study, incidence rates cannot be calculated because the subjects do not necessarily represent the population as a whole. However, an estimate of the *relative risk* is produced by the *odds ratio*. This ratio is constructed by dividing the odds of the case group having been exposed to the risk factor by the odds of the control group having been exposed (Table 2.6). The calculation of these indices and the statistical theory underlying them is beyond the scope of this book but they have been introduced in outline to give an insight into the way in which the results of these more specialised epidemiological studies may be presented and interpreted.

Aside from the relative risk, it is possible to calculate other measures of risk when examining associations between possible risk factors and diseases.

Table 2.6: The findings of a case-control study

Exposed to risk factor	With the disease 'Cases'	Without the disease 'Controls'
YES	a	b
NO	c	d
Total	a + c	b + d

The Odds Ratio is a measure of the association between the risk factor and the disease and is calculated:
Step one: Odds of a person in the case group having been exposed to the risk factor = a/c
Step two: Odds of a person in the control group having been exposed to the risk factor = b/d
Step three: Ratio of odds = $\dfrac{a/c}{b/d}$ = $\dfrac{a\,d}{b\,c}$

Attributable risk

An alternative approach is to examine the difference in disease occurrence between the exposed and unexposed groups rather than the ratio. Such an approach is used to construct the *attributable risk*.

Data from a cohort study could thus be analysed:

Incidence of the disease in the exposed group $= I_e$
Incidence of the disease in the non-exposed group $= I_n$
Attributable risk $= I_e - I_n$
If no association, attributable risk $= 0$

The attributable risk is useful in examining the absolute additional risk which individuals experience as a result of their exposure.

Population attributable risk

Another measure, the *population attributable risk* is a measure of the extent to which the amount of the disease which occurs in the population is due to the risk factor. The population attributable risk is useful in terms of assessing the public health impact of a risk factor and hence the benefits which could be obtained by preventive action.

It is calculated by multiplying the attributable risk by the prevalence (P) of the risk factor in the population:

$(I_e - I_n) \times P$

A relatively small excess (i.e. attributable) risk of developing a disease where a large number of people are exposed to the risk factor would yield many additional cases. The benefits of preventive action could be great. Alternatively an attributable risk which was large but where relatively few people were exposed to the risk would not produce a large burden of disease in the population and the scope for major preventive action would be limited.

Analysis of case-control study data

Table 2.7 shows data from an actual case-control study which investigated the relationship between the use of sunbeds and sunlamps and the occurrence of malignant melanoma.

The data are shown to illustrate the way in which such an analysis can be presented (not to describe the particular case-control study in detail). Nevertheless, as Table 2.7 shows, there was an elevated odds ratio in men and women who used sunbeds or sunlamps (though in the latter not quite achieving statistical significance because the lower confidence limit did not exceed 1). The authors concluded that the use of artificial tanning devices appeared to be a risk factor for melanoma.

Table 2.7:   *Analysis of data from a case control study to investigate the relationship between sunbed and sunlamp usage and malignant melanoma*

Males		Cases	Controls
Used sunlamps (exposed)		67	41
Did not use sunlamps (unexposed)		210	242
Total		277	283
Odds ratio	1.88		
95% Confidence interval*	1.20–2.98		

Females		Cases	Controls
Used sunlamps (exposed)		85	68
Did not use sunlamps (unexposed)		221	256
Total		306	324
Odds ratio	1.45		
95% Confidence interval*	0.99–2.13		

* 95% confidence interval is a measure which enables the statistical significance of the observed raised odds ratio to be assessed. Given that the odds ratio is estimated from a sample of a hypothetical whole population, we can be 95% confident that the true odds ratio (which we do not know) lies between the lower and upper limits. In this case, if the lower limit is above 1 (it is for males, not quite for females) then the odds ratio can be said to be significantly raised. Other confidence intervals (e.g. 99%) can be calculated if higher levels of significance are required.

Source: Adapted from: Walter SD, Marrett LD, From L, Hertzmann C, Shannon HS, Roy P. The association of cutaneous malignant melanoma with the use of sunbeds and sunlamps. American Journal of Epidemiology 1990; 131: 232–43.

Table 2.8:   Analysis of data from a cohort study investigating the association between oral contraceptive usage and the occurrence of chronic inflammatory bowel disease

Use of oral contraceptives	Woman years of observation	Ulcerative colitis		Crohn's disease	
		No. of cases	Incidence/1000 woman years	No. of cases	Incidence/1000 woman years
Never used	75,950	8	0.11	6	0.08
Ex-user	67,319	7	0.10	4	0.06
Current user	61,116	16	0.26	8	0.13
Total	204,385	31	0.15	18	0.09

Source: Vessey M, Jewell D, Smith A, Yeates D, McPherson K. Chronic inflammatory bowel disease, cigarette smoking, and use of oral contraceptives: findings in a large cohort study of women of childbearing age. British Medical Journal. 1986; 292: 1101–3.

Relative risk (RR)   = $\dfrac{\text{Incidence in exposed population } (I_e)}{\text{Incidence in non-exposed population } (I_n)}$

RR Ulcerative colitis   = $\dfrac{0.26}{0.11}$ =   2.36

RR Crohn's disease   = $\dfrac{0.13}{0.08}$ =   1.63

Analysis of cohort study data

Table 2.8 is an example of a different way in which data from a cohort study can be analysed. This is because it is only a comparison of incidence and there is no calculation of risk. However, the risk calculation is added to the table. The data are from a large study in which married women using different forms of contraception were followed up and information was gathered on a range of health outcomes. The aspect of the study shown in Table 2.8 examines the relationship between use of oral contraceptives and the subsequent development of two inflammatory bowel diseases (ulcerative colitis and Crohn's disease).

There was a higher incidence of both ulcerative colitis and Crohn's disease in current oral contraceptive users than in women who had never used the pill or had given up using it (Table 2.8). Whilst the difference did not achieve statistical significance for Crohn's disease, it did for ulcerative colitis. Incidences in those who had stopped using oral contraceptives were similar to those who had never used them.

The authors concluded that whilst the associations between oral contraceptive use and chronic inflammatory bowel disease could not be regarded as established, they provided important clues to its causation.

Establishing a causal relationship

As has been made clear, both cohort and case-control studies are observational in nature. To investigate hypotheses of cause and effect they rely on observing real life events: people who are exposed (or expose themselves) to risk factors and those people who develop disease. If an association is found it is probable that the relationship between exposure and disease is not, in fact, one of cause and effect.

It is important, therefore, to consider the possible explanations for any association between a risk factor and a disease, whether the association has arisen as a result of a descriptive epidemiological study or from carrying out a cohort or a case-control study.

Three possible alternatives for such an association should be reviewed before detailed consideration is given to establishing whether it could be causal. The three are either that the association has arisen by chance, or that it may be spurious, or that it may be a secondary association. A brief description of each follows.

Association is a chance occurrence

The association between the factor and the disease may be a chance occurrence which would generally not be found on another occasion. Statistical tests exist, however, to allow a statement to be made of the probability with which the observed association would have arisen by chance on the hypothesis that there is, in fact, no association between the factor and the disease.

Association is spurious

The apparent association between causal factor and disease may not be real, but a product of the way in which the investigation was carried out. For example, suppose that it was intended to investigate the association between place of delivery (cause) and perinatal mortality (effect). A comparison of two groups of women might show that the perinatal mortality for those delivered in consultant obstetric units was higher than for women delivered in general practitioner maternity units. It might be concluded that general practitioner units were safer places in which to have a baby. Such a conclusion is almost certainly fallacious, however. In general, consultant obstetric units, because of their special expertise and equipment deliberately select women at high risk for delivery in their units. Thus, the consultant unit might have a higher perinatal mortality rate than the general practitioner unit because of this fact alone, and not because the quality of care was inferior. This source of bias (selection bias) where like is not being compared with like is very important. Other sources of bias (such as those described in the section on case-control studies) can also yield spurious associations between risk factors and diseases.

Association is secondary

A factor and a disease may appear to be associated in a causal fashion when in reality the reason for their association is that both are related to a third factor. Thus, an association is found between countries with a high proportion of television owners and the frequency of coronary heart disease. The fact that these two factors are strongly associated does not mean that they are causally related and that television causes coronary heart disease. A more reasonable explanation is that television ownership is an indicator of societies with lifestyles which themselves are causally related to coronary heart disease.

Criteria which infer a causal association

If an association between a factor and a disease is found which probably did not occur by chance, is not spurious and not due to a secondary association, then this does *not prove* that the association is causal. However, six criteria, if present, help to infer that the association is causal:

(1) *Plausibility.* Greater weight is given to a possible causal factor if it seems to fit in with what is known about the pathology of the disease.

(2) *Consistency.* The association would, if causal, be expected to persist when studies were carried out by different investigators working in different populations at different times.

(3) *Temporal relationship.* Clearly to assess causality it is necessary to show that the factor preceded in time the development of the disease.

(4) *Strength.* A causal relationship is more likely to be present when there is a marked difference in frequency of the disease in people who have been exposed to the factor than amongst those who have not. An additional piece of evidence which is strongly indicative of causality is the presence of a dose-response relationship: with increasingly greater exposure to the risk factor the incidence of the disease rises.

(5) *Specificity.* An ideal finding would be that the postulated causal factor was related to the disease in question and no other. This is, however, not always the case since a factor may be causally related to more than one disease.

(6) *Change in risk factor.* If the factor is removed or reduced and the incidence of the disease falls, this strongly indicates that the factor is causal.

RANDOMISED CONTROLLED TRIALS

Another type of study design which is not observational in nature, as are cross-sectional studies, cohort and case-control methods, is the so-called 'intervention' design. This usually takes the form of *a randomised controlled trial (RCT)*.

In it, two or more groups are assembled. They receive defined interventions (for example, treatments, health education messages, dietary modification) which are controlled by the investigator and they are then monitored to detect events which are hypothesised to result from these actions (for example, relief of pain, improvement in health, loss of weight). The best established context of the RCT is the clinical trial in which new therapies are assessed in comparison with old methods of treatment or of placebos ('dummy' treatments).

Outline of methodology

The main feature of the *interventional* method, which sets it apart from observational studies, is the aim of producing groups of patients comparable in respect of features known to affect the outcome, except for the different interventions which it is planned that they will receive. Other unknown differences between such groups may, of course, still be present but the usual means of negating their effects and enabling valid inferences to be made is through introducing *randomisation*. This process involves dividing the group of subjects (or any subgroup or subgroups with particular characteristics) into two parts, one part becoming the 'experimental' or 'intervention' group and the other the 'control' group. The outcome or end-point of the study is then assessed as the two groups are followed up in an identical way.

Clinical trials of therapies are much more commonplace than RCTs evaluating preventive measures. This is, in part, because of the difficulty involved with large numbers of subjects being required for the latter and a long time span to await the appearance of outcome measures. Perhaps the most frequently occurring type of preventive trial is the trials of vaccines that have been carried out. However, a number of RCTs of coronary heart disease preventive measures have been conducted, as well as a small number in the field of screening (for example, for breast cancer). The importance of the RCT to the evaluation of health services, though infrequently applied, is also often emphasised.

Choice of a study population

The planning of a randomised controlled trial necessitates an early decision, in principle, on the number of groups of people which will comprise the study population. This in turn will depend on the number of interventions to be tested. In the simplest form of randomised controlled trial, there will be two groups, of which one receives the intervention and the other does not.

Having made this decision, the first stage in assembling the study population will be to identify a base population from which the study groups can be drawn.

The choice of this base population will influence the extent to which the findings of the investigation can be generalised to other populations. This is a factor which is sometimes overlooked in the eagerness of investigators to eliminate other (albeit equally important) sources of bias in designing the randomised controlled trial. However, it can be extremely important in determining the value of the findings of the investigation. In the evaluation of a therapy, it is commonplace to draw the study group from amongst the admissions to a hospital. If, for example, the hospital is a centre of excellence and admits only the most complex cases within a particular diagnostic category (say patients with hypertension) then the findings on the effectiveness of the therapy under study would not be generalisable to all patients with the disease (in this example hypertension) but only to those with the same degree of complexity.

Eligibility

The next step in the process of assembling the study population is to decide upon criteria for eligibility. These will include a precise operational definition of the disease status of the patients (for the disease under study); age, sex and possibly other characteristics; and, the presence or absence of other clinical features (such as complications of the disease or associated conditions).

Randomisation

Once patients have been found to be eligible for the trial on the basis of diagnostic and other criteria previously laid down, then, and only then, does randomisation take place. It is an essential requirement that after eligibility for the trial has been confirmed, no further influences can be brought to bear on whether patients are allocated to particular groups. Anything other than random choice (for example, the deliberate placing of very ill patients in a non-treatment group) will introduce bias.

There are various techniques through which randomisation can be accomplished: for example, the use of random number tables, the opening of sealed envelopes containing the treatment category, or computer randomisation methods.

The process of randomisation, thus involves placing individuals from amongst the eligible population into either 'intervention' or 'control' groups in such a way that they have an equal chance of ending up in either of the groups. Its purpose is to eliminate the effect of confounding factors which can influence the outcome of the study independently of the intervention. Randomisation probably never truly eliminates the effects of confounding but it does minimise its potential effect and is a more effective technique than those used in observational studies (for example, matching in case-control studies) to eliminate confounding.

Specification of the intervention

A very precise specification of the nature of the treatment or other measures to be used, is also necessary, together with rules for the method of administration or the conditions under which the treatment should be administered. For example, in the evaluation of a preventive measure, criteria might be laid down as to who is to administer say, a health education message, whereas with the treatment the route of administration of a drug must be specified.

Placebo effect

A further element of the investigation is to specify the conditions of the 'non intervention' group and it is here, in trials of clinical therapies, that the 'placebo' is brought into play. The so called 'placebo effect' is the change in a patient's outcome or health status which can be achieved simply by being given an inactive therapy or through being a participant in a study. The psychological processes involved in this phenomenon are not fully understood.

It is easier to correct for this influence in trials of therapies. In such cases, both groups of patients (the 'intervention' and the 'non-intervention' groups) are given tablets, one set containing the active treatment under investigation, the other pharmaceutically prepared to look, smell, and feel like the active treatment but which is, in fact, inert as far as the disease under investigation is concerned.

Patients are therefore 'blind' as to whether they are receiving the real treatment or the placebo. It is also better to keep the investigators in ignorance so that they do not use their knowledge of the patient's treatment category consciously or unconsciously to influence their assessment of the patient's status following intervention (a 'double blind' study).

It is much more difficult to use a placebo process in randomised controlled trials other than those evaluating drug therapies. For example, in a trial to test the effectiveness of an intra-abdominal surgical technique, it would almost certainly be unethical (as well as inappropriate) to anaesthetise patients in the control group, then open and close their abdomens as a placebo operation.

Assessment of the outcome or end-point

Very clear study rules need to be laid down to ensure that outcomes for the patients in the two groups of the trial are clearly defined, assessed and recorded in a standard way. The outcomes (or end points) which are the subject of the investigation, will vary according to its aims but might include: (in a trial of a new therapy) improvement or worsening in a patient's condition, death, length of survival or (in a preventive trial) the onset of disease, death, change in physical or physiological characteristics such as weight, serum cholesterol, fitness.

There is a danger of bias when either the patient, the clinician or investigator (who is responsible for assessing outcome) is aware of which groups have received the intervention as opposed to the non-intervention (control) measures. This source of bias can be minimised (as described above) by ensuring that neither the patient nor the investigator is aware of which experimental group is the intervention group. This is called a 'double-blind' study. The code identifying the two groups is only broken at the end of the study.

It is important to ensure that if patients drop out of the study, or fail to complete their treatment (non-compliance) that they are included in the analysis according to the randomised group to which they were originally allocated (on the basis that there was an intention to treat). To do otherwise would be to introduce potential bias.

ETHICAL ISSUES

In the conduct of a study involving human populations a strict ethical code must be obeyed. A number of organisations have laid down codes of practice for the conduct of research investigations involving people. Of particular importance are those which have been produced by the World Medical Association, the World Health Organisation and the Royal College of Physicians of London. Health Authorities are required to have Ethics Committees to which applications must be made for approval of research to be undertaken in their area.

INVESTIGATING HEALTH SERVICE PROBLEMS IN PRACTICE

The previous section dealt with the use of two major epidemiological methodologies (cohort and case-control studies) to investigate disease causation. It began by pointing out that these methodologies were infrequently used in day-to-day practice (aside from the use of the case control method in the investigation of communicable disease outbreaks). It was also emphasised that it is essential to have a good understanding of the methodologies. Their strengths and weaknesses must be fully appreciated, not just for the occasions when they are used, but to enable the published work of others to be properly evaluated. This is especially important if decisions about health care priorities and programmes are to be based upon such studies.

This section of the chapter contains a description of the kinds of investigation which might be carried out by those playing a part on a day-to-day basis in identifying the health problems within a population and ensuring an appropriate range and quality of health services is available to address them.

There is a great deal of misunderstanding about this area of public health practice and this seems to be for a number of reasons. Firstly, this field of investigation is seldom debated and certainly is not the subject of texts, such as those written about case-control or cohort studies, which deal with the possible approaches and methodologies systematically and in-depth. Secondly, and perhaps as a consequence of the first reason, health service problem investigation is often denigrated as flawed or unscientific, particularly by those investigators used to undertaking studies using the more formal epidemiological methods. Thirdly, the investigation of a health service problem usually leads to a report which is presented to a health service policy-making board or as an aid to decision-making at an operational level within the management structure of the service. All energies are usually deployed to this end and it is less common for the investigator to set aside the time to write up his study separately for submission to a journal.

The approach of investigators based in academic institutions is very different. A report will always be produced (or internally published) for the funding body and wider circulation but major emphasis will also be placed on identifying those aspects of the study which can be written up for submission to journals. This will often result in one or more publications in major peer review journals, all of which adds to the standing of this type of investigative work.

This debate is epitomised by the phrase which is sometimes used to describe the type of investigative work undertaken within the health service: 'quick and dirty'. As with any catchphrase, it is easy to see why it has gained widespread usage but the juxtaposition of these two terms 'quick' and 'dirty' when applied to any form of bona fide public health investigation is both inappropriate and unfortunate. The term 'dirty' is intended to convey the impression of crudeness or unreliability in either the study methods used or the findings. It is only necessary to think of a cohort study of disease causation, taking many years to carry out, with consequent consumption of resources, having had a seriously flawed design at the outset, to realise that 'dirtiness' can equally apply to large-scale investigation using methods traditionally associated with scientific purity.

The importance of this issue cannot be over-emphasised because it draws attention to fundamental principles which should apply equally to the investigation of a circumscribed and urgent problem in a health service as to the study of possible risk factors for the genesis of a disease which poses a large scale public health problem.

Whether using routinely available data on *ad hoc* and limited data gathering exercise, conducting a population survey, a case-control or a cohort study, the investigator should have a clear view of the aims of the investigation and the questions which need to be answered by it. He should choose the appropriate method to carry out the investigation (bearing in mind the prevailing constraints including time and money). He should be aware of the strengths and weaknesses of the approach chosen and, most importantly, should present the findings of the study in a way which makes clear the extent of the conclusions which can be drawn from them.

Thus, some studies are more limited in scope than others because of time constraints, the availability of resources or the quality of available data. Even in such circumstances, however, good investigations can still be carried out, provided that it is made clear precisely what conclusions can be drawn from them (bearing in mind the limitations of the data). This does not make them 'dirty'.

It is also worth bearing in mind that decisions about health service priorities and the allocation of resources are being made on a daily basis and, sadly, too often on purely subjective grounds. Even a limited investigation, if carefully carried out, potentially can improve the quality of decision making.

Examples of investigations of health service problems

This section of the chapter describes a small number of examples of investigations of health service problems which have been carried out as part of the practice of departments of public health medicine. Each was the subject of a comprehensive report with presentation of data and whilst they are too extensive to be described in full here, the main features of each, together with some illustrative data, are included.

It is important to bear in mind that any investigation, no matter how small scale must be carefully planned, the first stage of which is to clearly set out the aims or questions the investigators are seeking to address or answer. It is always surprising in reading reports of investigations in public health medicine, even those submitted to editors of journals for publication, to see that the aims of the investigation were not identified at the outset.

The main purpose of the examples, however, is not to describe investigations from start to finish in exhaustive detail (space alone would prohibit this). Rather it is to give the reader an understanding of some of the practicalities of designing and executing such investigations and, particularly, to show how they can be used to provide insights into, and solutions to, health problems and the working of health services.

A survey of the health and social status of elderly people in an ethnic minority group

This investigation set out to describe certain aspects of the health and social status of people aged 65 years and over belonging to the Asian population of a city in the East Midlands area of England. An Asian person was defined as a person not of United Kingdom descent originating from India or Pakistan or, of Indian or Pakistani descent, originating from East Africa.

Context and problem definition

The population in which the study was carried out was Leicester, a city in the East Midlands area of England, which at the time had a population in which approximately 1 in 4 people belonged to ethnic minority groups. The largest group of old people in the population of Leicester who belonged to an ethnic minority group were those born in India (mainly in Gujerat or the Punjab) although the majority had come to Britain via East Africa.

At the time of the investigation, a great deal of service provision work was being undertaken within the Asian community of Leicester by health, social services and voluntary organisations but there was little objective information on the pattern of health and social need.

Carrying out the investigation

The first step in this study of elderly Asians was to gain the co-operation of the local community to the investigation.

The Asian community has strong networks and relatively well defined leadership so that it was possible to gain agreement and support for a large exercise, of the sort which was being contemplated, by discussing it with a small number of people who then took on the responsibility to inform the local community so that they would be prepared for the approach by the investigators.

It is important at this stage in planning an investigation to strike a balance between keeping the population to be surveyed properly informed and conveying only so much information about the detail of the survey that their responses to particular questions will not become prejudiced by prior thinking about what responses are needed. Thus, in the Leicester survey, the community leaders offered to publicise the forthcoming field work by a series of radio programmes. This offer was declined in favour of a more low key dissemination of information to the community.

The next stage in the planning of the survey was to select a suitable sampling frame. A number of alternatives were considered. It was felt that the electoral roll could not provide satisfactory coverage of the elderly Asian population. The possibility of identifying elderly Asians by door knocking in known Asian areas was seriously considered but informal discussions within the Asian community indicated that this approach might run into serious difficulty. Asian people are often initially wary of enquiries which seem to be of an official nature and it was feared that the response of relatives, on the doorstep, might be to seek to protect the elderly by denying the interviewer access. A further factor was that there had been recent reports in the local newspaper of people posing as survey workers in order to try to rob Asian people. On balance, it was felt that the greatest degree of co-operation could be achieved if the individuals to be approached were identified in advance so that they could receive a personal letter which explained the aims of the survey before an interviewer called to see them.

The sampling frame eventually chosen was the central register of the Family Practitioner Committee (now called the Family Health Services Authority) and agreement was reached on this by seeking the permission of the Committee and its advisors.

The next major stumbling block was that the sampling frame did not categorise patients records by ethnic status (nor is this even now a routine variable recorded in health information systems). However, experience had been gained in using the Asian naming system to identify and classify Asian people into broad cultural and religious groupings. In this way, all the names of Asian appearance occurring amongst people of age 65 years and over (the elderly for the purposes of this investigation) were extracted from the sampling frame by trained staff and used as the basis for drawing the sample.

It is well documented that general practitioner registers are inflated above their true value by people whose names appear on them but who are no longer strictly members of them, having died or moved away. The Asian population was also a relatively highly mobile group which added to sampling frame inflation and made it particularly important to eliminate errors (which was done by checking against individual general practitioners' records when individuals could not be traced).

Those identified as members of the sample were written to in the Asian languages in order to seek their co-operation, and to indicate that an interviewer would be calling. Data were collected using a questionnaire which was administered by Asian language speaking field workers in the homes of the elderly people.

The areas of enquiry included demographic details (sex, date of birth, country of origin, religion, current and past employment status); family life and social contact; aspects of lifestyle; level of physical capacity; language and communication; knowledge and use of health and social services.

Findings and implications

Three illustrative examples from amongst the range of information yielded by this investigation are shown in Tables 2.9 to 2.11.

Table 2.9 shows that whilst 5% of elderly Asians lived alone and 13% with someone of their own generation, the most frequent household configuration for these old people was multigenerational. Overall, as Table 2.9 shows, 82% lived in a household with two or more generations and the most common type of household was that in which there were three generations (usually the elderly person, their children and their grandchildren). There was little variation in household composition between religious groups.

Table 2.9: *Composition of households in which elderly Asians lived, by religion – percentages*

Household composition	Hindu	Sikh	Muslim	All Religions
Lived alone	5	4	4	5
One generation	13	19	9	13
Two generations	23	17	31	24
Three generations	56	56	49	55
Four generations	3	4	7	3
With non-relatives	>1	>1	>1	>1
All households	100	100	100	100
N (100%) =	(510)	(73)	(138)	(721)

Source: Donaldson LJ. Health and social status of elderly Asians: a community study. British Medical Journal 1986; 293: 1079–82.

Further analysis (not shown in Table 2.9) revealed that of those old people who lived in multigenerational households, about one fifth, whether they were married or widowed, shared a bedroom with someone else, most commonly grandchildren.

This pattern of household structure of the elderly Asians was in marked contrast to that of the indigenous elderly where, for example, 46% of old people lived alone.

These data had major policy implications. Participation and acceptance within the family remained a key feature of old age in the Asian Community of Leicester (this was confirmed by other findings of the investigation, not just those relating to household structure). Whilst elderly Asians were at an advantage in having the immediate help and support of other household members, the implication for services was that the situation would be very sensitive to changes in kinship patterns. Furthermore, within existing households, the opportunities for privacy were diminished and there was no way of knowing how harmonious life was within these large multigenerational households. Organisations in Leicester providing sheltered accommodation at the time were seeing instances of family conflict leading to rejection of elderly members, and it was possible that this would become a larger problem.

Another very important aspect of the investigation related to the language skills of the old people. It was common for respondents to report that they could speak more than one language. Overall, half of the sample could speak a second language and almost a third could speak a third language. Almost all Hindus spoke Gujerati and a substantial minority Hindi, Swahili or English. Sikhs nearly all spoke Punjabi with English and Hindi being the languages next most commonly spoken. Muslims were the most diverse linguistically: after Gujerati, they were likely to speak Urdu, Kutchi and English.

It was in relation to English speaking ability that particularly important findings were made. As Table 2.10 shows, a fifth of the sample could speak English but the proportion speaking it was very low amongst elderly women (only 2%). Moreover, it was also found (not shown in Table 2.10) that 63% of women could not read in any language.

Table 2.10: *The percentage of elderly Asian men and women who said that they could speak, read or write English*

English ability	Males (N=389)	Females (N=337)	Both sexes (N=726)
Spoke English	37	2	21
Read English	24	<1	13
Wrote English	21	<1	11

Source: Donaldson LJ. Health and social status of Asians: a community survey. British Medical Journal 1986; 293: 1079–82.

Even for the old people who said that they could speak English, in three of six common social situations, more than half considered that they would have had difficulty making themselves understood without an interpreter (Table 2.11).

The investigation's findings in relation to language indicated the extent to which the old people were dependent on others for contact outside their community, particularly in health settings.

The finding that nearly two thirds of Asian women were illiterate, in all languages, was of immediate importance in that it implied that simply translating leaflets on health education or welfare benefits would not be adequate.

Table 2.11: *Elderly Asians' assessment of their own ability to use English in a range of everyday situations expressed as a percentage*

Situation	Ability to make themselves understood			
	Easily	With difficulty	Only with interpreter	Total (n = 145)
Asking for cost of fare on a bus	68	22	10	100
Asking for goods in English shop	64	27	9	100
Returning faulty goods to English shop	47	31	22	100
Telephoning to rearrange outpatient appointment	43	23	34	100
Giving directions to an English person	52	31	17	100
Explaining a problem to a doctor	41	21	38	100

Source: Donaldson LJ. Health and social status of elderly Asians: a community survey. British Medical Journal 1986; 293: 1079–82.

A useful alternative to the conventional approach to posters and leaflets was considered to be the Asian language radio programmes (which were listened to by a high proportion of the old people interviewed) and home videos (ownership of rental video recorders was also relatively high in the Asian community of Leicester).

The language findings of the investigation also emphasised the need for interpreters as an integral part of health and social service provision.

Comment and overview

The investigation yielded valuable information for policy makers and planners in the health, social services and voluntary sectors. As a type of investigation in public health, the study was of the cross-sectional type and the techniques adopted were generally those described in the section of this chapter dealing with such studies. However, as with any other such investigation carried out in practice, its design and conduct had a number of special features which were variations on the textbook account of the study methodology concerned. This was particularly so because there had been relatively few surveys which had set out to gather data directly from people belonging to this ethnic minority group. It was important to seek the co-operation of community leaders to ensure success in the fieldwork and to ensure that there were people skilled in interviewing in the Asian languages if valid information was to be obtained.

An investigation into the population's access to specialist services provided in a limited number of centres

The Northern Region is one of the English health regions. It has a population of approximately three million and stretches from the border with Scotland in the north down to Yorkshire in the south, over to Cumbria in the west and Cleveland in the east. The region is made up of health districts with resident populations of varying sizes.

Many services are present in every district general hospital but some, because of their high cost or highly specialised nature, are provided in one, or a small number of hospital centres within the region. At the time that the investigation (described in this section) was carried out, heart surgery was provided in only one centre in the Northern Region. Patients who were thought to require coronary artery surgery (and other open heart procedures) were referred to the specialist centre by general practitioners or consultants in other parts of the region. Ophthalmology and some other specialist surgical services were provided at a number of hospitals (but not all) so that a patient requiring cataract surgery, for example, would be treated by one of these services.

The investigation aimed to describe the extent to which patients in different parts of the region, particularly those outside the district in which the regional or sub-regional centres were located, received treatment.

Context and problem definition

At the time of the investigation, the changes to the organisation and funding of the NHS brought in during 1990 had yet to take place. There was no formal framework of contracting for clinical services. The Regional Health Authority had been concerned to examine the extent to which the population in different places received access to services which, though located in only some centres, were funded on the basis that they would be available to the whole population.

Carrying out the investigation

Data were assembled from routinely available hospital inpatient data. Patients treated by services provided on a regional (for example, cardiothoracic surgery) and a sub-regional (for example, ophthalmology) basis were classified according to health district of residence and to the smaller local government districts of residence.

The extent to which residents of these different populations were treated as inpatients or day cases by each of these regional or sub-regional services was then calculated.

A small number of local government districts were omitted from the analysis because they were served by hospitals in a neighbouring health region and therefore all possible hospital admissions from within the population could not be captured in the analysis.

Data were analysed in two main ways. Firstly, simple hospitalisation rates were produced for different operations in relation to the populations living in health or local government districts. This enabled the number of operations per thousand (or ten thousand) population to be examined and compared.

Secondly, standardised hospitalisation ratios (SHRs) were produced. The concept is similar to the standardised mortality ratio (SMR) which is described in chapter 1. It allows for differences in the age and sex composition of the resident populations and hence enables a more valid comparison to be made. For example, a district with a young age composition could be expected to record low rates for cataract operations (cataracts being more common in the elderly). SHRs enable a comparison of this district's operation rates with other districts' rates to be made allowing for the different age compositions. In the investigation described here, the regional SHR for each specialty was, by definition, 100 and SHRs for individual resident populations were compared to this regional average value. A figure above 100 denoted more hospital discharges, and a figure below 100 denoted fewer hospital discharges, amongst residents of a particular area, than might have been expected given the experience of the region as a whole.

Findings and implications

Two examples are given here to illustrate the findings and show the kinds of issues which were raised by the investigation. The first relates to cataract operations, the second to coronary artery by-pass operations.

Table 2.12 shows the SHRs for cataract surgery in relation to local government district of residence, together with information on the location of the sub-regional ophthalmology services which were undertaking the surgery. It can be seen that there was a two-fold variation in the likelihood of a person being admitted for cataract surgery according to where they lived. To some extent, the likelihood of being admitted was higher in resident populations with greater geographical proximity to the service but some local government districts with a service within their boundaries appear to have substantially lower admission rates than others. These lower rates often apply to adjacent local government districts predominantly served by this same service.

Table 2.12:   Extent to which residents of local government districts in the Northern Region received cataract operations

Place of residence	Standardised hospitalisation ratio (inpatients and day cases)
Castle Morpeth	128
Durham	127
Darlington	123*
Newcastle	122*
Gateshead	112
Derwentside	109
Stockton	107
North Tyneside	106
Blyth	103
Wansbeck	103
Sunderland	98*
Carlisle	96*
Copeland	95
Middlesbrough	93*
Tynedale	92
Sedgefield	88
Wear Valley	88
Berwick	85
Allerdale	81*
Alnwick	81
Easington	78
South Tyneside	76
Langbaurgh	75
Eden	71
Hartlepool	61
Chester-le-Street	60
Region	100

* Local Government Districts which have within their boundaries an Ophthalmology Unit.

Table 2.13 displays the data for coronary artery by-pass operations and clearly shows that the highest admission rate was for residents of the host district, with the lowest for a district (South Tyneside) some eight miles away. Other districts further from the host district (for example, North Tees, 36 miles away) had higher resident access rates.

The interpretation of data on the use of health services is made difficult by the absence of any general understanding of what constitutes need. Thus, when comparing admission rates to a particular hospital service from two or more populations, there is no way of knowing in any of the communities concerned the size of the pool of patients requiring treatment. Therefore, it is not possible to say what level of hospital admission would have been appropriate in the investigation described.

Demographic differences can account for some variation in admission rates when diseases are more common at certain ages. For example, coronary heart disease is more common in older males; if one district contains more older males

Table 2.13: **Extent to which residents of district health authorities in the Northern Region received coronary artery bypass surgery (1984/1985)**

Place of residence	Inpatient discharges per 1,000 resident population
Newcastle	0.27*
North Tyneside	0.22
Northumberland	0.20
North Tees	0.17
East Cumbria	0.16
Durham	0.16
Darlington	0.15
Gateshead	0.12
North West Durham	0.12
South Tees	0.12
Hartlepool	0.11
West Cumbria	0.11
South West Durham	0.11
South Cumbria	0.10
Sunderland	0.09
South Tyneside	0.07
Region	0.15

* District Health Authority with a cardiothoracic unit.

than another with the same total population, then it is to be expected that they will record higher admission due to this disease. This was tested as a possible source of variation in Table 2.13 where unstandardised rates are used but it was found to be a very minor source of variation. It cannot be responsible for any of the variation documented in Table 2.12 however, because there the data are presented as SHRs which allow for any demographic differences between the districts.

It may be wondered why SHRs were not also the method of presentation of the data for the coronary artery by-pass surgery analysis. They could equally well have been. The reason they were not was concerned with the potential impact of the presentation of the findings of the investigation on a health authority which included lay members.

SHRs (or SMRs for that matter) are usually quite well understood by people without a background in public health if the concept is simply explained as part of the presentation of data. Their power of impact is as a comparative measure, showing the extent of variation between populations. Used alone, however, they can sometimes have reduced impact with the lay person because of the abstract nature of a relative measure.

Therefore it is sometimes important to give the target audience a feel for absolute values. There is additional impact in being able to picture the number of people being admitted for every thousand or ten thousand in the population.

Whilst such data must be interpreted cautiously, it is unlikely that differences of the size in the examples described could have resulted from limitations in the data (considerable validity checks were in any case carried out).

As was indicated earlier, broad knowledge of the population and its pattern of disease and mortality does not suggest that the variation could have arisen from differences in morbidity and demography. The cataract data were in any case standardised to eliminate the effect of differences in age-structure, the strongest correlate with incidence. Mortality rates from coronary heart disease in the Northern Region were amongst the worst in the country and districts such as South Tyneside (with low access to coronary artery by-pass surgery) were amongst the worst within the region. There was no evidence either that Newcastle's population was being over-treated (another theoretical explanation for the differences).

Thus, the investigators felt it a fair assumption that the variations represented the differing extent to which need was being recognised and acted upon by patients and doctors.

The underlying factors which determine the extent to which a given level of need is translated into inpatient care include: patient consultation rates (with general practitioners); general practitioner referral rates (to hospital consultants); availability and accessibility of hospital facilities; thresholds for admission and treatment (by individual consultants); secondary referral rates (from one hospital consultant to another).

Tentative ideas about the main sources of the variation in the investigation described here, were that the differential coronary artery by-pass admission rates may have partly been explained by the availability, in district services, of physicians with expertise in cardiology who were able to recognise and refer appropriate cases. This certainly seemed to fit with existing knowledge of the pattern of district service. For example, in Newcastle, a specialist cardiology team was in place and many general practitioners would refer cases to them as a first choice. The North Tees physicians also had expertise in the specialty which may explain higher access rates in a more geographically remote population.

The data for rates of cataract extraction seem to be more closely related to geographical proximity to a service providing centre. Beyond this, descriptive data like these can only be used for discussion and exploration of issues and not to draw conclusions.

Comment and overview

This investigation used routinely available data and hence was relatively rapidly carried out and limited in its scope. Nevertheless, it stimulated a debate at the time, at the highest policy-making level within the region and one which ranged across issues such as: the siting of specialist services; the level and distribution of consultant posts in particular specialties; resource allocation policy; general practitioner referral patterns and the prioritisation of patients on waiting lists.

An investigation into variations in clinical practice in an aspect of health service provision

The majority of the clinical work of consultants employed by the National Health Service is carried out within a hospital setting (either on an inpatient, outpatient or day case basis). The main elements of clinical care of patients outside hospital is provided by general practitioners. In certain specific circumstances, however,

National Health Service consultants can provide care in a patient's home and receive additional payments for doing so. The pattern of usage of this domiciliary consultation service is variable and is responsible for substantial health service expenditure. The investigation, described as an example here, sought to establish the pattern of practice, examine its relationship to contractual entitlement and, through a process of peer review, to explore its appropriateness.

Context and problem definition

The domiciliary consultation, in which a hospital consultant travels out into the community to provide specialist advice in the patient's home setting at the request of a general practitioner, has been a feature of the National Health Service since its inception.

A consultant's entitlement to be paid extra for such a home visit is based upon a clause in the Terms and Conditions of Service for Hospital Medical Staff in the National Health Service in which a domiciliary consultation is defined as "... a visit to the patient's home, at the request of the general practitioner and normally in his company, to advise on the diagnosis or treatment of a patient who on medical grounds cannot attend hospital".

At one end of the spectrum of medical opinion, (at the time of the investigation), domiciliary consultations seemed to be regarded as purely a contractual entitlement able to be claimed when indicated by the professional judgement of the requesting general practitioners. At the other, they were viewed as an outmoded concept which was rarely justified within a modern specialist service.

Yet, for the individual consultant undertaking the maximum number of visits permitted contractually, fees for domiciliary consultations (and associated investigations and procedures) could add a salary supplement of around 25%. Expenditure on domiciliary consultations in the Northern Region before the investigation started amounted to around £1.3 million.

Carrying out the investigation

The study population was 15 of the 16 health districts of the Northern Region, in which an estimated 2.8 million people were resident during the period of investigation. One district (population approximately 280,000) was excluded because, as a teaching district, consultant contracts were not held by the Regional Health Authority and, hence, the monitoring of the domiciliary consultation service was carried out separately.

No routine data were available on the pattern of usage of the domiciliary consultation service at the time the investigation started, except for financial data arising from the claims made for payment by the consultants undertaking the visits.

It was decided to build the gathering of data around the claim forms. This enabled the whole population of domiciliary consultations to be captured comprehensively at a single source. Moreover, it was possible to ensure completeness of data by linking processing of forms for payment to completeness of the claim forms themselves. Patient identification details were not included in the analysis (although they were clearly necessary for administrative purposes). It is important to ensure complete anonymity in such circumstances.

Where the collection of data relies largely on the clinician, as in this example, its completeness and accuracy are very dependent on the extent to which the data required are those which would be recorded also as part of the clinical process (and in this case as elements of the payment claim system). Where requests for additional data are introduced, compliance in completing such sections of a proforma by clinicians is often poor. This is not surprising given the pressure of time on most clinical consultations and it is, therefore, better in such an investigation to err on the side of requesting a limited core of information (sufficient to address the main aims of the investigation) which is collected to a high standard rather than a more extensive range where completeness and accuracy may be patchy.

Data from the investigation into the domiciliary consultation service were made available to senior medical staff so that they could examine the pattern of usage of the service between and within specialties. This led to the whole subject of domiciliary consultations, their appropriateness, and the indications for them, being actively discussed by consultants at regional and hospital level throughout the Northern Region over a period of several years. The impact of this peer review process on the overall level of service, and expenditure on it, was observed by data for overall service usage which were routinely collected by the Health Authority for monitoring purposes.

Findings and implications

Some of the main findings of the investigation are described here for a sample time period for illustrative purposes.

There was marked variation in the use which was made of the domiciliary consultation service by general practitioners on behalf of their patients. Whilst 86% of general practitioners requested ten or less consultations in the study period, a small number of general practitioners made heavy use of the service (Table 2.14).

Table 2.14:   Requests for domiciliary consultations made by
              general practitioners in Northern Region, 1988–9

Number of domiciliary consultations	Number of requesting general practitioners
0	367
1–10	1073
11–20	148
21–30	41
31–40	17
41–50	7
51–100	10
101–150	3

Source: Donaldson LJ, Hill PM. The domiciliary consultation service: a time to take stock. British Medical Journal 1991; 302: 449–51.

Similar variation occurred amongst consultants (Table 2.15). The distribution of consultations undertaken within specialties was broadly similar to the all specialty data. However, certain specialties made a disproportionate contribution to the total domiciliary consultations which took place, with the highest proportions of all consultations being carried out by consultant geriatricians (25%) and consultant psychiatrists (23%). Consultants in one of a number of specialties (geriatrics, psychiatry, general medicine, general surgery and rheumatology) carried out 84% of all domiciliary consultations.

The general practitioner was recorded as accompanying the consultant in 635 out of 10,516 domiciliary consultations (6%) which took place during the sample time period.

An analysis of diagnostic information showed little major illness amongst the patients who received domiciliary visits from consultants. For example, one general practitioner requested 38 domiciliary consultations for paediatric patients. Diagnoses for these included feeding problems, rash, vomiting, secondary milk intolerance, an unsettled baby and a child with sexual obsession.

The findings in relation to the low level of general practitioner attendance at domiciliary consultations, together with the pattern of diagnoses in sample specialties (indicating that patients who could have attended hospital were being seen at home instead), suggested that custom and practice had considerably departed from the original concept of the domiciliary consultation and upon which entitlement for payment was based. It should be remembered that the regulations stated that the visit made by the consultant should "normally be in [the general practitioner's] company" and that the patient who was the subject of the visit should be someone "who on medical grounds cannot attend hospital".

Table 2.15: **Domiciliary consultations undertaken by consultants in Northern Region, 1988–9**

Number of domiciliary consultations	Number of consultants
0	297
1–10	249
11–20	66
21–30	44
31–40	17
41–50	21
51–60	16
61–70	5
71–80	7
81–90	7
91–100	6
101–150	18
151–200	4
201–250	1

Source: Donaldson LJ, Hill PM. The domiciliary consultation service: a time to take stock. British Medical Journal 1991; 302: 449–51.

Viewing the issue purely in financial terms, it seemed that substantial sums of money might have been disbursed under a budget heading without all relevant criteria being fulfilled. However, this is an extraordinarily difficult issue for management to address when arguments about clinical autonomy are vociferously invoked in response to routine monitoring enquiries about the validity of claims.

Each of the patients had a stage of care identified for each day of the hospital stay using a methodology adapted from one developed by North American investigators. This was based on the application to each day of care of the question: 'why is this patient in hospital now?'.

After discussion with the clinical team, each day of each patient's stay was assigned to one of the following categories:

A. Preoperative, no perceived problems, awaiting surgery.
B. Preoperative, awaiting medical assessment or therapy before surgery.
C. Postoperative, condition improving, no complications.
D. Postoperative, complications of surgery have developed and are prolonging stay.
E. Postoperative, medical difficulties have developed which would have required hospital admission regardless of surgery.
F. Medically and surgically fit for discharge, but hospital stay continues for other reasons (e.g. awaiting geriatric assessment or bed, arrangements being made for domiciliary services, arrival of caring relatives awaited).
G. Receiving conservative therapy, no operation.

As Table 2.17 shows, almost all the bed-days were spent by the patients awaiting a theatre session (10%), recovering from surgery without complications (51%) or waiting to leave the orthopaedic ward despite being medically and surgically fit to do so (28%). Other analyses (not presented here) were performed on the number of days spent in each stage.

Table 2.17: **Number of patient days spent in each stage of acute hospital care by people with fractured neck of femur**

Stage of care*	Number of patient days	% of total stay
A	492	10
B	141	3
C	2690	51
D	59	1
E	56	1
F	1437	28
G	292	6
TOTAL	5167	–

* See text for definition of stages
Source: Robbins JA, Donaldson LJ. Analysing stages of care in hospital stay for fractured neck of femur. Lancet 1984; 1: 1028–9.

It was calculated that, if all patients who were fit for surgery had been taken to theatre without delay, 492 hospital days could have been saved. Moreover, if it had been possible to discharge or transfer patients when they no longer needed to remain in hospital for medical and surgical reasons, 1437 hospital-days could have been saved.

It was further estimated that by combining both of these strategies, the average duration of stay could have been reduced by eight days.

Comment and overview

The methodology adopted contained elements of the cohort study approach, the study population being a consecutive group of patients admitted to hospital and then followed up during their hospital stay. Whilst the period of the year chosen to recruit the cohort could have been unrepresentative of all patients' experience (for example, if there had been strong seasonal differences), there was no evidence that overall length of stay varied markedly at different times of the year. The use of caring staff to contribute to the classification of the days of care, is open to the criticism that through the knowledge of being studied they could have modified their assessment of each patient. However, one of the senior investigators was in active clinical practice and had made his own baseline assessment of the patients and review of the medical records. Thus, a more independent judgement was also available.

The investigation provided a focus for policy discussion. It pinpointed and addressed the problem of extended hospital stay in this group of elderly patients and provided the focus for in-depth review of the whole issue, including the timing of surgery (with implications for out of hours staffing of operating theatres, the availability of on-call radiographers) and arrangements for assessment, rehabilitation and future placement (with implications for greater involvement of geriatricians and social workers earlier in the acute hospital stay).

An investigation to describe rapidly an emerging problem for which little information was available

From time to time, a health, or health service problem will suddenly come to the attention of the public through critical comment in the local or national media in such a way that there may be a high level of disquiet or a loss of confidence in services. Just such a major crisis was caused when a sudden increase in the number of children suspected of having been sexually abused, were taken into local authority care in Cleveland, a county in the north east of England, over a three-month period in the summer of 1987. As is sometimes the case in such circumstances, little information was available to be able to define the size or nature of the problem so that it could be discussed rationally and objectively. This example describes an investigation which was carried out very rapidly to provide such information.

Context and problem definition

The Cleveland crisis came about because of a number of factors. Firstly, there was a sharp rise in admissions of children with a diagnosis of suspected sexual abuse to one of the main hospitals in the county (Middlesbrough General Hospital). Many of these children were then made the subject of court orders (under the then child protection legislation) which led to them being retained in the hospital as a 'Place of Safety' for further assessment and investigation.

The presence of these additional children who were physically active, boisterous and, in some cases behaviourally disturbed, placed enormous pressure on the physical facilities available and on the nursing staff who were also trying to care for acutely ill children. The Social Services department (as the lead agency in child protection services) did not have the resources, in terms of skilled social work staff, to respond to this rapid increase in cases referred to it.

The presence of large numbers of parents whose children were being kept largely in one place, focused parental anger and led to involvement of Members of Parliament who publicly and effectively articulated the collective sense of indignation and concern. Finally, the open airing of professional differences of opinion on the validity of the diagnoses led further to the impression of confusion. In the first few weeks of the crisis, the services underwent a period of major instability and perceived loss of public confidence.

Much of the prevailing media comment led the public to believe that the number of cases being diagnosed was large and unprecedented (amounting to 1 in 10 of the population). This added to the sense of incredulity and the impression that a wholesale mistake had been made by the professional staff involved.

At this stage, however, no firm data were available on the numbers of children involved. Therefore, numbers could not be related to the population of origin or valid comparisons made with elsewhere in the country or with other countries. In addition, many professionals expressed public disquiet at the frequency of anal abuse diagnosed, particularly in very young children and in girls. Thus, part of the initial controversy resulted from a failure to be able to quantify and describe the problem in population terms. Coupled with this, the perception that parents were being denied their rights, that social workers and paediatricians had acted over-zealously (apparently seeking out abuse where it did not exist), that undue reliance had been placed on an unproven diagnostic technique (the reflex anal dilatation test) added to the sense of public concern and turmoil.

A Judicial Inquiry was established by the Minister for Health, for which evidence was prepared on a wide range of aspects on the background to the problems in Cleveland. As part of this evidence, information was gathered to describe the population of children who were the subject of the diagnosis of suspected sexual abuse.

Carrying out the investigation

The investigation began by assembling all cases of sexual abuse or suspected sexual abuse in children coming to the attention of paediatric services or of the social services department over the three month period. These cases were identified by searching hospital records of all paediatric admissions (sexual abuse was not a diagnosis recorded in routinely available hospital inpatient data) and the cases referred to the social services department over the same period.

A precoded structured pro-forma was designed to record data extracted from the children's records. The main areas of data recording were: demographic and administrative; mode of presentation; main clinical findings; subsequent management; details of referral for other medical opinion (where this occurred).

High standards of confidentiality were observed when extracting the data. Medical staff undertook the work personally. Analyses were carried out on an aggregated and anonymised basis only so that no children or families could ever be identified.

Cases were classified into three categories according to the way in which they came to light:

 a. Index cases – the child in a family (or group of children) who, on presentation, first gave rise to the suspicion that sexual abuse may have occurred.
 b. Sibling of index case – brother or sister of index case, who was examined because of the suspicion of child sexual abuse in the index case.
 c. Contact of index case – a child connected with the index case (but not a brother or sister), who was examined because of the suspicion of child sexual abuse in the index case.

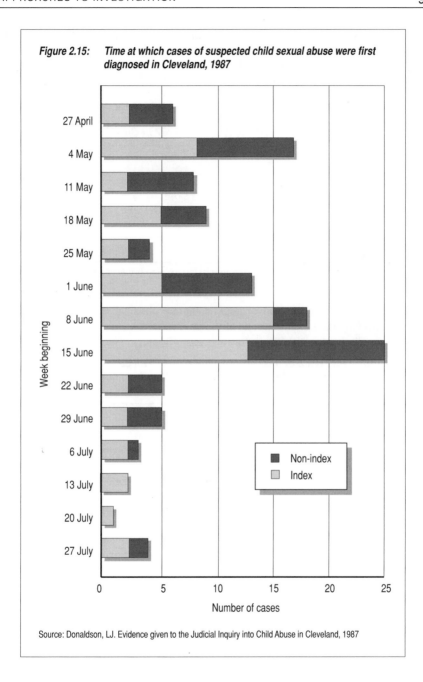

Figure 2.15: *Time at which cases of suspected child sexual abuse were first diagnosed in Cleveland, 1987*

Source: Donaldson, LJ. Evidence given to the Judicial Inquiry into Child Abuse in Cleveland, 1987

Findings and implications

Figure 2.15 shows the time at which children were diagnosed over the three month period. The crisis broke publicly following the peak of diagnoses in the week commencing 15 June 1987.

Table 2.18 shows the overall rate for the three month period was 9.8 per 10,000 population, which is equivalent to approximately 1 case in 1,000 children (aged 0 –14 years). The rate for girls of all ages was approximately twice that for boys and the highest rate was in girls up to the age of 4 years.

Table 2.18: *Age and sex specific rates of occurrence for cases of suspected child sexual abuse per 10,000 population during the three month period May to July 1987 in Cleveland*

Age group (years)	Male	Female	Both sexes
0–4	5.4	19.2	12.2
5–9	8.9	17.7	13.2
10–14	4.4	4.2	4.3
0–14	6.2	13.7	9.8

Source: Donaldson LJ. Evidence given to the Judicial Inquiry into Child Abuse in Cleveland 1987.

Table 2.19 shows an analysis of anal or vaginal physical signs recorded by the doctors following their examinations of the children.

Table 2.19: *Presence of anal and vaginal signs in all cases with suspected child sexual abuse diagnosed in Cleveland May/June 1987: percentages*

Physical signs	Male	Female	Both sexes
Anal only	100	28	51
Vaginal only	N/A	9	6
Both	N/A	60	41
Neither	0	2	2
Not stated	–	1	1
Total	100 (N=38)	100 (N=82)	100 (N=120)

N/A = Not applicable.
Source: Donaldson LJ. Evidence given to the Judicial Inquiry into Child Abuse in Cleveland 1987.

The figure and the two tables show only a small selection of the analyses. Nevertheless, they illustrate the role in which simple descriptive data can play in throwing light on a problem. In this investigation, they illustrated that the problem was far less common than some of the exaggerated early impressions had suggested. Furthermore, they emphasised that part of the numerical problem arose from children who had been examined because they were siblings or contacts of children suspected of being sexually abused. On the other hand, the doctors' findings of signs of anal abuse even in very young children emphasised the centrality of these physical signs to the debate and demonstrated the need to address issues of 'normality' and 'abnormality'.

Many of these issues were the subject of extensive scrutiny by the Judicial Inquiry.

Comment and overview

The study could not, and did not purport to, provide a definitive estimate of the size of the problem of sexual abuse in the population concerned. Neither did it set out to examine the validity of the diagnoses made. It also used a retrospective method of enquiry whose primary source of data, medical and social services records, was not created specifically for investigative purposes. Nevertheless, a prospective study would probably have proved impossible in the light of the attention which had been focused on the issue, circumstances would have certainly influenced the way in which information was recorded.

However, given that its limitations were made clear (which they were at the time) the investigation fulfilled a useful purpose in helping to correct a misleading anecdotal impression. This can be an important and useful role for investigations in public health medicine in a situation where absolutely no data are available, and when decisions are being made and conclusions drawn on purely subjective grounds. The investigation also proved invaluable in designing a conceptual framework for categorising the cases (index, non-index) so that the size of the problem which arose from children being diagnosed at presentation could be distinguished from the extent to which children contributed who were only included by virtue of their association with other cases. This approach was subsequently adopted by the Judicial Inquiry in its own case analysis.

The investigation also highlighted the need for further study: in particular for population based studies of the size and distribution of sexual abuse using agreed criteria for their case definition and to improve the quality of routinely collected statistics held on child protection registers.

An investigation to examine the implications of the phasing out of large mental hospitals

It has been long established policy of British Governments in the field of services for people with mental illness to shift the balance of care from hospital to community. An important element of this policy has been to provide care for mentally ill people in need of hospital care in facilities which are integrated within district general hospitals.

The most visible manifestation of these policies has been the closure (or re-designation), in many parts of the country, of the past cornerstone of care for the mentally ill: the large mental hospitals, many of which are buildings which housed Victorian asylums.

The investigation described here set out to identify some of the practical problems of implementing these policies by assessing the levels of physical, mental and social functioning of mentally ill people in institutional care within a large health district in the East Midlands part of England.

Context and problem definition

One of the key determinants of the success of the policies described above, was the ability of local psychiatric services satisfactorily to reduce the number of patients requiring nursing care on a longer-term basis. In practice, this was, and still is, an issue about suitability for discharge of patients who have already spent much of their lives in a psychiatric hospital setting. It is also about preventing the accumulation of a 'new' long-stay group arising from younger patients who are admitted for what are intended as short spells of hospital inpatient care.

Further key factors for policy success were, and also still are: the adequacy of community-based psychiatric services to care for mentally ill people who would previously have ended up in hospitals and to have adequate ways of helping elderly, severely mentally ill people, whose physical and mental frailty make it extremely difficult for them to be returned from hospital to the community.

The investigation set out to evaluate each patient within psychiatric inpatient hospital care facilities in the health district of approximately 850,000 population and to assess their level of physical, social and mental capacity relevant to care requirements.

Carrying out the investigation

The method chosen for the investigation was a one-day census in which each patient was identified and the assessment carried out. With over one thousand beds or hospital places in psychiatric facilities in the district, the investigation was a very major exercise and required careful planning and detailed preparatory work in advance of the date which was agreed for the census.

Nursing and medical staff completed a 47 item assessment schedule on each patient in their care, the assessment covering eight main areas: demographic and administrative; current diagnoses; ward behaviour and nursing problems; current treatment; employment status and occupational therapy; contact with the outside world; rehabilitation prospects; and, family dependants.

In many of these areas of assessment, standard scales or measures were used which had been validated in earlier studies (these will not be described in detail here).

Findings and implications

At census point, there were 1,087 inpatients of whom 1,052 (96%) were resident in two large mental hospitals.

Table 2.20 shows that the largest group of psychiatric inpatients was the very elderly. Thirty seven per cent of patients were 75 years or older, a much greater proportion than the very elderly population of the health district as a whole (5% were aged 75 years and over). The table also indicates that whilst the proportion of very elderly people was lower amongst those who had been resident for the shortest and longest times, even in these length of stay groups it was still very substantial.

Comparing the bottom row of figures in Table 2.20 gives an impression of the relative sizes of the different length of stay groups. Whilst the largest proportion (413 out of 1086, or 38%) of patients had been in hospital for less than one year, 26% were inpatients of more than ten years standing, and more than half this latter group were elderly (65 years of age or older). The remaining group of patients, whose stay had extended beyond a year but was less than ten years, made up 36% of all inpatients; a third of these were under 65 years of age.

Table 2.20   Cumulative percentages of psychiatric patients in different length of stay groups who were a given age or older

Age (years)	Length of current stay (years)					
	<1	1–2	2–5	5–10	10 and over	All lengths of stay
85 and over	8	17	19	15	7	11
75 and over	29	56	51	39	31	37
65 and over	45	70	70	57	59	56
55 and over	58	82	80	78	82	72
45 and over	67	88	88	88	92	81
35 and over	78	92	96	94	98	89
25 and over	88	97	100	100	100	95
15 and over	100	100	100	100	100	100
(n=)	(413)	(174)	(92)	(121)	(286)	(1086)

Source: Levene LS, Donaldson LJ, Brandon S. How likely is it that a district health authority can close its large mental hospitals? British Journal of Psychiatry 1985; 147: 150–5.

Dementia was the most common diagnosis in patients of all lengths of stay, except the very long-stay group, amongst which schizophrenia predominated.

The social withdrawal rating scale used in the investigation provided an indication of patients' level of social functioning within the hospital, and gave an indication of their chances of discharge. The possible score derived from this rating scale ranged from a minimum of zero to a maximum of 16 points. A score in the 0-4 range had been shown from previous studies to indicate that psychiatric inpatients have the potential for discharge.

Overall, more than half of all patients had scores above the 0–4 range. However, the patterns were so different for elderly, compared to younger patients, that data are presented for the two groups separately (Tables 2.21 and 2.22).

Table 2.21:   Percentage of psychiatric inpatients aged under 65 years with different social withdrawal (SW) scores by length of stay

SW score[+]	Length of current stay (years)					
	<1	1–2	2–5	5–10	10 and over	All lengths of stay
0–4	81	46	61	86	65	72
5–9	12	28	28	10	28	19
10–14	4	20	11	4	6	7
15–16	3	6	0	0	1	2
All scores	100	100	100	100	100	100
(n =)	(220)	(50)	(28)	(51)	(117)	(466)

+ Higher scores denote more severely incapacitated patients
Source: Levene LS, Donaldson LJ, Brandon S. How likely is it that a district health authority can close its large mental hospitals? British Journal of Psychiatry 1985; 147: 150–5

Of patients under the age of 65 (Table 2.21), almost three-quarters, regardless of length of stay, had low social withdrawal scores, but less than half of those with a duration of stay of 1–2 years had such scores. Furthermore, another finding of the study (not tabulated here) showed that one-quarter of patients aged under 65 years old with a 1–2 year length of stay were not fully continent of urine. These findings strongly suggest that disability in this group was intrinsic to the disorder, rather than a consequence of institutionalisation and that major efforts at treatment, rehabilitation or training would need to be directed at these patients.

The patients under 65 years of age with a length of stay of ten years or more (comprising a quarter of all patients aged under 65 years) were people in the main with low social withdrawal scores, but it is this group who are most used to institutional life and therefore potentially the most difficult to return to the community.

Three-quarters of all residents in the over 65 year age group (Table 2.22) had substantial social withdrawal and two-thirds were not fully continent of urine. The group of patients aged over 65 years who had been in hospital for less than one year had lower social withdrawal scores overall and therefore seemed to have greater potential for discharge.

Table 2.22:   Percentage of psychiatric inpatients aged 65 years and over with different social withdrawal (SW) scores, by length of stay

SW score*	Length of current stay (years)					
	<1	1–2	2–5	5–10	10 and over	All lengths of stay
0–4	28	14	19	15	41	26
5–9	37	30	31	29	37	34
10–14	28	44	34	30	20	30
15–16	7	12	16	26	2	10
All scores	100	100	100	100	100	100
(n =)	(185)	(122)	(64)	(69)	(168)	(608)

* Higher scores denote more severely incapacitated patients
Source: Levene LS, Donaldson LJ, Brandon S. How likely is it that a district health authority can close its large mental hospitals? British Journal of Psychiatry 1985; 147: 150–5.

Overall, the investigation clearly showed that the presence of large numbers of elderly patients was the most important feature of the short, intermediate, and long-stay groups of patients in psychiatric hospitals. Those elderly patients who had been in hospital for longer than ten years were less incapacitated, both socially and physically, than their shorter-stay counterparts, though they clearly exhibited much higher levels of incapacity than younger patients. Nevertheless, it seemed possible that for a proportion of this group of very long-stay elderly patients some alternative less dependent form of care could have been provided. However, prolonged exposure to an institutional way of life, coupled with advancing years, made it likely that this care would need to continue to be provided in a very protected environment.

It was noted that whilst the elderly group amongst the long-stay patients would dwindle (because of deaths), this could be a slow process and optimism about reduction of numbers in this category needed to be tempered by the observation that there were substantial numbers of elderly mentally ill people in the intermediate-stay groups. Moreover, the continuing demand for hospital places from patients in the community and the possible development of a younger long-stay group would create further pressure on the same facilities.

Comment and overview

The findings of an investigation such as the one described here could not provide a blueprint for future services, but they did identify several key issues.

Firstly, the large existing number of elderly disabled patients, together with the expectation of a further increase in their numbers, presented the most serious obstacle to hospital closure. It was noted that alternative facilities would take time to develop and were likely to consume even more resources than currently being expended. If admission and treatment facilities were to be transferred to general hospital units, whilst the existing mental hospitals remained open, they were in danger of becoming repositories for the disabled elderly, with consequent major problems in maintaining staff morale and high standards.

A second issue identified by the investigation was the high disability scores amongst patients with a duration of stay exceeding one but less than two years. This suggested that services were focused upon the acute episode or on the rehabilitation of long-stay patients and that the needs of medium-stay patients were being comparatively overlooked. The transition from acute admission to long-term resident is often insidious, and concentration on treatment issues may delay efforts at social rehabilitation.

The findings on aspects of physical disability (although not discussed in detail here) were also of major policy importance. Incontinence, for example, is a significant impediment when alternative accommodation is being sought. The substantial number of patients, even in the younger age-groups, who were incontinent of urine suggested this as a target symptom demanding special attention. It also pointed the way for studies to examine the role of medication in causing and reducing incontinence, the development of behavioural programmes in incontinence management, and the criteria for more vigorous intervention with this problem.

The investigation as a whole exposed a wide range of policy issues relevant to the organisation of psychiatric services in the health district concerned. Many of the issues raised by this investigation remain topical in the 1990s.

CONCLUSIONS

This chapter has described an important facet of public health medicine, namely, the study methodologies and investigative approaches which must be mastered if the full range of health and health service problems are to be addressed. The practice of clinical medicine is often compared to a series of detective stories in which the clues to the diagnosis of a patient's clinical problem are investigated. In population medicine, the mysteries of health and disease in entire populations, some extremely complex, are also very challenging. The benefits of solving these problems in terms of delaying death, preventing disease and improving the quality of health care are enormous. To develop the analogy, whilst the clinical detective is pursuing the ordinary criminal, the public health investigator is on the trail of the Godfathers of syndicated crime.

3 The promotion of health

INTRODUCTION

As the 20th Century moves towards its conclusion, concern amongst the population living in Britain and other industrialised nations, about health and its relationship to individual lifestyle, and to the environment, has never been greater.

This is evident not just in the behaviour of individuals but also through shifts in societal attitudes as reflected, for example, in the response of major manufacturers to consumers' wishes and expectations as well as in the increasing preoccupation of mass media with health issues.

Examples which illustrate this greater health consciousness are numerous. They include the widespread adoption of jogging and other forms of regular aerobic exercise amongst the adult population; the removal of artificial substances from foodstuffs and the resultant marketing success of manufacturers promoting products which are additive free. There has been a growth in the number of public places where cigarette smoking is not permitted and a major increase in sales of low alcohol drinks. In the workplace, more and more companies have adopted stress-reduction and other health programmes for their employees.

All these are welcome signs that individuals and societies are now more receptive than at any other time to initiatives which will promote health and prevent disease. Yet, the challenges remain formidable. The leading causes of death and disability in Britain remain: heart disease, stroke, cancer, chronic bronchitis and accidents. Knowledge about the causation of these problems should be sufficient to provide the potential for a major impact to be made on them through health promotion programmes. Despite this, consistent success in reducing the burden of illness and premature death from these causes has remained elusive, whilst inequalities in disease experience between different social strata are wider than ever.

Drawing on the great success of preventive medicine in the past, the United States Surgeon General, in his 1979 report *Healthy People*, set in context the need for a modern impetus for health promotion and disease prevention:

'Not to find and employ those [preventive] strategies would be irresponsible – as irresponsible as it would have been for our predecessors merely to alleviate the ravages of smallpox and polio and cholera, without attempting to eradicate them.'

Health services should have as their major aims to reduce the amount of illness, disease, disability and premature death in the population and also to increase the numbers of people who spend a high proportion of their lives in a state of health rather than ill-health. Health services do not have direct control over all the factors which can influence these aspects of the health of the population but the design and implementation of health promotion strategies is one of their major functions.

This chapter describes the main strategies available to promote health and prevent disease, beginning with an historical account of the development of thinking about the causation of disease.

ORIGINS OF DISEASE AND ITS CAUSATION

Early concepts

The writings and teachings of Hippocrates had an impact far beyond his lifetime, which began on the island of Cos near the Ionian coast of Asia Minor, about 460 BC and ended (legend has it) when bees swarmed on his grave producing a special honey: the cure for stomatitis in infants. Hippocrates is regarded by many as the father of medicine, although medicine was practised before this time. Indeed writings on such matters date back to the earliest civilizations. In Hippocrates' time, however, there were no boundaries between medicine, art, religion or philosophy.

One of the main contributions of the Hippocratic School lay in focusing intellectual attention on medicine in its own right, a science, founded on the observation of facts and the recording of clinical experiences. One of the major teachings was that the body contained four humours: blood, black bile, yellow bile and phlegm. In health, the humours mingled together and were in harmony or balance; in disease there was a derangement of this mixture.

Hippocrates was the first to seek to explain the origins of disease and in so doing he put forward many observations which do not seem out of place even today. He distinguished between diseases which were endemic (always present in a given area) and those which at times become excessively common (epidemic). In suggesting a role for exercise, diet, climate, water and the seasons, he fore-shadowed modern views of the importance of the interrelationship between man and his environment in the causation of disease.

Many of his aphorisms resonate with modern causal thinking, for example:

'Those naturally very fat are more liable to sudden death than the thin.'

During the time of the Roman Empire which eclipsed its Greek predecessor, it is the name of another Greek, Galen, who lived in the second century AD, which stands out in the history of medicine. He is said to have cured the emperor Marcus Aurelius of abdominal pain. Whilst his observations on the nature and cause of disease added little to the Hippocratic writings, he did much to advance knowledge in relation to anatomy and physiology. It was also the Roman Empire which introduced sanitation and domestic water supplies, thereby making a significant contribution to public health.

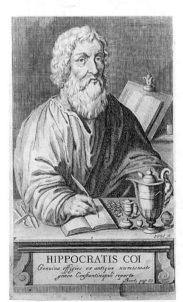

HIPPOCRATIS COI
Genuina effigies ex antiquo numismate
greco Constantinopoli reperto

Hippocrates. Engraving, 1665.

Throughout the Dark and Middle Ages, Europe was ravaged by disease and pestilence: the plague, smallpox, diphtheria, tuberculosis and leprosy. Millions of lives were lost to these scourges of mankind. It is clearly apparent from reading about the measures which were adopted at the time to combat these diseases that they were understood to be contagious. For example, sufferers from leprosy were isolated and required to carry bells to warn of their approach. However, there was no suggestion at this time of a contagious agent; rather, such diseases were held to be caused by changes in the composition of the atmosphere ('bad air') arising from stagnant or decaying organic matter.

Fracastorius (1478–1553), a Veronese poet and physician, is best remembered for writing a long poem about syphilis or the 'French disease'. His views on the general nature and cause of infectious diseases were, however, remarkable and were expressed some 200 years before such ideas were embraced as new and revolutionary. Fracastorius compared contagion in disease to the putrefaction that passes from one fruit to another when it rots. Moreover, when he referred to the essential nature of infection he suggested that minute particles or seeds were conveyed from person to person and propagated themselves. This first mention of the possibility that diseases are caused by specific germs attracted little attention at the time it was published.

The Miasma

Thomas Sydenham (1624–1689) was essentially a practical physician who regarded experimental physiology, so much in vogue at the time, with contempt. His philosophy was to set aside all theory and begin by observing and recording symptoms and signs and their progression (march of events) in the sufferer from the particular ailment. He is greatly revered for his classical descriptions of diseases such as gout, measles, scarlet fever and pneumonia. He is often called the English Hippocrates because his observational method had many similarities with his distant Greek predecessor. Yet, despite his genius in this respect, Sydenham added little to the understanding of why people became ill. But because of his stature, his miasmic theory of the causation of disease – little more than a re-expression of earlier ideas – was much more influential than it deserved to be. The miasma was an unidentified vapour believed to result from mysterious changes in the air. It is easy now to scoff at such an apparently preposterous suggestion. Nonetheless, as recently as the second half of the last century, many medical officers of health in their annual reports still related epidemics of infectious diseases to bad odours arising in a locality.

However, the fact that the true nature of infectious disease had not been revealed, did not impede progress.

Bills of mortality

An important, though less spectacular contribution to this progress, was the start of mortality data gathering. Before causes of disease can be investigated or preventive measures initiated, it is essential to have an indication of the size of the problem. Statistics which would allow the various outbreaks of infectious diseases to be traced, originated from the work of a man who died in impoverished circumstances towards the end of the seventeenth century. This man, John Graunt (1620–1674), analysed the statistics which he gleaned from the Bills of Mortality. These Bills were broadsheets issued weekly, and listed for the London parishes, the numbers and (in a crude fashion) causes of death. They were purchased by well-to-do people who could forewarn themselves of an outbreak of the plague and forsake the city for less hazardous surroundings.

Graunt laid the foundation for the work of his illustrious successor William Farr (1807–1883), whose statistical writings from the office of the Registrar General served as the basis for the great sanitary reforms.

The Broad Street pump

There is one episode on the road to the discovery of the true nature of infectious disease which has assumed almost romantic proportions to students and practitioners of public health medicine: that of the investigation of the London cholera outbreak of 1854. John Snow (1813–1858), apprenticed as a doctor in Newcastle upon Tyne could justifiably have settled for one claim to immortality when he later became the first man to introduce anaesthesia in childbirth. He used chloroform in the delivery of two of Queen Victoria's children. Yet, it was his interest in cholera and his painstaking investigation of an outbreak of this disease which earned him a further place in medicine's Hall of Fame.

Cholera is a major infectious disease which spreads rapidly and causes death by the gross fluid depletion that results from the intense diarrhoea produced by the infection. It is rare today in the Western world, but is still a serious cause of mortality in some developing countries. During the early nineteenth century, however, epidemics of cholera swept through London killing thousands of people.

Snow's own words best describe the outbreak in 1854:

'The most terrible outbreak of cholera which ever occurred in this kingdom is probably that which took place in Broad Street, Golden Square and adjoining streets, a few weeks ago. Within two hundred and fifty yards of the spot where Cambridge Street joins Broad Street, there were upwards of five hundred fatal attacks of cholera in ten days. The mortality in this limited area probably equals any that was ever caused in this country, even by the plague; and it was much more sudden as the greater number of cases terminated in a few hours. The mortality would undoubtedly have been much greater had it not been for the flight of the population.'

By plotting the geographical location of each case Snow deduced that the deaths had occurred amongst people living in close proximity to the Broad Street pump (many families at this time had no water supply in their own homes but used such a communal supply). There were one or two pieces of evidence, however, which did not at first seem to fit Snow's theory of the complicity of the pump. Firstly, a workhouse with 535 inmates in the street very close to the Broad Street pump experienced only five deaths from cholera amongst its population. Secondly, a brewery in Broad Street itself, had no fatalities amongst its workforce. Snow investigated these differences and found that the workhouse had its own pump on the premises whilst the workers in the brewery never frequented the Broad Street pump. Finally, Snow turned his attention to a woman and her niece living at a considerable distance from Broad Street who, nevertheless, died of cholera during

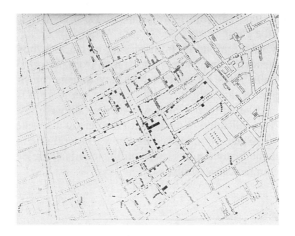

Snow's map of Soho with black units indicating deaths from cholera.

the epidemic. As a result of his interview with neighbours and next of kin, Snow ascertained that the woman had a particular liking for the flavour of the water of the Broad Street pump and sent her son to it every day for a bottle to drink.

On completing his enquiries Snow sought an interview with the Board of Guardians of St James' parish (who were in charge of the pump) and as a result of his representations the pump handle was removed and the epidemic which was already declining came to an end.

The importance of the removal of the pump handle was symbolic of a new understanding of the nature of the disease, for Snow had demonstrated that disease can be conveyed by water and specifically that cholera is a waterborne disease.

In a less dramatic but similarly painstaking series of other investigations, Snow further clarified the mode of transmission of cholera. In London, at that time, a number of private companies supplied water to its residents and Londoners paid for their supply. Snow turned his attention to the water supplies of two of these companies: the Lambeth company and the Southwark and Vauxhall company which both supplied similar areas of London. The pipes of both companies in some cases went down the same street, so that it was possible to. identify individual households supplied by one or other company. The death rate from cholera in the areas of London supplied by these two water companies was much higher than it was in places supplied by other companies. Both obtained their supply from the lower part of the Thames which was, then, the one most greatly contaminated by sewage.

A chance occurrence in 1852 provided Snow with a marvellous opportunity for a natural experiment. In that year the Lambeth water company changed its intake to another source which was free from sewage. Snow obtained the addresses of all people dying of cholera and sought information on the source of the water supply to each household. During the epidemic in the year 1853 Snow found that there were 71 fatal attacks of cholera per 10,000 households supplied by the Southwark and Vauxhall company, compared with only five per 10,000 in those supplied by the Lambeth company. In other words, people getting their water from the polluted part of the Thames had 14 times more fatal attacks of cholera than those getting their supply from the purer source.

Snow's theory of the mode of transmission of cholera then appeared to be vindicated. He considered that cholera was spread from person to person, the sick to the healthy, rather than by contact with any miasma or similar substance. Moreover, he deduced that this spread took place via morbid material from the alimentary canal of the sufferer which was then swallowed by other people and had the power of multiplication in the body of the person it attacked.

Even so clear an explanation, backed by Snow's careful scientific observations, failed to convince the many doubters who still categorically rejected the idea of a specific contagion in the cause of disease.

The germ theory

The invention of the microscope around 1670 had allowed living organisms to be seen for the first time. Leeuwenhoek (1632–1725), a Dutchman, examined a range of materials such as saliva, blood, water and faeces and made drawings of micro-organisms including what are now clearly recognizable as bacteria. No attempt was made, however, to associate these living organisms with disease in man. For example, there is no evidence that Snow saw them as the morbid material he suggested as a cause of cholera. Indeed, a separate controversy existed as to the origins of these micro-organisms themselves. Some scientists believed that they arose *de novo* (by spontaneous generation) from the fluids in which they were discovered.

Two names stand out as those who transformed causal thinking and finally gave birth to the germ theory of disease which had been so slow in its gestation: Louis Pasteur (1822–1895) and Robert Koch (1843–1910).

Pasteur firmly rejected the idea of spontaneous generation, a longstanding theory which held that tiny particles were present in the air which formed into living material. He believed that micro-organisms came from the air and settled on the culture media in which they were found. To prove his theory, he conducted an experiment in which he filled two flasks with suitable culture medium. These flasks were then heated to kill any organisms that were likely to be present in the medium; one was covered and the other left open. Bacteria quickly appeared in the uncovered flask but not in the covered one, thus firmly refuting the idea of spontaneous generation.

Development of preparation and staining techniques allowed Robert Koch, a doctor working in the town of Wollstein, Germany, to isolate the tubercle bacillus (1882) and the cholera vibrio (1883). In a very short period of time a wide range of organisms were identified and linked to disease in man: *Bacillus anthracis* (anthrax), *Corynebacterium diphtheriae* (diphtheria), *Mycobacterium leprae* (leprosy) and *Salmonella typhi* (typhoid fever). The practical applications of the work were not slow to be realised. Joseph (later Lord) Lister took up Pasteur's ideas and using carbolic acid during surgery founded the modern methods of antisepsis that transformed the nature of the hospital wards from places where virtually every post-operative case became septic and developed fever.

There are many other examples of the growing understanding of the ways of combating sepsis. Ignaz Philipp Semmelweis (1818–1865) was born in Hungary,

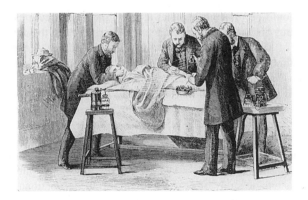

Lister carbolic spray in use. Engraving from W W Cheyne, Antiseptic surgery, 1882.

trained as a doctor in Vienna and became an obstetrician. In his early career he took an intense interest in the high rates of sepsis in the lying-in hospitals. Many women in these times died from puerperal fever.

Semmelweis conducted careful epidemiological research in which he observed the incidence of puerperal fever in different settings. He noted that medical students came from the dissecting room and, with only a cursory washing of hands, examined the women in labour.

Semmelweis made his students scrub up carefully and as a result mortality in the labour wards fell dramatically.

Such was the enthusiasm with which the medical establishment now embraced the germ theory of disease that attempts were made to link virtually every known disease to a specific causal contagious agent. Claim and counterclaim abounded. It was left to the Nobel laureate, Robert Koch, who had begun his career as a general practitioner in Germany, to impose a scientific discipline to check this bandwagon effect in which the hunt for micro-organisms in diseases led to causal inferences being made on very flimsy grounds.

Koch's postulates, sometimes also referred to as the Henle-Koch postulates (Koch was Henle's pupil), may be summarised as follows:

- The organism should be isolated in pure culture from each case of the disease.
- It should not occur in any other disease as fortuitous and non-pathogenic occurrent.
- Once isolated it should be grown in a series of cultures.
- This culture should reproduce the disease on inoculation into an experimental animal.

It is clear today that Koch's postulates, if interpreted literally, are too rigid and would exclude most viral diseases and also many bacterial diseases from having a proven causative agent. Nevertheless, they served as an important landmark at the time.

The search for other causative agents

Almost at once, the germ theory of the causation of disease dispelled myths, superstitions and ill-conceived quasi-scientific theories which had stood for centuries. It should be remembered that at that time, the infectious diseases were the major killing diseases, so the excitement produced by the revelation of the causative role of micro-organisms was quite understandable. Nevertheless, there were other landmarks in causal thinking in which specific agents other than micro-organisms were linked with diseases.

The possibility that factors in Man's occupation could be a cause of illness and disease was largely ignored in ancient writings, despite the grim and inhuman working conditions which often prevailed, for instance, in the quest for valuable metals in the mines of ancient Egypt, Greece or Rome. After the Renaissance, there emerged a man who is generally regarded as the father of occupational medicine: Bernardin Ramazzini (1633–1714). His *De Morbis Artificium*, published in about 1700, was a systematic study of diseases arising from occupational factors. When in his writings he recommended that, in addition to other questions and examinations, the doctor should ask the question 'What is your occupation?', he could scarcely have realised the enormous importance of his words.

Subsequently, occupational medicine has had a long and distinguished history. Discoveries such as Percival Pott's observation in 1775 of the occurrence of scrotal cancer in chimney sweeps as a result of persistent contact with soot or the cerebral effects of mercury poisoning in the hat-making trade (the basis of Lewis Carroll's *Mad Hatter*) opened new vistas when considering possible causes of disease.

Role of diet

Another field of study in disease causation is to be found in those conditions which arise because of lack or excess of some specific substance in the diet. A classic account is to be found in the work of James Lind, a surgeon in the Royal Navy at a time when long voyages were commonplace and provisions taken on board were those that could withstand such voyages without perishing. Sailors were afflicted after a time at sea by a strange malady: lethargy, and weakness, pains in the joints and limbs and swelling of the gums. This was scurvy and it cost many thousands of lives on the great sailing ships of the time. In 1747 Lind performed an experiment in which he added different substances to the diet of 12 sailors on such a voyage. He divided his patients into pairs and supplemented the diets of each pair with: cider, elixir vitriol, vinegar, sea water, a mixture of nutmeg, garlic, mustard and tamarind in barley water, and two oranges and one lemon daily. Only the sailors given oranges and lemons recovered. Thus, long before vitamin C was isolated, Lind had determined the cause and instituted preventive measures to redress the dietary deficiency. Sailors on long voyages took supplies of fruit juice and the tendency to use limes led to the nickname 'limeys' for British sailors.

The importance of the host

In parallel with the development of the concept of a contagion in the cause of infectious diseases, attention was also being directed to the capacity of the person to resist infection. It had been known since ancient times that people who had suffered from certain diseases and survived, rarely contracted the same disease a second time.

This observation led to the practice in smallpox of deliberate inoculation with material from a diseased person, in the belief that a milder infection would ensue than from a natural infection. The risks were great since the people being inoculated were acquiring a real attack of smallpox. Smallpox was one of the major scourges of the past, often called the 'minister of death'. It is estimated that during the eighteenth century 60 million people died from the disease in Europe alone.

Towards the end of the eighteenth century Edward Jenner (1749–1823), a country physician in Gloucestershire, decided to investigate a piece of local folklore relating to the disease. It was well-known by country people that milkmaids often acquired from infected cows, a disease called cowpox which gave rise to a pustule on the finger or crop of pustules on the body. It was believed that girls who contracted this mild disease would not contract smallpox when they were exposed to it. This observation is probably the origin of the rhyme:

'Where are you going my pretty maid?'
'I'm going a-milking, Sir', she said.
'What is your fortune my pretty maid?'
'My face is my fortune, Sir', she said.

In 1779, Jenner took material from the sore of a milkmaid called Sarah Nelmes who had cowpox and scratched it on to the arm of a boy, James Phipps. In an experiment which would be considered quite unethical today, the boy was later inoculated with smallpox. He did not develop the disease and Jenner's experiment was repeated on others with similarly successful results. Thus, the practice of vaccination became widespread, although it was a very different procedure from that practised today. Material was scratched from arm to arm amongst vaccinees without any antiseptic precautions and complications were thus common.

Despite its obvious historical importance and success in retrospect, it is surprising that Jenner's discovery was not universally accepted at the time. In many quarters of the medical establishment he was bitterly denounced as a charlatan. Jenner had earlier been elected to the Royal Society as a Fellow following the publication of a treatise on the Natural History of the Cuckoo. Yet, The Royal Society showed little interest in his cowpox discovery and it was many years before Jenner received his just professional and public acclaim for a discovery which effectively began one large element of preventive medicine, immunisation.

Almost a century later, a further great advance was made in knowledge of how to protect the host against disease. On this occasion, Louis Pasteur who had developed techniques of immunisation of animals against anthrax, turned his attention to rabies in humans. Rabies, a disease of the dog, was one of the most feared diseases because of its universal fatality. At different periods in history it had been attributed to the sun, the

Hand of Sarah Nelmes. Cowpox pustule. From Jenner's Inquiry, 1798.

weather or the dog star. Although existing technology meant that he could not see or produce a free culture of the rabies virus, Pasteur reasoned that it existed in the saliva and nervous system of infected animals and was the mode of transmission of the disease. He injected material from infected animals attenuated by desiccation into other animals and protected them against the disease.

In July 1885, a nine-year-old boy from Alsace, Joseph Meister, was brought to Pasteur's laboratory by his mother. The child, whilst walking to school on his own, had been pounced on and bitten 14 times by a mad dog before it was beaten off by a labourer. Pasteur was a chemist, not a physician, and consulted with his medical colleagues as to whether his success in the immunisation of animals against rabies justified using it on a human being. It was decided that the child faced almost certain death and thus a course of immunisation was begun which lasted ten days. The child survived and Pasteur allowed himself the following excess of emotion when he wrote to his family[1].

> '... perhaps one of the great medical facts of the century is going to take place; you would regret not having seen it!'.

Pasteur had further success with another celebrated case. A shepherd boy, Jean-Baptiste Jupille, had fought off a rabid dog which had been terrorising a group of children. He had been badly mauled. Six days after the attack, Pasteur treated him with his new vaccine. The fourteen year old shepherd boy survived.

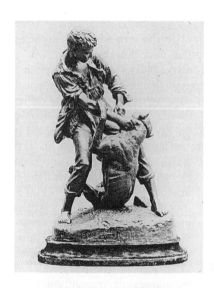

Jean-Baptiste Jupille (b 1871) being attacked by a rabid dog. Statue in the Institut Pasteur, Paris.

Pasteur was the subject of criticism from many sections of the scientific and medical establishment who did not accept his claims. But as with Jenner, Pasteur's contribution to public health would turn out to be lasting and immense. A new era in preventive medicine had dawned.

Despite the attention which was directed towards producing specific immunity in the host to allow a person to resist disease, concern with other more general factors was singularly absent. Apart from the investigation of specific dietary problems like scurvy, the relevance of nutrition to health was largely ignored. This was despite the fact that the majority of the population at most periods of history was seriously undernourished. Such a state limits the individual's ability to resist infection, and compounds the sequelae of the disease. Even so, this was not recognised and measures against under-nutrition were not taken until well into the present century.

The multifactorial concept of cause

The concept of cause embodied in the germ theory is of a one-to-one relationship between causal agent and disease. It was soon realised however, that a more complicated relationship existed for most diseases. For example, it is only possible to develop pulmonary tuberculosis by being infected with the tubercle bacillus. Yet, not everyone who is exposed to it becomes infected and only a minority of cases will proceed to pulmonary tuberculosis. Thus, the realisation that some people developed the disease because of their nutritional status or their genetic make-up led for a time to a 'seed and ground' model of causation, in which there was seen to be an interplay between causal agent and host. This was quickly superseded by the modern view of cause, which is the multifactorial one. It is now recognised that a disease is rarely caused by a single agent alone, but rather depends on a number of factors which combine to produce the disease. These factors may be grouped together under three main headings:

(a) *Agent*

A specific agent may be recognised or presumed depending on the level of current knowledge. It may be a micro-organism, a chemical or physical agent, or the presence or absence of a particular dietary substance.

(b) *Host*

The involvement of the host in the causation of disease is today a much wider concept than it was in the past. Constitutional factors such as genetic make-up and general nutritional status are still important. More recently, however, the behaviour or lifestyle of an individual, whereby he sets out on a road which will end in disease or ill-health, is seen to be of growing importance. A true understanding of the cause of many diseases means appreciating the complexity of factors (such as education, family and social background, occupation, economic status) which lead people to behave in a particular way.

(c) *Environment*

Similarly the concept of environment does not merely encompass physical, chemical and biological elements which have a bearing on health, but also the socio-cultural milieu in which the person lives. In this way, many factors can be seen as implicated in the causal pathway of many of the common diseases. On the larger scale, the political and economic climate can have a distinct bearing on health. Moreover, the general attitudes and expectations of society through stress and many other manifestations, can become part of the web of causation.

This classification considerably simplifies what for many diseases is a highly complex inter-relationship.

HEALTH PROMOTION STRATEGIES

Extensive debates have taken place and a great deal has been written about the concept of health and how it should be defined. One early formal definition was produced by the World Health Organisation in 1946:

'Health is a state of complete physical, psychological and social well-being and not simply the absence of disease or infirmity.'

Over the years which followed the promulgation of this concept of health, the definition was considered too idealistic, and just too difficult to convert into operational goals upon which action could be based. However, the World Health Organisation's post-war definition was seen to be in harmony with a modern concept of health. Programmes to improve health have become much more wide ranging. They have placed greater emphasis on individuals' perceptions of their own health status and have stressed the importance of psychological, social and environmental measures in achieving true health improvement in populations.

This more profound view of health, whilst acknowledging the importance of improving lifestyles, health services and environment, sees even more fundamental conditions as needing to be met if high levels of health in populations are to be achieved (Table 3.1).

A modern public health movement began to take shape in the early 1970s based upon ideals of improving health and tackling some of the seemingly intractable problems of chronic disease and its consequences.

Table 3.1:   ***Pre-requisites for health***

- Peace
- Shelter
- Education
- Food
- Income
- A stable ecosystem
- Sustainable resources
- Social justice
- Equity

Source: Ottawa Charter for Health Promotion, 1986.

Probably the main turning point in focusing attention on prevention, after many years of relative neglect, and introducing the concept of health promotion, was the publication in 1974 of a report by the Canadian government. This report, written by the Canadian Minister of Health (Marc Lalonde), 'A New Perspective on the Health of Canadians'[2], can be viewed in retrospect as a major international breakthrough, which placed health promotion high on the agenda of governments across the world. In Lalonde's 'health field concept', health was recognised as being a function of lifestyles and the environment, as well as being influenced by human biology and health care provision.

'Healthy People', a report by the Surgeon General of the United States of America was a further landmark in the development of modern health policy.[3] It set out a clear and structured commitment to health promotion and disease prevention through the identification of priorities and the specification of measurable goals.

Of particular significance to health worldwide, was the resolution of the thirtieth World Health Assembly at Alma Ata in 1977 that:

'The main social target of governments and of the World Health Organisation (WHO) in the coming decades should be the attainment by all citizens of the world by the year 2000 of a level of health that will permit them to lead a socially and economically productive life.'

The adoption of the *'Health for all by the year 2000'* theme led to many initiatives around the world and has been specifically developed by the WHO European Region of which Britain is a member state. This has resulted in the formulation of targets across a broad range of health promotion and disease prevention fronts addressing two main issues: firstly, to reduce health inequalities between and within countries and, secondly, to strengthen health as much as to reduce disease. Four principal areas of action were identified as part of the Health for All in Europe[4] process:

- **Ensure equity in health** by reducing the present gap in health status between countries and groups within countries.
- **Adding life to years** by ensuring the full development and use of people's integral or residual physical and mental capacity to derive full benefit from and to copewith life in a healthy way.
- **Add health to life** by reducing disease and disability.
- **Add years to life** by reducing premature deaths and thereby increasing life expectancy.

The publication by the British Government in the early 1990s of a White paper called 'The Health of the Nation'[5] further raised the profile of health improvement as a national priority. It firmly established that the health of the population as well as the care of patients is something to be specifically addressed. Although the initiative was led by the Department of Health, it drew together other Government departments with duties and responsibilities which have the potential to contribute to the improvement of health. 'The Health of the Nation' set out a broad national strategy for health improvement with health authorities being required to produce their own local strategies.

It is a popular misconception that efforts directed at promoting health and preventing disease have a limited overall impact on health care. Some people argue that they merely create a larger number of elderly people who then require expensive forms of care. This overlooks the fact that many diseases caused by preventable factors do not lead to sudden death, but they do produce a chronic lingering state of ill-health during which time the person involved will be a major consumer of health and social services. Whilst the human life span will probably only increase very slightly in the foreseeable future, the aim should be to secure a maximum period free of ill-health. This could enable individuals' levels of health and functional status to be improved considerably in their later years, so that the elderly do not become dependent until much nearer the ends of their lives. This approach has become known as the 'compression of morbidity'.

The approaches used in the promotion of health are somewhat different from those used in the diagnostic and therapeutic branches of medicine.

Firstly, relatively little evidence is available to inform decisions about which interventions are likely to be effective, for example, in changing the population's behaviour in the direction of healthier lifestyles. Secondly, there is seldom any single measure which will be effective alone. It is usually necessary to consider a range of approaches as part of a co-ordinated programme if there is to be any genuine impact on the health status of the population. Moreover, many of the actions which can bring about improvement in health are not those over which health services have direct control. Increasingly, it is being recognised that to be effective, health promotion programmes must be multisectoral in nature and involve the active participation of the public.

In practice, the term health promotion used alone or in combination with disease prevention, embraces a wide variety of perspectives from preventing premature death, to legislative and fiscal measures to improve health, the promotion of individual responsibility for the maintenance of healthy ways of living and to mobilising the support of communities as part of health improvement programmes.

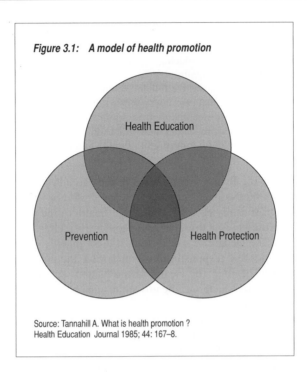

Figure 3.1:   A model of health promotion

Health Education

Prevention

Health Protection

Source: Tannahill A. What is health promotion ?
Health Education Journal 1985; 44: 167–8.

The activities within the field of health promotion can be grouped into three overlapping spheres: prevention, health education and health protection (Figure 3.1).

This model recognises that there are distinct aspects to the health promotion process and at the same time, acknowledges their mutual interdependence. Thus, for example, the successful implementation of a motor vehicle seat belt programme is aimed at reducing death and injury in road accidents (*prevention*). It resulted from the passage of legislation (*health protection*) but, for its success the programme relies upon the public understanding the benefits of the protective measure and adopting health orientated behaviour (*health education*). This particular example would fall in the area where the three circles in Figure 3.1 overlap. The following sections deal with health promotion under these three broad headings but it must be remembered that a combination of approaches is invariably required.

PREVENTION

Reducing the risk of disease, premature death, illness or disability or any other undesirable health event is the orientation of preventive activity within the health promotion process. Traditionally, prevention has been classified into three types (Table 3.2).

(a) *Primary prevention*

This approach seeks actually to prevent the onset of a disease. The ultimate goal of preventive medicine is to alter some factor in the environment, to bring about a change in the status of the host, or to change behaviour so that disease is prevented from developing. Many of the triumphs of public health in the past relating to the infectious diseases, were brought about by primary prevention.

(b) *Secondary prevention*

This level of prevention aims to halt the progression of a disease once it is established. The crux, here, is early detection or early diagnosis followed by prompt, effective treatment. Special consideration of secondary prevention aimed at asymptomatic individuals is necessary. This subject is covered later in the chapter in the section on screening. Whilst it may seem to be merely a logical extension of good clinical practice, careful evaluation is necessary before early disease detection is carried out on a population scale.

(c) *Tertiary prevention*

This level is concerned with rehabilitation of people with an established disease to minimize residual disabilities and complications. Action taken at this stage aims at improving the quality of life, even if the disease itself cannot be cured.

Table 3.2: **Spectrum of health and disease with the main strategies for prevention at each level**

	Stages			Outcomes		
	Health	*Asymptomatic*	*Symptomatic*	*Disability*	*Recovery*	*Death*
Intervention strategies	Health Education*, Immunization, Environmental measures and Social policy	Pre-symptomatic screening	Early diagnosis and prompt effective treatment	Rehabilitation		
Levels of prevention:	Primary	◄——— Secondary ———►			Tertiary	

* Some of these strategies, particularly health education, can also operate at other levels.

A preventive component of a population-based health promotion programme can involve specific interventions or procedures to reduce the risk of disease occurrence. Immunisation and vaccination programmes are an example of a primary preventive approach to reduce or eliminate the infectious diseases of childhood (such as whooping cough, measles, rubella, poliomyelitis, mumps) which can still have serious consequences. In practice, specific preventive techniques will often be used in combination with another element of health promotion. In this example, health education would be an essential element in order to raise parents' awareness of the benefits of immunisation and encourage them to bring their children into the programme.

The field of secondary prevention is an important one for health services and public health practice and is therefore dealt with at greater length in the remainder of this section on prevention.

SCREENING: THE DETECTION OF DISEASE IN ITS PRESYMPTOMATIC PHASE

In its widest sense the term 'screening' implies the scrutiny of people in order to detect the presence of disease, disability or some other attribute which is under study. There are a number of kinds of screening, each of which is carried out for a particular purpose. These can be summarised as follows.

Protection of the public health

This type of screening has its origins in long established methods to control infectious diseases. For example, people entering a country are often subjected to tests or examinations designed to detect the presence of infectious diseases or a carrier state. An immigrant in this category would be judged as a potential risk to the indigenous population and might be refused admission altogether or only admitted after appropriate treatment. Mass chest radiography was originally introduced in Britain to identify cases of tuberculosis which could then be isolated from the rest of the population.

Prior to entering an organisation

It is a universal requirement that all potential recruits to the armed forces should undergo screening by medical examination. This practice dates from the time of the Boer War when a similar screening exercise revealed the high levels of ill-health which so shocked the government and resulted in a wide range of measures aimed at improving the health of the nation. In addition to the armed forces, industry may use the medical examination as a screening tool in the pre-employment context. In some cases, this may also serve to protect the public (for example, in the case of airline pilots or train drivers), but its essential purpose is to benefit the organisation so that it recruits a healthy workforce.

Protection of workforce

In addition to the pre-employment medical which is compulsory in certain occupations, many industries have a statutory obligation to screen their workforce. This is usually for the protection of workers in industries which have a high risk of disease due to hazards in the working environment (for example, ionising radiation).

For life insurance purposes

Most life insurance companies screen prospective policy holders, either by a questionnaire about their health or by direct medical examination. Their aim in so doing is to allow them to load the policy against high-risk clients.

The early diagnosis of disease

This form of screening, often called 'prescriptive screening', is concerned with the detection of disease in its early stages so that early treatment for that disease may be started. With chronic degenerative disorders like cancer, often first seen in their later stages, this may seem to be a logical extension of clinical practice. This argument, coupled with the fact that many population surveys showed a high frequency of previously unrecognised abnormalities, led in the early 1960s to the advocacy of presymptomatic screening for disease on a large scale.[6] It does not follow that population screening should be carried out whenever technology allows a disease to be detected in its presymptomatic phase. A number of criteria must first be considered.

Is the disease an important health problem? Before channelling resources on a large scale the problem must be deemed to be a serious one. Nevertheless, importance is, of course, a relative concept. Some health problems may be important because they are very common. Others, although rare, may have serious consequences for the individual or Society as a whole.

Is there a recognisable latent or early symptomatic stage? In order to detect a disease in its early stages there must be a reasonable time period during its natural history when symptoms are not manifesting themselves.

Are facilities for diagnosis and treatment available? If a screening programme were to reveal large numbers of patients with a particular disease, facilities to provide the necessary follow up investigation and treatment would have to be available.

Has the cost of the programme been considered in the context of other demands for resources? At no time in the foreseeable future are there likely to be unlimited resources that would permit every proposal to be followed through. Proposed expenditure on any one health option must, therefore, be weighed against other proposals.

Is there an agreed policy on whom to treat as patients? This brings in the question of borderline cases. In any population, disease exists in a spectrum of severity. At the less severe end of the spectrum, there is a problem of differentiating people with the disease from normal people. Strict criteria must be laid down, therefore, about what constitutes the particular disease, before screening is carried out.

Does treatment confer benefit? This is perhaps the most important consideration of all and it raises fundamental ethical principles. The presymptomatic screening of people for the presence of disease differs from normal medical practice. In the usual situation the patient makes contact with a doctor because he has recognised that he is ill and in need of medical care. The doctor attempts to formulate a diagnosis and give the best treatment available to the patient, based on his experience and current medical knowledge. In the screening situation the 'patient' has not recognised that he is ill. In fact he probably believes himself to be healthy. The doctor (or screener), in offering him the opportunity to be screened, implies that a health benefit will result, i.e. the early treatment of the disease (if present) and favourable outcome. The reality is that only in a few diseases is there any convincing evidence that striving for early diagnosis on a total population basis, and hence early treatment, affects the outcome for the patient. Thus, it is essential, before embarking on a screening programme for a particular disease, to review all the evidence and decide whether early diagnosis and treatment will truly benefit the person being screened. Or whether, on the other hand, the outcome is no different for a person detected through screening than for someone who is treated at such time as the condition manifests itself clinically.

Choosing the screening test

Having decided to embark on a programme to screen for the presence of a particular disease in a population, the next issue centres on which test to choose for the purpose. Usually those proposing to carry out the screening will have a particular method in mind for detecting the disease, whether it is a blood test, a urine test, an examination or a questionnaire. When making the choice, however, a number of general criteria should be borne in mind. The test should be *cheap* and one that can be carried out *rapidly* by trained non-medical personnel. It should be *acceptable* to the majority of people and this usually rules out very painful or time-consuming procedures. The test should be *reliable*. In other words, the same result would be expected if it was repeated by a different observer altogether or by the same observer on a number of occasions.

Finally, and most importantly, the *validity* of the test must be known. By validity is meant the test's ability to measure or discover what the investigator wants to know. How good is the test at discriminating between people who have the disease and people who are healthy? Validity is usually expressed in terms of *sensitivity* and *specificity*.

Applying a screening test to a population may divide people into four possible types (Figure 3.2). Firstly, there may be people who have the disease and give a positive result on screening (*true positives*); secondly, people who are healthy, or

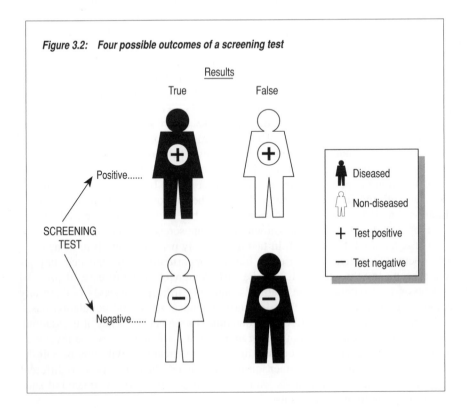

Figure 3.2: Four possible outcomes of a screening test

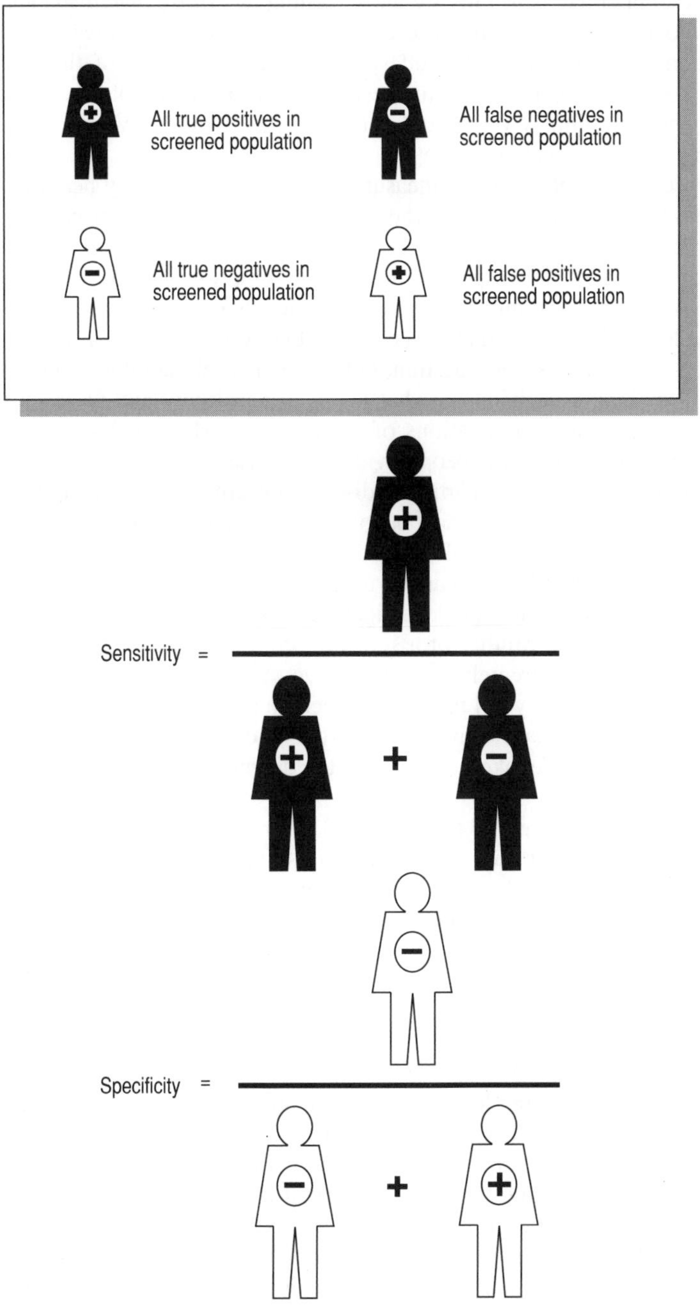

Figure 3.3: Results of a screening test showing sensitivity and specificity

non-diseased, and give a negative result on screening (*true negatives*). If a screening test was ideal, these are the only categories of people who would exist. No test is perfect. So, two further categories are possible: people who, despite having the disease, are classified as healthy by the screening test (*false negatives*) and healthy people who are classified by the screening test as diseased (*false positives*).

The concepts of sensitivity and specificity take account of these problems (Figure 3.3). The sensitivity of the test is a measure of its ability to detect the disease when present. A very highly sensitive test would have no (or very few) missed cases (false negatives).

The specificity of the test is a measure of its ability to identify healthy people as non-diseased. A test of high specificity would have no (or few) people wrongly labelled as diseased (false positives). It is seldom possible to have a test which is 100% sensitive and 100% specific. Usually a compromise level must be agreed. Figure 3.4 shows diagrammatically different levels of sensitivity and specificity. Clearly, a level of 60% would never be acceptable. A level of 90% might possibly be, depending on the diseases in question, but a higher level than this would usually be sought. In making a decision on what levels of sensitivity and specificity will be accepted, the practical implications of the choice must be realised. A sensitivity below 100% means that some people with the disease will be missed and the consequences of this depend on the particular disease concerned. A specificity below 100% means that some healthy people will be told that they might have the disease, with the ensuing anxiety that might result from this. It is important to stress that screening tests cannot be regarded as diagnostic and those people with positive results must undergo further examination and investigation to establish a definitive diagnosis.

The question of the validity of a screening test, as expressed in sensitivity and specificity, is thus an extremely important issue. A knowledge of these principles is, however, of value far beyond the arena of screening. Great benefit would result to the patient, to the standard of medical practice and to the health service, if such a scientific approach were taken to many of the diagnostic tests and examinations in common use today.

For example, if we are told that duodenal ulcer is diagnosed by barium meal we might not accept that at face value without asking 'how good is barium meal at diagnosing duodenal ulcer? ... how does it compare with other diagnostic techniques? ... how many cases of duodenal ulcer do I fail to identify if I investigate them only by doing a barium meal?'.

Example of a population screening programme in current use: pre-symptomatic breast cancer screening

Breast cancer is one of the leading causes of premature death amongst women in many Western countries. In the absence of individual risk factors on which to base a strategy of primary prevention, the main issue in this disease relates to presymptomatic screening. An early important study on the impact of screening apparently healthy women for breast cancer was a randomised controlled trial of women enrolled in the Health Insurance Plan of New York.[7] Two groups of 31,000 women were assigned either to annual screening (in the form of breast palpation and X-ray mammography) or to routine medical care with no such annual screening. Follow-up over a number of years showed a lower mortality from breast

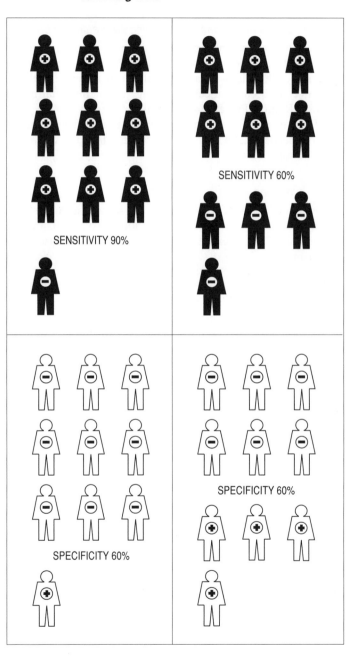

Figure 3.4:   Differing levels of sensitivity and specificity of screening tests

cancer in the screened group, but only amongst older women. There was no apparent benefit from screening younger women.

Introduction of a national breast cancer screening programme in Britain

In 1987 the British Government launched a national programme to detect breast cancer in its early stages. The decision to adopt a population screening approach to reduce the impact of this disease was taken after consideration of the report of an expert committee on breast cancer screening[8] under the Chairmanship of Sir Patrick Forrest, Regius Professor of Clinical Surgery at the University of Edinburgh. The committee, having evaluated the evidence for and against screening, recommended that a national programme should be established and laid down an organisational model.

Organisation of screening

Breast cancer screening involves the use of low dose x-ray of the breast (mammography) to detect small cancers in previously asymptomatic women.

The programme of breast cancer screening operating in Britain contains the following elements.

The offer of screening. Eligible women in the target age group (50–64 years) are identified through a computerised population listing based upon Family Health Services Authorities' patient registers. Automated systems then enable a computerised call and recall system to operate so that women can be mailed with invitations to attend initial screening or follow-up visits. Each woman receives a personalised letter of invitation mentioning that her general practitioner endorses the screening programme and is being kept informed.

The initial screen. Women who are called for screening attend a conveniently situated centre (often in a local hospital) or a mobile facility (used in parts of the country with rural or widely dispersed populations). The initial screening procedure involves a single view low dose x-ray (mammogram) being taken of the breasts. This technique is capable of detecting abnormalities as small as 1–2 mm in diameter. The method needs careful technique by the radiographers who take the mammogram and skilled interpretation by radiologists. Following the initial screen, some women will be recalled for further assessment. Approximately 10% of women will be recalled for further assessment after the initial screen, though many will be cleared following this second assessment.

Further assessment. Women who undergo further assessment following the initial screen will typically have further mammographic views taken of the suspicious area of the breast and may also have ultrasound examination. After this, or directly following the initial screen (depending on the nature of the abnormality), some women will have an examination by a specialist team usually comprising a surgeon, a radiologist and a pathologist, all of whom are skilled in the diagnosis of breast abnormalities. The nature of the examination at this stage of the screening programme will vary according to the clinical circumstances but can involve a fine needle localisation in which the needle is guided to the abnormality under direct x-ray visualisation of the breast. A surgical biopsy follows this process.

Approximately 2% of women who have attended the initial mammographic screening will eventually proceed to a surgical biopsy. Specialist assessment teams of the type described are not provided in all local hospitals. There are a limited number in each region serving larger populations. This may be inconvenient for some of the small number of women who need the service and have to travel further afield but it is essential if quality control is to be maintained. Specialist skills can only be kept at a high standard if staff see sufficient diseased people to remain experienced.

Treatment. Definitive treatment of a breast malignancy may involve simple removal of the breast lump ('lumpectomy') or more extensive surgery by removal of the breast with or without radiotherapy. Although radical treatments were clinically fashionable in the past, there is little scientific evidence to show that they improve survival or reduce the rate of recurrence of the cancer. Early detection of very small cancers allows the use of techniques which conserve the breast and is more likely to remove the abnormality at a pre-invasive stage. It is thus less mutilating to the patient and more likely to be successful.

Counselling. It is important that all women who attend screening should understand the basic screening process and why they are being offered screening. They are also informed that most women who have to undergo a second assessment do not have cancer. This considerably reduces the anxiety of women who have screening. Finally it is important that adequate counselling is available for women who do have cancer both pre- and post-surgery.

Health education. Education of the public about the availability of presymptomatic screening and its purpose is an essential and integral part of the programme. This helps to gain the maximum uptake of the invitation to be screened and ensures that women who need to be followed up comply with the necessary arrangements.

Screening frequency. Present national policy is that the interval between mammographic screening should be three years.

Screening of women outside the target age groups. There is no scientific evidence, as yet, that screening of women in the population who are under the age of 50 years reduces mortality from the disease. This is an issue which has caused controversy in some localities because the public and media have presumed that younger women are being discriminated against or that insufficient resources have been made available to offer them the service. It is important that the public understands the reasons for this policy decision which is in line with one of the key principles for embarking on a presymptomatic programme (does the treatment confer benefit?). National policy is to provide screening only if it is specifically requested by women over 65 years. Women under 50 years do not have access to screening on demand, but may be referred by a general practitioner if there is a particular personal or family history of the disease.

Evaluation and quality control

Whilst presymptomatic screening for breast cancer has been successful in reducing mortality amongst study populations, the ultimate test of its efficacy is in the impact it makes on the disease in a general population. It is too early to assess the effect of the national breast cancer screening programme in the population of Britain. However, the potential benefits of the screening programme, which will be achieved if the results of the trials are translated to the national programme, have been estimated (Table 3.3).

These benefits are most likely to be achieved if the programme is strongly rooted in quality. This means achieving the highest possible uptake of invitations to be screened and ensuring that staff involved at all levels in the screening process are highly skilled. It also requires the establishment of systems and standards for continuous improvement in call and recall arrangements, radiology and radiography, pathology, surgical treatment, health education, and communication with the women being screened.

Table 3.3:   Expected impact of the British breast cancer screening programme

- By the year 2000, 25% of deaths from breast cancer prevented in the population of women invited for screening
- On average each of the women in whom death from breast cancer is prevented will live about 20 years more
- By the year 2000, about 25,000 extra years of life gained annually in the United Kingdom

Source: Department of Health. Breast Cancer Screening 1991: evidence and experience since the Forrest Report. London. Department of Health, 1991.

OTHER EXAMPLES OF SCREENING PROGRAMMES IN CURRENT USE

Many screening tests are already a firmly established part of medical practice. Most of them were introduced at a time when new proposals were not subject to the kind of rigid scrutiny which preceded the introduction of the British national breast cancer screening programme.

Clearly it would be unrealistic as well as unethical when a screening programme is well-established (and perhaps of benefit) to begin again and withhold screening from some individuals in order to carry out an evaluation. Some examples of screening tests in common use are shown in Table 3.4. They have found a definitive place in public health practice and are likely to remain there for some time to come. There can be little dispute about the value of establishing the presence of serious congenital abnormalities (such as congenital heart defects or congenital dislocation of the hip) by screening all newborn children by physical examination. Effective surgical procedures exist to deal with such disorders which, if left untreated, can cause serious disability and even death. Critical appraisal of such screening programmes revolves around other issues (such as the choice of the most appropriate method and the best time at which to carry them out).

Screening programmes for detecting disease in later life are more controversial. Doubts have been expressed about the value, for example, of population screening for hypertension or the screening of elderly people in the home. Some believe that

Table 3.4: **Examples of screening programmes in common use**

Group screened	Disease or abnormality detected	Test and by whom carried out	Aim
Neonates	Structural abnormalities (e.g. congenital heart disease, spina bifida, congenital dislocation of the hip)	Physical examination by doctor/midwife/health visitor	Prevention of death or handicap by early correction
		Ultrasound by radiologist	
	Functional abnormalities (e.g. cerebral palsy, visual and hearing defects)	Physical examination by doctor/midwife/health visitor	Prevention of handicap or educational impairment by early treatment
	Metabolic disease (e.g. phenyl-ketonuria)	Special test (e.g. Guthrie test) by midwife/health visitor	Prevention of handicap by dietary modification
Pregnant women	Adverse factors in pregnancy (e.g. anaemia, raised blood pressure, proteinuria)	History taking/physical examination/special tests by doctor/midwife	Prevention of death or disability in mother or fetus
	Fetal abnormalities (e.g. neural tube defects, mongolism)	Serum or amniotic fluid test	Prevention of birth of abnormal or handicapped fetus by offering abortion
Middle-aged men and women	Hypertension	Blood pressure reading by doctor / nurse	To prevent premature death or disability from complications
	Cervical cancer	Papanicolaou smear by doctor	To prolong survival from the disease
	Breast cancer	Mammography	To prolong survival from the disease
Elderly people	Disease, disability or social isolation	General practitioner or health visitor making regular visits/examinations	To delay onset of dependency

these activities are best left to case-finding within general practice rather than being mounted and organised on a total population basis.

HEALTH EDUCATION

Expressed most simply, health education seeks to improve health and to prevent ill-health by enabling people to follow and sustain particular actions and choices. Such a broad definition, however, has little utility since it conceals an enormous variety of aims from the general to the very specific. Health education may, for example, seek to: promote regular exercise in a population; ensure that hypertensive patients adhere to their prescribed treatment schedule; get more pregnant women to attend antenatal care at an earlier stage of their pregnancy than hitherto; and to achieve high uptake of immunisation programmes.

Table 3.5: Health education defined in terms of its possible purposes

Model	Purpose
Educational	To provide information and create well-informed people
Self empowerment	To empower choice and foster personal growth
Preventive medical	To prevent disease by persuading people to adopt medically approved behaviours
Radical-political	To raise awareness of the need for health policy, to stimulate people to tackle the social, environmental and political influences on health

Source: Adapted from: Whitehead M, Tones K. Avoiding the Pitfalls. London: Health Education Authority, 1991.

Health education concepts

One way of definining health education is in terms of its purpose. Table 3.5 summarises four different ways of conceptualising health education activity. The first is to inform people so that they understand the basis of health risks and the nature of disease causation and are in a position to make informed choices (*the educational model*). The second way of viewing health education (the so-called *health improvement model*) is concerned not just to inform people but to equip them with practical skills to exercise choice and resist pressures to conform to particular social pressures. The *preventive medical model* sees health education as a process through which people are persuaded to pursue medically approved behaviours, whilst the fourth approach is a *radical-political model* of health education. It seeks to achieve fundamental change in social and economic policy through education about the social, environmental and political influences on health.

Process of health education

The process of health education is complex, but it is often viewed in three phases:
- Imparting knowledge
- Changing attitudes
- Altering behaviour

This used to be seen as a sequence in which people are first provided with information which emphasises the benefits and risks of following particular courses of action. As a result of this, a change in attitude results in a change of behaviour in the direction required to achieve the particular health education goal.

However, this simple sequential process is now largely discounted as a basis for action. For example, behavioural change can occur without alteration of attitude. A motorist may wear his seat belt to conform with the law, even though he maintains a negative attitude towards its use. This should not detract from the importance of imparting knowledge about health, whether it is with the intention of changing behaviour, or for other reasons.

Each of the phases of health education is very complex and much is still unknown. The supplying of information to increase an individual's knowledge about a particular health risk is not a straightforward proposition to be embarked upon without careful research. The source of the information is important. It has been said in the past that more credence is usually given if a message comes from a member of the health professions than a lay person or government spokesman. In this context the cynical observation, attributed to a member of the tobacco industry, that a doctor or nurse who smokes is worth £50,000 to them, is of particular relevance.

It is by no means certain, however, that messages emanating from purely professional sources are always the correct approach, particularly, for example, when addressing the process of health education in young people. It is important that young people receive both formal and informal education about health issues. One fundamental approach which provides a long-term strategy for health education is to incorporate health-related messages into a person's value system during primary socialisation. Children are born with certain basic patterns of behaviour which are genetically determined. However, during early life they learn skills, attitudes and values which determine how they will function and interact with other members of society. This process of socialisation is not influenced solely by parents, although the family is clearly central to it. A number of other influences directly affect the process such as, school, peer groups, youth organisations and the mass media. The potential for health education to inculcate its messages as part of this process of socialisation is clearly enormous since, by this means, attitudes to health and health-related behaviour are established from a very early age.

The inclusion of health education themes within the National Core Curriculum in schools is an important development. Nonetheless it is also important that, whether in the school setting or in other contexts, health education in childhood does not just involve the imparting of knowledge. It must also seek to equip children with the ability and skills to understand and cope with influences such as peer pressure, the media, product promotion and advertising.

Approaches to achieve change

At a broader population level, health education is not simply a way of conveying information about health and risks. It must seek to influence young people's values towards healthy options in ways which have as much appeal and attraction as the allure of the risk taking alternatives. For example, in considering health promotion programmes to cut down the incidence of unprotected casual sex in young people, traditional approaches which centre on urging general sexual restraint, are unlikely to be successful. Such approaches fail to address the reality and motivation of risk-taking behaviour in young people. Researchers who have worked extensively in the field of health education and health promotion of young people have identified ten points which should be borne in mind when directing health messages at young people (Table 3.6). Although the example is taken from the field of HIV infection and AIDS, these pointers have a more general applicability.

Table 3.6:   Designing health promotion programmes for young people: 10 key points

- Clear, realistic and measurable objectives
- Start with what young people already know and think
- Convey clear and accurate information
- Challenge and correct misinformation and prejudice
- Avoidance of over-reliance on mass media methods
- Use the language and imagery of youth
- Education sensitive to individual background and culture
- Personalise the risks
- Use fear appeals with caution
- Encourage appropriate use of legislation and political measures

The process through which attitudes are changed is one which has stimulated a great deal of research, particularly by social psychologists. It has been suggested, for instance, that a change in attitude (resulting in consequent health behaviour) will occur if the individual's perception of the benefits of the action (in terms of the seriousness of the disease and his susceptibility to it) outweigh his perception of the barriers to his taking this action. Any individual's belief system is likely to result from a vast complexity of factors, which may be cultural, social, familial, formally educational or experiential. Health education must attempt to come to grips with these issues if the process of behaviour change is to be successful.

Resources allocated by health authorities for health education tend to be relatively small and they must therefore be used wisely. This means that every health education programme should seek to evaluate itself. In other words, it should seek to determine how successful it has been in achieving its declared objectives. Steps forward will only be made by building on scientifically established foundations. It cannot be assumed, for example, that a television commercial is effective merely because it has been shown at peak viewing time.

One important aspect of health education in the process of helping people to adopt and sustain healthy lifestyles is direct contact with a person skilled in risk assessment and counselling. At present, it appears that the majority of people who could be helped in this way do not receive any service and this in turn is almost certainly a reflection of the lack of any systematic way of identifying those who are at risk, a lack of evidence on effectiveness of the approaches which should be adopted and lack of sufficient number of people with the necessary skills to deliver the service.

HEALTH PROTECTION

The question of using legislative means to secure health goals is an issue which often provokes bitter controversy. The counter argument usually hangs on the immorality of removing the individual's freedom to choose. The relationship between the State and the individual as expressed in law is a major theme in political philosophy. Although much has been written since, the major reference is still an essay published in 1859 entitled 'On Liberty' by the British philosopher, economist and author John Stuart Mill (1806–1873), and generally regarded as his masterpiece. In it he states that:

'the only purpose for which power can rightfully be exercised over any member of a civilised society is to prevent harm to others. His own good, either physical or moral, is not a sufficient warrant.'

Measures which prevent the spread of disease are accepted without question, for example, legislation to ensure adequate standards of hygiene by food producers and handlers, or to maintain a pure water supply. Other proposals which affect individual freedom such as the wearing of seat belts, or restriction on smoking, cause controversy.

Similar arguments are raised about fluoridation of drinking water. This measure is well researched and is safe and effective in preventing dental caries, yet action to introduce it is opposed by some as an infringement of individual liberty.

Influencing individuals' choices

In addition to measures which seek to prohibit or enforce a particular action, another approach which may or may not involve legislation, is to attempt to channel an individual into a particular action. The consumer's choice may be influenced by economic means, for example, increasing taxation on cigarettes and alcohol or by subsidising products thought to be beneficial, like polyunsaturated fats or wholemeal bread.

Other approaches seek to limit choice other than by economic pressures. An example of this is the restriction of smoking in public places.

The introduction of such measures can result in complex reactions, so they need to be carefully monitored to see if they produce the desired effects. There is evidence to support the approach of increasing the price of alcohol in order to achieve reduction in consumption. On the other hand, if the price is too high it could encourage people to make alcoholic drinks at home.

Modifying the environment

Another way in which policy changes can influence the health of individuals and the community is by action taken to adjust the environment. For example, measures which control atmospheric pollution and noise levels, or those which limit the effect of radiation and other environmental hazards are contained within a legal framework which acts to modify the environment in such a way as to meet health aims. These are issues discussed fully in Chapter 10 but it must be remembered that this is not just an issue of ecology in the sense that it is usually understood. The home, the workplace and places where the public gather are linked to health in a complex range of ways. Designs for safety, policies on matters such as smoking and drinking, and the prevalence of product advertising can affect people's outlook and influence the choices which they make.

The health service alone, is relatively limited in influencing these matters within the general population, although, in terms of its own premises and workforces it is considerable. The scope for the health service working in a concerted way with business and commerce, and other public bodies is enormous and, as yet, largely unexploited.

An emphasis on multisector collaboration is likely to be a common feature of successful health promotion programmes in the future. For example, in the area of health risk-taking amongst young people, which is discussed in other sections of this chapter, there could be important roles for the drinks and leisure industries in creating and promoting attractive and acceptable, alcohol and drug free environments and in extending the range of recreational and leisure opportunities available to young people.

Modifying individuals' risks and resistance

Another example of a preventive measure to modify individual's risk status or resistance to disease is the use of drugs to lower blood cholesterol in individuals with high levels on testing (for example, people with familial hypercholesterolaemia). It is likely that, as scientific advances in human genetics progress, the scope for prevention through changing an individual's risk status will greatly widen. These developments in genetics already have a wide range of applications. In future, there are likely to be greater opportunities to avoid or modify environmental mutagens, thus reducing the incidence of many diseases. Prevention or better treatment of communicable diseases will occur as further effective vaccines are developed and antiviral agents come into wider use. Many more conditions will be detectable antenatally and whilst this may lead to an increase in the number of pregnancies being terminated, it is also likely that gene therapy applications will widen.

Protective technologies

In some fields of health protection, goals are achieved through the development and application of technology. Some examples in the field of accident prevention are discussed later in the chapter. The use of cycle helmets by children to reduce the impact of head injuries, the use of speed ramps around schools to slow traffic and the design of motor vehicles are all measures with the potential to contribute to the reduction in mortality and morbidity from accidents. Technological solutions are also widely used in the food industry to prevent the transmission of communicable diseases caused by micro-organisms and their toxins.

SOME HEALTH PROBLEMS

To illustrate the public health challenges faced by those concerned with promoting health, some examples of health problems relevant to the population of Britain are discussed in the sections which follow.

Coronary heart disease and stroke

Coronary heart disease results from total or partial occlusion of the coronary arteries. This is brought about by deposits of a fibrofatty substance, called atheroma, in the inner part of the coronary arteries which, as a result, become thickened so that the space through which the blood flows is narrowed. This process of narrowing of the coronary arteries can be added to by deposits of blood clot.

These changes in the coronary vessels produce a number of main clinical manifestations: sudden death, heart attack (acute myocardial infarction), angina pectoris, heart failure and abnormal heart rhythms.

The impact on the population is major in terms of deaths, years of life lost prematurely, hospital bed-days used, major surgical procedures performed and working days lost to the economy (Table 3.7).

Table 3.7: The impact of coronary heart disease, England 1991

- Causes 26% of all deaths.
- Accounts for 2.5% of total NHS expenditure.
- Results in 35 million lost working days.

Source: The Health of the Nation. London: HMSO, 1992.

Stroke or cerebrovascular disease results from reduction in the supply of arterial blood to the brain. The pathological basis of stroke is more diverse than that of coronary heart disease. Atheroma of the cerebral arteries with thrombus formation is one of the common underlying processes. Haemorrhage from a cerebral vessel either associated with atheroma or a ruptured aneurysm is a second mechanism. A third is through an embolism lodging in a cerebral artery and obstructing it.

The clinical manifestations of a stroke are often devastating: loss of consciousness (from which the person may not recover), weakness or paralysis (usually) of one side of the body (arm, leg, face), loss or impairment of speech, emotional lability, loss of other functions (such as continence of urine or faeces). Cerebrovascular disease can also result in loss of function without the acute occurrence of a stroke. Of particular importance is its role in the causation of one of the forms of dementia. Dementia varies in the way in which it affects mental, physical and social functioning but (as is discussed in chapter 8) it can affect all three.

As with coronary heart disease, stroke has a major impact on the person concerned and on the family. If the person survives, he or she will often be seriously impaired and unable to function independently. A spouse, or a middle-aged son or daughter (with children of their own) may then have to assume the burden of care.

The impact in population terms is also considerable. The large number of deaths, the demand for hospital care during the acute episode, the need for rehabilitation, and longer term residentially based care, and the pool of chronic disability created, make stroke a major public health problem.

Coronary heart disease and stroke remain leading causes of premature death, illness and disability in many of the developed countries of the world. Moreover, when the experience of Britain is compared to other countries, it fares badly.

During the period spanning the 1970s and 1980s, mortality from coronary heart disease declined in many parts of the world (Table 3.8). This included countries (such as the United States, England and Wales, New Zealand) where rates had peaked in the previous two decades and in Japan where it had previously been lower. In some Eastern European countries death rates increased. As Table 3.8

shows the downward trend was not as great in England and Wales over this period as in some other countries.

Table 3.8: *Change in mortality from coronary heart disease in selected countries 1970 to 1986*

	Men	Women
Finland	−27.5	−30.6
United States	−52.2	−50.4
New Zealand	−32.2	−30.7
England and Wales	−13.9	−4.7
Sweden	−7.2	−27.7
Hungary	+38.6	+14.0
Poland	+78.5	+65.9
Japan	−43.6	−56.6

Source: Beaglehole R. International trends in coronary heart disease mortality, morbidity and risk factors. Epidemiologic Reviews 1990; 12: 1–15.

It is difficult to be certain about the reasons for these changes but reduction in the amount of saturated fat consumed in the diet and cessation of smoking appear to have been the major contributors for the countries in which reductions have occurred.

Rate of death from stroke has declined in Britain and some other countries, particularly during the 1970s and 1980s (Figure 3.5) but along with coronary heart disease, it remains an important cause of death from middle age onwards (Figure 3.6).

Risk markers for coronary heart disease

The causation of coronary heart disease has been the subject of extensive epidemiological investigation over many years and the evidence relating to markers of risk is well established.

Whilst it is clear that the causation of the disease is multifactorial, it is possible to identify and quantify individual risk markers. The three major independent factors are:

(a) **Cigarette smoking**
   The main data regarding smoking and coronary heart disease may be summarised as follows:

   (i)   Autopsy studies have shown that cigarette smoking increases the extent of atheroma formation in the coronary arteries.

   (ii) Cigarette smoking is a major risk factor in the genesis of acute myocardial infarction (AMI) in both sexes and is dose-related (i.e. increases with the amount smoked). The greatest risk of AMI in smokers compared to non-smokers is in the youngest age groups, the differences decrease in the older age groups. This age-related effect could be due to the elimination (by death) of susceptible individuals at younger ages or probably, more importantly, the greater influence of risk factors other than smoking in the older age groups.

   (iii) Although cigarette smoking is an independent risk factor in AMI, it may also act in a synergistic fashion with high blood pressure and raised blood cholesterol.

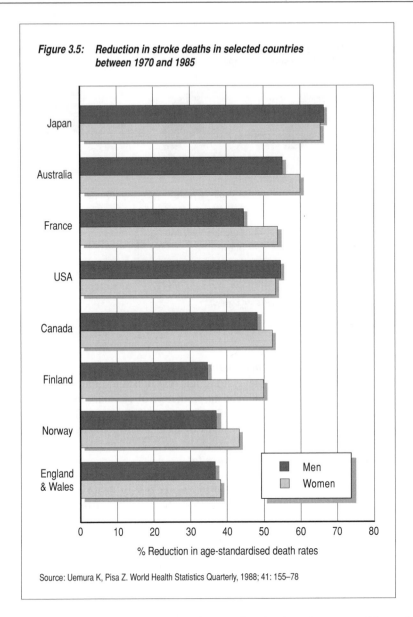

Figure 3.5: *Reduction in stroke deaths in selected countries between 1970 and 1985*

% Reduction in age-standardised death rates

Source: Uemura K, Pisa Z. World Health Statistics Quarterly, 1988; 41: 155–78

(iv) The occurrence of sudden death is strongly related to cigarette smoking and though the risk for smokers compared to non-smokers decreases with age, it persists even into the older age groups.

(v) Cigarette smokers (compared to non-smokers) are at greater risk of developing angina pectoris, but the relationship is weaker than for the other forms of coronary heart disease.

Thus, smoking is a major risk marker for coronary heart disease in both men and women. Coronary heart disease mortality is lower in ex-smokers than in those who continue to smoke.

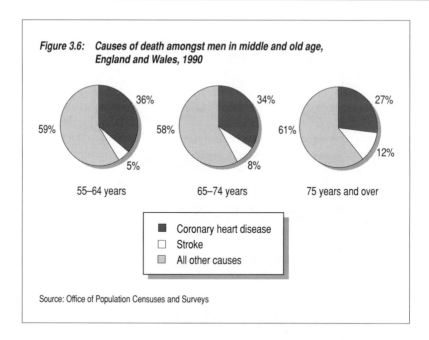

Figure 3.6:   Causes of death amongst men in middle and old age, England and Wales, 1990

55–64 years   65–74 years   75 years and over

- ■ Coronary heart disease
- □ Stroke
- ▨ All other causes

Source: Office of Population Censuses and Surveys

(b) *Raised blood pressure (hypertension)*

Increased levels of both the systolic and the diastolic components of blood pressure are both strong independent predictors of coronary heart disease risk. Those who have high levels of blood pressure have three to four times the chance of developing coronary heart disease when compared to those with normal blood pressures.

(c) *Raised blood cholesterol and dietary fat*

There is little doubt about the importance of raised serum cholesterol as a risk marker. Higher concentrations lead to greater risk of death and this has been demonstrated in all populations which have been studied. Broadly, people with the highest cholesterol levels have four times the risk of death from coronary heart disease as do those with the lowest. A more sensitive marker of risk can be derived by measuring the high-density lipoprotein (HDL) and low-density lipoprotein (LDL) fractions of cholesterol. High levels of the latter (LDL) increase the risk of coronary heart disease whilst the former (HDL) appears to be protective.

The link between raised serum cholesterol and intake of dietary fat is complex. It is true that in countries where the diet is usually high in saturated (mainly animal) fats as opposed to polyunsaturated (mainly vegetable) fats, rates of coronary heart disease are high. Similarly, national average saturated fat intakes are strongly correlated with average serum cholesterol levels in those same populations. However, it has been more difficult to demonstrate unequivocally a relationship between individual dietary intakes of fat and coronary heart disease, since individual people vary greatly, in how dietary intakes of various compositions affect their blood cholesterol levels. Nonetheless, in cohort epidemiological studies of male populations, reduction of serum cholesterol in the study populations through diet or drugs have been shown to lead to reduction in the occurrence of coronary heart disease. There are two other major strands to aetiological research on diet and coronary heart disease. The first puts forward evidence of influences in early life being a determinant of coronary heart disease in adulthood and the second postulates a role for an insulin resistance syndrome (syndrome X). Diet and metabolism will remain an important area for research into coronary heart disease causation.

Beyond these three major risk markers for coronary heart disease, a number of others have been implicated in its causation:

(d) *Physical inactivity*

Regular and vigorous physical activity confers protection against coronary heart disease. Physical inactivity increases the likelihood that a person will develop coronary heart disease. The level of physical activity required is not sufficiently well defined to enable estimates of risk reduction to be calculated but broad guidelines on the amounts and type of beneficial exercise are available. However, if other adverse factors are present then the beneficial effect of exercise may be lost.

(e) *Obesity*

Risk of coronary heart disease is higher amongst individuals who are above the average weight for their height. Whilst obesity is a marker for coronary heart disease, it is often present with other risk markers such as hypertension and raised serum cholesterol. When these and other factors are controlled for during analysis of survey data, it is not identified as an independent marker of risk. Nevertheless, it is a marker which is amenable to preventive action even though its mechanism of risk is not fully understood.

(f) *Genetic predisposition*

The increased occurrence of coronary heart disease in close relatives, particularly of a person who has developed the disease at a young age, is well recognised. Much of the association is explained by inheritance of two risk factors: hypercholesterolaemia and hypertension.

(g) *Stress*

In the minds of the public and in media coverage, stress often seems to be a major risk marker for coronary heart disease. There is little evidence that this is the case. Stress is difficult to define and measure and thus studies to elucidate its role have been inconclusive. There is some evidence that particular personality types have an excess risk. When explaining risk to the public it is important that discussion of stress does not obscure the importance of the major risk markers (such as cigarette smoking).

(h) *Diabetes mellitus*

The presence of diabetes mellitus increases a person's risk of developing coronary heart disease.

Risk markers for stroke

The predominant risk marker for the development of stroke is raised blood pressure. Linear increases in the frequency of stroke occur with rises in both systolic and diastolic blood pressure. Numerous controlled trials of hypertension have shown that a reduction in the occurrence of stroke can be achieved in treated compared to control groups. As a consequence, factors (such as obesity) which contribute to hypertension are also risk markers in stroke. Risk is also increased with pre-existing heart disease, diabetes mellitus and previous stroke or transient cerebral ischaemic attacks. Alcohol intake above recommended safe levels increases the risk of stroke. Serum cholesterol and cigarette smoking are associated with increased risk of stroke though the relationship is not as strong as for coronary heart disease. People with sickle cell anaemia are also at increased risk of stroke.

Prevention and control

Strategies to reduce the impact of coronary heart disease as a public health problem must be based largely on primary preventive measures aimed at the principal risk factors. There is little evidence that the more effective clinical treatment of people with the established disease has made any major contribution to the fall in mortality from the disease which has occurred in the populations of some countries over the last two decades.

It remains to be seen what the impact will be, in population terms, of the therapeutic approaches such as thrombolytic therapy administered immediately after an acute myocardial infarction or the revascularisation techniques (coronary artery by-pass graft and angioplasty).

Past experience has shown that, certainly as far as acute myocardial infarction is concerned, people do not interpret the symptoms and summon medical help immediately, so that a substantial proportion of fatalities occur before patients are in a position to receive therapy. Some element of public health education should be devoted to raising people's awareness of the early symptoms of heart attacks so that they present more quickly. However, there are difficulties with this approach, not least in raising public anxiety.

Health promotion strategies directed at the principal risk markers for coronary heart disease are discussed in other parts of this chapter. It is important to emphasise the multifaceted nature of such programmes, the need for coordination, and the key role for multisector collaboration.

Scope for the prevention of stroke lies with reducing risk factors which are important in the production of hypertension (including the reduction of obesity), smoking cessation policies, and strategies to increase safer levels of drinking in the population.

Aside from these primary preventive measures the other major control measure in stroke is to recognise and effectively treat established hypertension. Rapid advances have taken place since the 1960s in the development of anti-hypertensive drugs which are effective without having the severity of side effects of earlier drugs. The step from clinical trials, demonstrating control of hypertension and hence reduction of stroke, to advocating population detection on a wide scale is not a straightforward one. Many complex issues are raised. First is the question of screening an apparently healthy population to detect abnormality (and the principles here are discussed fully later in this chapter). In the case of hypertension, the benefits of reducing or delaying death and disability from its sequelae must be balanced against the physical, social and psychological impact of putting a sizeable proportion of the population on therapy for life. This is in addition to the direct financial consequences. Secondly, there are other important practical issues raised by the population approach. Even if cases of hypertension are detected, to bring their blood pressure under control, would not be easy to achieve across a whole population. Non-compliance with therapy by patients, particularly those with mild hypertension, is an important cause of failure of anti-hypertensive therapy. It may be difficult to persuade people who do not experience symptoms to remain diligently on therapy over a period of many years. Similarly, some individuals may experience side effects which may lead to them discontinuing therapy.

For these reasons, identification and treatment of hypertension on a case-finding rather than a population basis is the preferred strategy. Such an approach can be carried out effectively in general practice with the back up of hospital specialist departments in the management of the patients detected.

Accidents

The word accident implies an event which happens purely by chance but accidents do not occur at random. Some groups of the population, for example, children, the elderly or those in particular occupational groups, are at much greater risk than others. The perceived inappropriateness of the term accidents has led some researchers to call them unintentional injuries. However, here the term accident is adopted because of its widespread every day use.

Age is a powerful influence in determining the risk of accidents in a number of ways. Firstly, it influences the degree and nature of exposure to particular hazards. Secondly, it is related to skills, competence and attitudes in particular activities. The young child and the elderly person, although for very different reasons are at greater risks as pedestrians and fall more often than do others in the population. Young children are still developing physically, mentally and socially and are unaware of dangers such as speeds or distance, and their attention easily wanders. The elderly person may have limited mobility and failing vision or eyesight. Thirdly, age may influence the ability of a person to withstand injuries sustained in an accident.

Accidents account for approximately 13% of years of life lost under the age of 65 years and they are a particularly important cause of preventable death in the younger age groups. They also result in substantial numbers of non-fatal injuries each year and considerable health service expenditure. Accidents occur as a result of road traffic accidents, falls, poisoning, drowning and fires (Figure 3.7). They occur in the home, on the roads, in a variety of outdoor locations and in the workplace. Particular categories of road users (for example, pedestrians, motor cyclists, pedal cyclists, car drivers) have differing risks of dying or being injured in an accident.

Accidents as a cause of death in Britain have declined over recent years and are at lower levels than many other countries (Figure 3.8) but still represent an unacceptably large public health problem.

For many young people, car driving and motorcycle riding represent two ways in which they can experience the thrills of risk-taking. Most studies of young

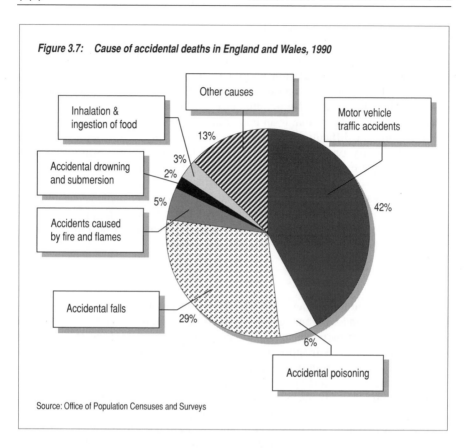

Figure 3.7:   Cause of accidental deaths in England and Wales, 1990

Other causes

Inhalation &
ingestion of food

13%

Motor vehicle
traffic accidents

3%

Accidental drowning
and submersion

2%

5%

42%

Accidents caused
by fire and flames

Accidental falls

29%

6%

Accidental poisoning

Source: Office of Population Censuses and Surveys

motorcyclists have found that excitement and adventure are the prime motivating forces behind their behaviour on the road and this is often reinforced by motorcycle manufacturers' advertising. The risk of serious injury or death from motorcycling is estimated to be 100 times greater than the safest form of travel by road (bus) and 25 times greater than driving a car.

At the same time car advertising reflects an increasing concern about safety features. Rigid passenger compartments as well as front and rear crumple zones are almost standard, whilst seat belts fitted both in the front and back of new cars are now a legal requirement. Furthermore, even more sophisticated safety features are appearing such as anti-lock brakes, collapsible steering columns and inflatable driver crash air bags. However, despite improvements to car design, travelling in motor vehicles still accounts for a substantial number of deaths each year. The largest proportion of these deaths occur to those between 15 and 24 years of age and are probably connected to young people's relative lack of driving experience and also to the element of risk-taking. An additional and extremely worrying aspect of this behaviour by young people on the roads is the rising incidence of joyriding in stolen cars, with sometimes fatal consequences.

An important aetiological factor in road accidents is alcohol. It is present in about a quarter of fatal accidents involving car users and pedestrians. Misuse of

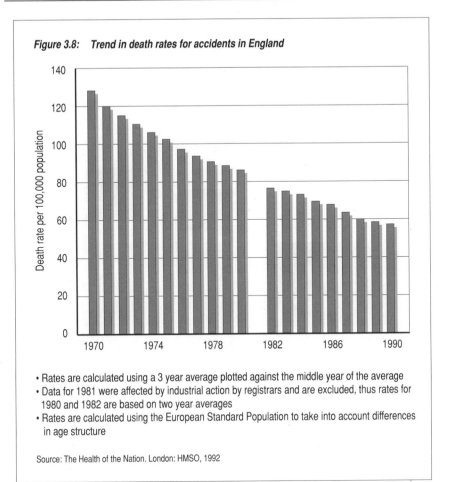

Figure 3.8:   Trend in death rates for accidents in England

- Rates are calculated using a 3 year average plotted against the middle year of the average
- Data for 1981 were affected by industrial action by registrars and are excluded, thus rates for 1980 and 1982 are based on two year averages
- Rates are calculated using the European Standard Population to take into account differences in age structure

Source: The Health of the Nation. London: HMSO, 1992

alcohol is also implicated in other types of accidents such as falls, fires and drowning. Smoking is an additional important factor in fires which start in the home.

The importance of road traffic accidents as a cause of death and serious injury in childhood is emphasised by the fact that they account for about a quarter of all deaths of children under the age of 15 years. Overall, the rate of deaths and serious injuries in road accidents is lower in Britain than most other European countries but the rate of pedestrian deaths amongst children are at relatively high levels in Britain. Indeed, pedestrian road accidents are the single commonest cause of accidental death in children, accounting for 40% of all accidental deaths in the 5 to 14 year old age group, and over 20% of accidental deaths in the younger and less mobile children from 1 to 4 years of age.

The impact of children's use of pedal cycles in the older age group when they start to go on to the open roads is also evident in the rate of occurrence of death and severe injury (Figure 3.9).

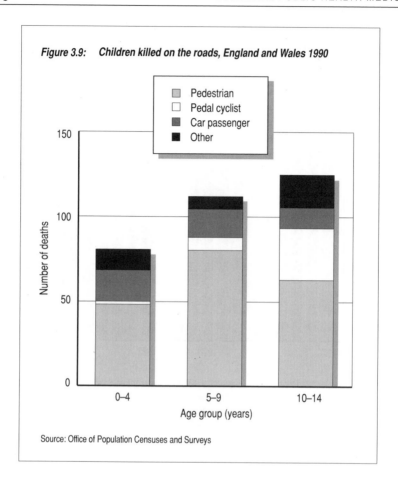

Figure 3.9:   Children killed on the roads, England and Wales 1990

Source: Office of Population Censuses and Surveys

Data on the true occurrence of home accidents which do not result in death cannot be routinely obtained. Many such accidents are self-treated or are treated by a general practitioner. However, a surveillance system which examines a sample of accidents in the home which are then treated in hospital, shows that the commonest mechanism was fall, accounting for half the accidents in children and nearly three quarters of those in elderly women.

Accidental deaths occurring in occupational settings have declined substantially since the 1960s.

Prevention and control

As a public health problem, accidents have been the subject of detailed study internationally, particularly in North America, where a great deal of work has been undertaken to develop ways of classifying them in a form which helps consideration of how they can be prevented. Fundamental to this is the view that the agent which produces an accident is energy in one of its five forms, that is, mechanical, chemical, thermal, electrical or various forms of radiation (for example, ultraviolet rays, x-rays). It is the sudden and harmful transfer of these

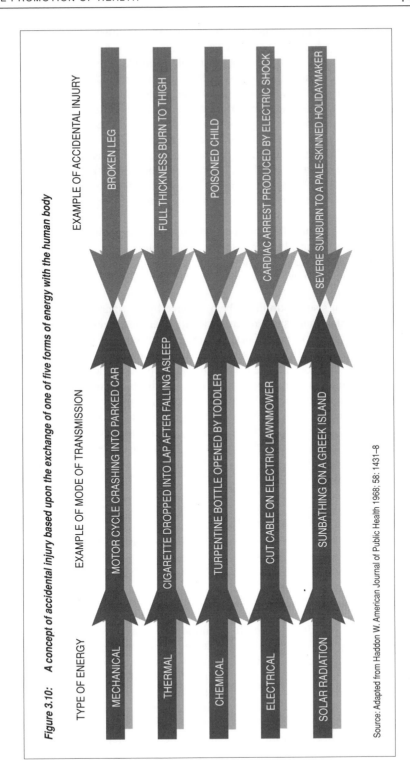

Figure 3.10: **A concept of accidental injury based upon the exchange of one of five forms of energy with the human body**

TYPE OF ENERGY	EXAMPLE OF MODE OF TRANSMISSION	EXAMPLE OF ACCIDENTAL INJURY
MECHANICAL	MOTOR CYCLE CRASHING INTO PARKED CAR	BROKEN LEG
THERMAL	CIGARETTE DROPPED INTO LAP AFTER FALLING ASLEEP	FULL THICKNESS BURN TO THIGH
CHEMICAL	TURPENTINE BOTTLE OPENED BY TODDLER	POISONED CHILD
ELECTRICAL	CUT CABLE ON ELECTRIC LAWNMOWER	CARDIAC ARREST PRODUCED BY ELECTRIC SHOCK
SOLAR RADIATION	SUNBATHING ON A GREEK ISLAND	SEVERE SUNBURN TO A PALE-SKINNED HOLIDAYMAKER

Source: Adapted from Haddon W. American Journal of Public Health 1968: 58: 1431–8

types of energy to human beings which causes the injury (Figure 3.10). For instance, a teenager might get on a friend's motorcycle without any lessons or instruction and crash into a parked car breaking his leg (mechanical energy); a toddler might open and drink from a bottle of turpentine which his mother is using for decorating and be poisoned (chemical energy); an elderly woman might drop a smouldering cigarette into her lap after she has fallen asleep in her chair and sustain a deep burn on her thigh (thermal energy); a middle-aged man might cut through a cable on his lawn mower and receive an electric shock (electrical energy); the pale-skinned holidaymaker from Britain, with little previous exposure to the sun, might sunbathe on a Greek Island beach and be seriously sunburned (solar radiation). The size of the transfer of energy, its duration, its distribution and the body's ability to resist it are all factors which determine the type and severity of the resulting injury.

All these are examples of incidents which would be readily acknowledged by most people as accidents. In each case, the energy source has caused the injury to the person concerned through a transmitting agent or vector. In the examples given here, the agent was the motorcycle, the turpentine, the smouldering cigarette, the electrical cable and the sun's rays.

The individual's susceptibility to being injured by the transmission of the energy is always an important aspect of an accident. Everyone, every day, is in contact with or is using many forms of energy. If the energy source is under control then it is not usually harmful. However, when it exceeds the ability of its user to control it, then an accident can occur. The balance between an energy source and the human being controlling it is therefore a crucial one. The balance can be tipped in favour of the energy source when it suddenly becomes stronger or more difficult to control. For example, a car skidding on an icy road surface risks causing the driver or the passengers injury as mechanical energy source becomes more powerful and gets out of control. The balance can also be altered if the person controlling the energy source lacks sufficient skill, the necessary physical attributes or relevant experience to exert full control over it. An elderly woman with arthritic hands who picks up a frying pan full of hot oil risks a scald injury due to her reduced capacity to exert full control over a source of thermal energy. A young, physically able person would not find such difficulty.

This description of accidents as interchanges of energy between their source and a man, woman or child is not just an interesting theoretical idea. It has proved to be an excellent basis for planning comprehensive action to minimise the unfortunate consequences of such impacts.

Many of the approaches used in the past to prevent accidents, and which are often still used today, are based upon the concept of accidents arising from acts of carelessness or stupidity. Successful solutions are therefore seen as those which ensure that people take a much greater degree of personal responsibility for their actions and adopt behaviour which appears less likely to result in accidental injury. Education, particularly of young children, regarding individual behaviour and road safety still remains an important component of accident prevention strategies. Yet, additionally, today's thinking places greater emphasis on safer product and environmental construction, drawing upon methods of research, innovation and design from within fields such as science, engineering and psychology.

This stems from a recognition that if a major proportion of crashes cannot be prevented, then structural modifications to reduce and distribute impact forces might at least minimise injuries and enhance the chances of survival.

This approach has been developed to identify three critical stages to an accident: pre-event, event and post-event. The factors which determine whether an accident will occur and what its impact will be are influenced by the interplay between a diversity of elements at each of these stages. This concept has been developed into a matrix which can help in understanding the causes of injuries arising from accidents and, even more importantly, can assist in designing prevention and control measures.

These ideas can be illustrated by considering such a matrix when it is applied to a car crash (Figure 3.11). The pre-event stage (in this example 'pre-crash') involves all the influences which determine whether the accident will occur in the first place, including the human factors (for example, how good the driver's eyesight is, how experienced and skilled a driver he is, and whether he has been drinking alcohol). Other important pre-crash factors will include the functioning state of the vehicle as well as aspects of the physical and socio-cultural environment (for example, tyre pressure and tread, effectiveness of brakes, provision of zebra crossings and adequacy

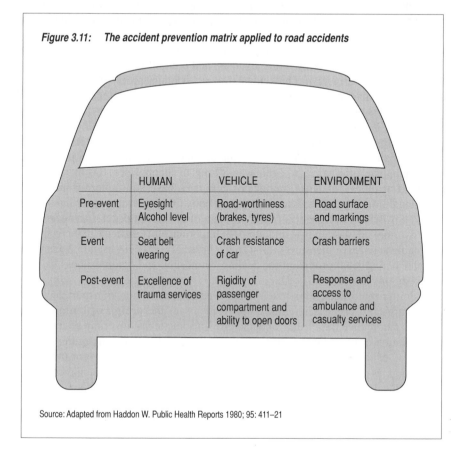

Figure 3.11:   The accident prevention matrix applied to road accidents

	HUMAN	VEHICLE	ENVIRONMENT
Pre-event	Eyesight Alcohol level	Road-worthiness (brakes, tyres)	Road surface and markings
Event	Seat belt wearing	Crash resistance of car	Crash barriers
Post-event	Excellence of trauma services	Rigidity of passenger compartment and ability to open doors	Response and access to ambulance and casualty services

Source: Adapted from Haddon W. Public Health Reports 1980; 95: 411–21

of road surface). Once the accident has taken place, its seriousness and the severity of injuries sustained by those people involved through the transfer of mechanical injury to their bodies will also be determined by the same groups of influences: human (for example, whether a seat belt was worn), vehicular (for example, how crash resistant the car body shell was), physical environment (for example, whether crash barriers were present alongside the road), socio-cultural environment (for example, attitudes to seat belt wearing). Post-crash, a range of factors will determine whether those injured survive the crash and, if they do, how well they recover or are free of long-term disability. It is here that vital issues such as rapid response by the trauma services come into play.

It will be clear from this illustration that a comprehensive strategy to reduce the toll of injury, disability and premature death arising from car crashes should not just involve measures directed at drivers themselves. It should also include targets for improved vehicle construction and design so that, as far as possible, drivers and passengers are 'packaged' to withstand the mechanical energy released if the car should crash. Similarly, roads which permit clear visibility, which have well-constructed surfaces, good signposts, clear lane markings and adequate crash barriers are also factors which, if targeted in an accident prevention programme, would contribute to the saving of lives and serious injuries.

Health education of children and parents in restricting the areas of mobility of young children, teaching them road safety procedures and imparting knowledge about the dangers are also important components of strategies to reduce accidents to children in traffic. Legislative measures in Britain have included the mandatory wearing of crash helmets by motor cyclists, and compulsory wearing of front and rear seat-belts by drivers and passengers in cars. A major problem in road accident prevention is alcohol. The Road Safety Act 1967 made it an offence to drive with more than the prescribed limit of alcohol in the blood. During the 1980s, the number of deaths on the roads associated with drinking and driving fell substantially. The introduction of the roadside breathalyser test and its use by the police initially received widespread media attention and has done so periodically since then. The original legal limit was 80 mg of alcohol per 100 ml and it has remained at this level but a number of countries have subsequently introduced lower legal limits than this. There is a strong body of opinion that more lives would be saved if Britain followed suit. The problem of alcohol in pedestrian accidents is often overlooked, though it is undoubtedly important. It is difficult to envisage any acceptable legislative measure similar to the breathalyser being used in pedestrians, though existing legal provision for dealing with drunk and disorderliness has little impact on this problem.

A similar multifaceted approach is required to prevent non-transport accidents. For example, in home accidents, improvements in the design of buildings and products can reduce the chance of accidents. In some areas, this may be backed up by legislation or by voluntary codes of practice agreed with manufacturers. Public awareness of these hazards has helped to encourage action to prevent the sale of such things as dangerous toys and to introduce the childproof medicine container. Health education also has an important part to play in preventing home accidents by making people aware of the dangers.

Strategies to reduce deaths and injuries in the workplace rely on a strong legislative framework. Appropriate training is an important element in workplace safety. Unlike health education aimed at the general public to prevent accidents in the home or on the roads, education of the person at work can be a mandatory component of training programmes in which knowledge and skills are formally assessed. As such, it has the potential to be more effective than population health education programmes. Factory design operating procedures and adequate maintenance of machinery are also important measures in preventing accidents in the workplace. Special measures are required for occupations or processes where there are particular hazards. The most successful programmes are undoubtedly those where an organisation's management demonstrates a strong commitment to occupational health and safety.

Sometimes a major accident and its subsequent investigation can lead to accident prevention measures being introduced. This has occurred following airline and other transport disasters and also following other forms of accidents where there was major loss of life.

The transfer of energy idea has been used to provide a comprehensive accident prevention framework. In it (Table 3.9), there are ten types of strategy for intervening to control the release or impact of energy. This approach is extremely

Table 3.9:   Accidents as energy forces: countermeasures to prevent injury

	Counter measure	Accident type	Example
1	Prevent the creation of a form of energy in the first place	Poisoning caused by chemical agent	Stop production of the agent
2	Reduce the amount of energy marshalled	Hot water scald	Limit temperatures in hot water systems
3	Prevent the release of the energy	Mauling by wild animals	Caging tigers
4	Modify the rate of release of energy from its source	Fire started by electric kettle boiling dry	Shut-off valve on the kettle
5	Separate in space and time the energy source from the individual who might be harmed	Burn from hot fat in frying pan	Keep toddlers out of kitchen when cooking
6	Interpose a barrier between the energy source and the susceptible individual	Child poisoned by tablets	Child-proof medicine container
7	Modify the basic structure of the hazard	Strangulation of baby in cot sides	Narrow space between bars in cots
8	Strengthen the resistance of the susceptible individual	Head injury in child cyclist	Widespread use of cycle helmet
9	Counter the damage done by the energy source	Lacerating wound due to broken glass	Apply first aid to stop further loss of blood
10	Stabilise and rehabilitate the person damaged by the energy	Multiple injuries in car crash	Rapid transfer to major accident and emergency department and provision of care

Source: Adapted from Haddon W. American Journal of Public Health 1970; 60:2229–34.

valuable, not necessarily in applying all measures to every accident prevention programme but in allowing all options to be carefully thought through prior to designing the particular programme.

The misuse of substances

One of the most important influences on health is behaviour associated with the use and misuse of substances such as alcohol, drugs and tobacco.

Whilst the use of these substances occurs at all stages of life, their adoption in childhood and adolescence poses a particular problem to the health of young people. Moreover, such patterns of behaviour established early in life can carry forward into adult life with long-term consequences in terms of dependency, illness and premature death.

Alcohol

There are three main spheres of behaviour associated with alcohol use: intoxication, excessive use and dependence (Figure 3.12). A spectrum of health and social consequences is associated with each.

Drinking patterns vary greatly internationally (Table 3.10). In Britain, drinking

Table 3.10:   The 25 countries with the highest alcohol consumption (Litres of alcohol per capita)

Country	Litres per capita
France	13.4
Luxembourg	12.5
Spain	12.0
Germany – DR	11.1
Switzerland	10.9
Hungary	10.7
Germany – FR	10.4
Portugal	10.4
Austria	10.3
Belgium	9.9
Denmark	9.6
Italy	9.5
Bulgaria	9.3
Czechoslovakia	8.7
Australia	8.5
Netherlands	8.3
Romania	7.9
New Zealand	7.8
Canada	7.7
Finland	7.6
United Kingdom	7.6
USA	7.5
Argentina	7.1
Cyprus	7.0
Poland	7.0

Source: Tables for World alcohol consumption in 1989 (except Canada). Extracted from World Drinks Trends 1991 Edition.

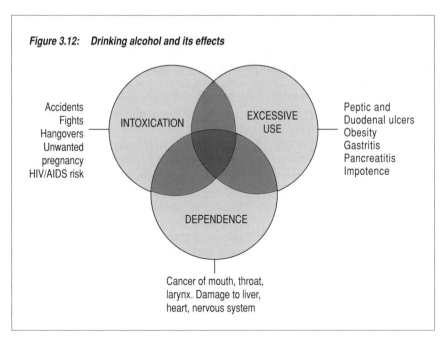

Figure 3.12:   **Drinking alcohol and its effects**

Accidents
Fights
Hangovers
Unwanted
pregnancy
HIV/AIDS risk

INTOXICATION

EXCESSIVE
USE

Peptic and
Duodenal ulcers
Obesity
Gastritis
Pancreatitis
Impotence

DEPENDENCE

Cancer of mouth, throat,
larynx. Damage to liver,
heart, nervous system

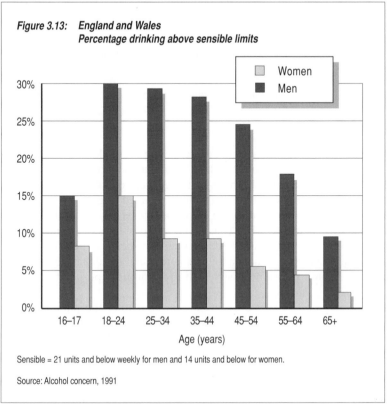

Figure 3.13:   **England and Wales**
             Percentage drinking above sensible limits

Women
Men

Age (years)

Sensible = 21 units and below weekly for men and 14 units and below for women.

Source: Alcohol concern, 1991

levels also vary between regions with the most damaging patterns of alcohol use being seen in the Northern parts of England and Scotland.

Amongst men in Britain, the highest proportion drinking above the sensible drinking level of 21 units per week were in younger adult age groups. The proportion of women drinking over the corresponding limit for their sex (14 units per week) was lower than for males, but was similarly the highest for young adults (Figure 3.13).

For some people, alcohol use occurs early. Although true dependence on alcohol is rare amongst young people, problems with intoxication are not. Intoxication raises short-term risks such as: accidents, anti-social behaviour, casual sexual relationships, vandalism, joy riding, theft and damage to property.

Surveys of young people who have tried alcohol or who drink it often have shown that whilst they know about the risks of dependence on alcohol, they are not aware of the risks associated with intoxication and excessive consumption in the short-term.

Table 3.11 shows findings from a survey of young people's drinking habits and presents a disturbing picture of the central part which alcohol plays in some young people's lives and the reasons why it is important to them.

Table 3.11: Some findings from surveys of drinking amongst young people in the Northern part of England

70% of children under age for legal drinking were developing a regular pattern of consumption

26% of 16 to 20 year olds were heavy drinkers

37% of young people drank alcohol because it made them feel good

29% of young people drank alcohol to get drunk

45% of young people who drank excessive amounts of alcohol said they did so because they had nothing else to do

The central thrust of strategies to reduce the impact of alcohol as a public health problem is in encouraging more people in the population to adopt sensible patterns of drinking. Such strategies are built on the concept of safe and sensible alcohol intake expressed in terms of units of alcohol consumed (Figure 3.14).

This poses an enormous challenge for those addressing the health needs of the population. Particularly so when considering the problems of communities where drinking patterns are set at levels determined by social and cultural norms and expectations. Issues such as unemployment and social disadvantage can also turn a reliance on alcohol into a necessity of life providing a purpose and continuity which is otherwise lacking.

Thus, strategies can rely only in part on educating the public on safe and sensible drinking levels. They must also provide practical help and support to people who need it. They must provide opportunities for local communities to develop programmes which will produce change in attitudes and behaviour. The fundamental aim is to shift the overall population pattern of alcohol use to safer and less damaging levels. There are many other important ways and contexts in which initiatives can be taken (for example, programmes centred on the workplace, in the

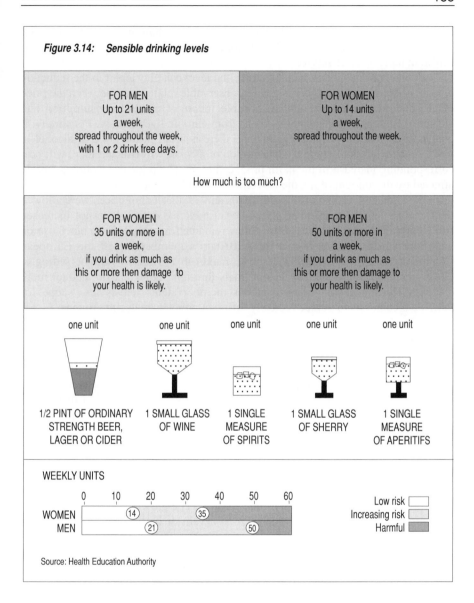

Figure 3.14: Sensible drinking levels

FOR MEN
Up to 21 units
a week,
spread throughout the week,
with 1 or 2 drink free days.

FOR WOMEN
Up to 14 units
a week,
spread throughout the week.

How much is too much?

FOR WOMEN
35 units or more in
a week,
if you drink as much as
this or more then damage to
your health is likely.

FOR MEN
50 units or more in
a week,
if you drink as much as
this or more then damage to
your health is likely.

one unit — 1/2 PINT OF ORDINARY STRENGTH BEER, LAGER OR CIDER

one unit — 1 SMALL GLASS OF WINE

one unit — 1 SINGLE MEASURE OF SPIRITS

one unit — 1 SMALL GLASS OF SHERRY

one unit — 1 SINGLE MEASURE OF APERITIFS

WEEKLY UNITS

0 10 20 30 40 50 60

WOMEN (14) (35)
MEN (21) (50)

Low risk
Increasing risk
Harmful

Source: Health Education Authority

prisons or associated with probation services, within ethnic minority communities and with homeless people).

There is also a narrower but very important role for health services and other organisations in the provision of help for people who have become dependent on alcohol or are suffering serious effects because of excessive use. These include the creation of day centres in which skills training, counselling and befriending services can be provided. They also include treatment services (inpatient, residential, out-patient, day care) which can provide detoxification programmes, family therapy and other specific treatment and support services. Few local services are based upon health service initiatives alone. The most successful are those in which the emphasis is on close collaboration between health, local authority and voluntary organisations skilled in these areas of service.

Action at national policy and governmental level can play a part in the reduction of alcohol consumption. There is a close, observable relationship between the price of alcohol relative to personal disposable incomes, alcohol consumption and alcohol-related harm indicated by deaths from chronic liver disease. Put simply, if people have more disposable income and there is a fall in the price of alcohol in real terms, then it is likely that consumption of alcohol will rise and there will be a corresponding increase in the harm produced by it. The price of alcohol is largely affected by the amount of tax the Government decides to put on it.

In the United Kingdom during the 1970s and 1980s alcohol prices were allowed to rise more slowly than other prices because excise duties were not increased sufficiently. The real value of beer duties remained roughly stable, but those on wine and spirits fell by over a third. Britain's membership of the European Community and the advent of the single market in 1992 has made the setting of Government policy to achieve health goals through higher tax on alcohol more difficult. Harmonisation of duty across member states leaves less scope for individual countries to pursue radically different policies on health grounds.

Drug misuse

The proper initial focus for consideration of the problem of the misuse of drugs in the population is on young people. For them, there are many paths leading to experimentation. Most accept their first offer of drugs from a friend or member of their peer group and not, as is popularly imagined, from the stereotypical drug pusher skulking by the schoolgates or in a darkened alley.

The inhalation of solvents remains a significant and relatively common aspect of substance misuse amongst young people in their adolescent years.

In adult life, cannabis smoking represents many people's only involvement with drug misuse. Cocaine, a well established drug taking behaviour in North American cities (particularly in its freebase form as 'crack') is a growing problem in Britain. The intravenous injection of drugs such as heroin or barbiturates is a sustained behaviour in a smaller hard core of the population, whilst the illicit use of hallucinogenic drugs is also a problem, particularly amongst young people.

There has been an increasing recognition of the problems of people who have become dependent on drugs (such as tranquillisers) which they are prescribed.

Routinely available information is very limited on the frequency of occurrence of various forms of drug-taking in the population. The nature of the activity, the fact that relatively few people are in contact with statutory services and the fear of detection or prosecution means that data are very difficult to obtain. Surveys properly designed and carried out to establish patterns of behaviour in local populations can be very valuable. They are likely to yield up-to-date information which has an immediate relevance to decisions on policy, service provision or preventive programmes.

In the past, the main national data system was based on drug addicts notified to the Home Office in accordance with the Misuse of Drugs (Notification of and supply to Addicts) Regulations 1973. The Regulations required doctors to notify cases of opiate or cocaine addiction and to re-notify cases which they were still attending after 12 months.

Regional Health Authorities are now responsible for setting up a regional database on drug misuse which includes data from specialist agencies and other services such as police, probation and social services. In time, it is intended that such databases will take over the Home Office notification process, increase compliance from data contributors and provide a more accurate picture of prevalence and trends.

The categories of drugs which most people associate with drug misuse or addiction comprise a wide range of substances, some of which have a bona fide therapeutic role and others which do not.

Cannabis ('marijuana', 'pot', 'grass', 'hashish') whose active ingredient is an extract of the flowers and leaves of a plant known as *Cannabis Sativa* is not a new discovery. Known for 2000 years, it was brought into Europe during the Napoleonic Wars becoming, at the time, fashionable with influential authors. Many young people today experiment with it whilst adults use it in a more controlled way socially for pleasure, much in the same way as alcohol is used. Cannabis is a mood-altering drug which tends not to cause dependence or aggressive anti-social behaviour. Most commonly, it gives rise to feelings of relaxation, talkativeness, hilarity and heightened appreciation of sensory experience. It has been suggested that use of this soft drug can lead to harder drug use but there is no firm evidence to support this. Nor is there evidence which proves that long-term cannabis use causes lasting physical or mental damage, although it is likely that frequent inhalation of cannabis smoke over a period of years will contribute to bronchitis, respiratory disorders and possibly lung cancer.

Hallucinogenic drugs were a major source of interest during the 'flower power' era of the 1960s when their ability to induce altered states of perception led to them becoming an integral part of the youth culture. Many will remember their principal exponent, Timothy Leary's celebrated phase: 'turn on, tune in, drop out'. The best known example is the synthetic drug LSD (lysergic acid diethylamide) although psilocybin and psilocin occur naturally in Liberty Cap, and are known as magic mushrooms. Hallucinogenic drugs cause an altered state of mind which may involve perceptual disorders, hallucinations and delusions. Through paranoia or panic, the individual can deliberately harm himself or others, although in practice this happens infrequently. There is no physical dependence as tolerance develops rapidly. Adverse psychological effects are possible, especially among regular users, and some prolonged serious psychological reactions have been reported. These usually occur in individuals with existing or latent mental illness.

Heroin is one of a group of opiate drugs which also includes codeine, morphine, pethidine and methadone. The drugs are mainly used therapeutically to produce pain relief. They have psychological effects such as reduced sensitivity to and emotional reaction to pain. Dependency withdrawal symptoms may be severe. Misuse of narcotics is a major health, social and legal problem worldwide. A major risk to people injecting drugs, particularly those using shared needles or equipment, is becoming infected with the Human Immune Deficiency Virus (HIV) which causes the Acquired Immune Deficiency Syndrome (AIDS). Similarly, intravenous drug misuse can lead to Hepatitis B infection.

Cocaine is another drug whose misuse is on a worldwide scale. It acts as a nervous system stimulant and increases alertness, delays sleep and diminishes fatigue. Tolerance and physical withdrawal symptoms do not occur although users may develop strong psychological dependence on the heightened feelings of physical and mental well-being induced by the drug. A common route of administration is by inhalation or sniffing which makes it convenient to take. Although sometimes associated with the lifestyle of the rich and famous, it is a strong feature of drug taking in poor inner city areas, particularly in North America, where in its freebase form (cocaine freed from the acid hydrochloride) it is called 'crack'.

Drug misuse fashions and designer drugs are a feature of the drug scene at street level amongst the young. It is a rapidly changing and quickly evolving world. The drugs which are sold and used vary from month to month and year to year in what they contain, what they are called, how they are packaged and in the way in which they are taken. The extent to which such drugs can insidiously become a dangerous component of an otherwise harmless craze was shown in the North East of England in the early 1990s through the creation and sale of tabs. These were small pieces of blotting paper impregnated with LSD bearing pictures of Teenage Mutant Hero Turtles and Viz comic characters. So-called designer drugs also come and go. Ecstasy (or 'E'), containing a mixture of stimulant and hallucinogen, was also a popular form of recreational drug use amongst young people in England in the early 1990s. Similarly, the types of drugs which are injected can rapidly change depending on availability, price and prevailing fashions.

Benzodiazepines (**tranquillisers**) may only be supplied through a doctor's prescription but prescribed or stolen benzodiazepines are available on the illicit market. They are commonly prescribed drugs in Britain and are primarily used in cases of anxiety, other kinds of psychological disturbance or for sleeping problems. They are manufactured in different potencies to be effective over different time spans: long, medium or short acting.

All benzodiazepines produce feelings of tranquillity at low to moderate doses because they depress mental activity and alertness. If continued for longer however, the therapeutic effect fades and the individual becomes tolerant to the drug. There is a risk of drug dependency if the drug dosage is increased by either the doctor or the patient without the doctor's knowledge.

Dependence is mainly psychological, as the drug is relied on to help the individual cope with situational pressures or psychological problems, although there are a range of physical symptoms associated with withdrawal. These include headache, dizziness and blurred vision through to incontinence, vomiting and severe stomach cramps. Although not life threatening, the symptoms can be extremely distressing and tend to be more noticeable with the short acting drugs. The withdrawal syndrome can closely resemble the original complaint, tempting both the doctor and patient to continue the treatment or even increase the dose.

As benzodiazepines do not tend to produce positive feelings of pleasure, euphoria or well-being, they are not especially popular as recreational drugs. They may be used however when the main drug of choice is not available or to enhance the effects of other depressant type drugs such as alcohol or opiates. They can also be used to offset the effects of amphetamine sulphate (speed) and there is increasing evidence of them being used illicitly in injectable form.

Solvents inhaled as vapours from glue, paint thinners, nail varnish remover, typewriter eraser fluid, cigarette lighter fuel and a wide variety of other substances, remain a serious problem amongst children and adolescents. Solvent sniffing can be a solitary or a group activity. The solvent is usually placed in a small plastic bag or often in an empty crisp packet which is then held over the nose and mouth. Although this has caused few deaths directly in the United Kingdom, more deaths have been associated with aerosol or butane gas inhalation or plastic bags placed over the head. Fortunately, these practices are much less common.

The effect produced by solvent misuse is one of dizziness, unreality and euphoria, although some experimenters feel nauseous or drowsy. Pseudo-hallucinations commonly occur and the effects can last from 15 minutes to three quarters of an hour after inhalation stops.

The behavioural signs in young people are similar to those produced by use of other drugs: aggression and irritation, lowering of inhibitions, secretive behaviour and poor performance at school. Physical signs such as anorexia, vomiting, skin rash, irritation of the eyes or nasal passages may occur in children who sniff frequently. Solvent abuse is a classic example of experimentation and risk taking behaviour amongst children and young people. Often responding to curiosity or the pressure of peers they form a habit. Very rarely does the behaviour carry on into adult life. Tragically, some children die each year because of solvent abuse, either through behaviour which leads them to have an accident or due to the toxic effect of the solvent itself (this is more likely to occur when inhalation occurs in a confined space).

Prevention and control

Illicit drug use and the harm it causes, can be prevented or reduced, and problems can be treated. Rehabilitation of drug users can be achieved and social dysfunctions may be improved or eliminated. Health services can develop multi-disciplinary prevention strategies aimed at both the primary prevention of drug misuse and harm reduction in cases where individuals are already using drugs. With the additional risks of HIV infection for injecting drug users, clean needles and syringes can be provided either as a service from specialist agencies or by arrangement with local pharmacists. Every opportunity should be taken to offer information on health, injecting techniques and safer sexual practices to service users.

Confidential counselling, advice and information services should be available and easily accessed by drug users, relatives and friends. Detoxification pro- grammes, maintenance schedules and other prescribing regimes to reduce the effects of dependency can be provided in the community with close co-operation from general practitioners. Heavily dependent individuals and those with polydrug problems need access to specialist services and may require inpatient admission and extended support through rehabilitation and aftercare.

In many parts of Britain a key role is played by voluntary organisations with expertise in the drug misuse field and it must be acknowledged that many people who have problems are more comfortable in using these informal, non-statutory services. Moreover, voluntary organisations and their staff may also have more credibility with young people in relation to relevant health promotion and disease prevention programmes.

It is very important that regional and local services develop in an integrated and coordinated way, making use of the expertise of health, local authority, other statutory services and these voluntary organisations.

Tobacco

Cigarette smoking is the commonest preventable cause of death in Britain. It is estimated that smoking is responsible for 110,000 premature deaths in Britain each year. Smoking is implicated in the causation of cancer of the lung, coronary heart disease, stroke, peripheral vascular disease, diseases of the lung (such as bronchitis and emphysema), cancer of the larynx, oesophagus, pharynx, oral cavity, pancreas and bladder. Women who are smokers have more low birthweight babies and more thrombo-embolic disease (particularly if they are taking the oral contraceptive pill).

There are potential risks to non-smokers through passive smoking (inhalation of the components of cigarette smoke in the environment). Apart from the smoking related diseases described above there is an increased risk of upper respiratory disease in children living in a household where the adults smoke.

The widespread adoption of tobacco use in England is usually attributed to Sir Walter Raleigh. When first introduced it was claimed to have beneficial and therapeutic properties. Although the adverse effects of smoking have mainly been elucidated in the second half of the twentieth century, as is so often the case in the history of public health, when looking back, islands of enlightenment can be recognised, which did not gain acceptance at the time.

James I mounted a sustained campaign against tobacco. In a treatise called *Counterblaste to Tobacco*, he observed:

'a custom loathsome to the eye, hateful to the nose, harmful to the brain, dangerous to the lungs.'

In the middle of the nineteenth century, James Copland, a Fellow of the Royal College of Physicians, observed:

'there is no vice that visits its sins on the third and fourth generations more completely than smoking; it is seldom that smokers have great-grandchildren or grandchildren.'

The smoking of tobacco in cigarettes increased rapidly from the turn of the century. Before then pipes, snuff, cigars and chewing were the main methods of use.

The total number of cigarettes sold each year in the United Kingdom (Figure 3.15) increased steadily during the present century reaching a peak at the end of the Second World War and then increasing again during the late 1950s through into the mid-1970s. From the late 1970s through the 1980s consumption began to decline. The economic implications of smoking remain major (Table 3.12).

Table 3.12:   The economics of smoking in Britain: some facts

---

- 50 million working days lost to industry because of smoking-related illness
- £500 million spent by the National Health Service each year in treating diseases caused by smoking
- £6,040 million earned by the Treasury in 1988/89 from tobacco duty and value added tax
- £600 a year spent by a 20 per day smoker
- £90 million a year spent on cigarettes by children aged 11 to 16 years

---

Source: Data extracted from fact sheets 1 and 6. Action on Smoking and Health. London, 1990 and 1991.

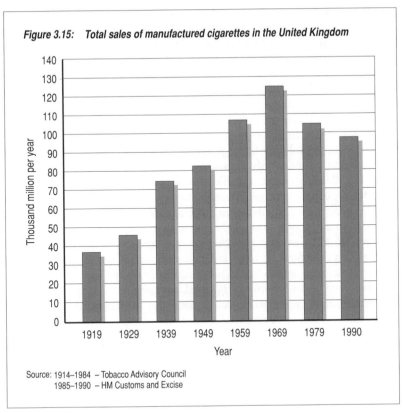

Figure 3.15:   Total sales of manufactured cigarettes in the United Kingdom

Source: 1914–1984 – Tobacco Advisory Council
        1985–1990 – HM Customs and Excise

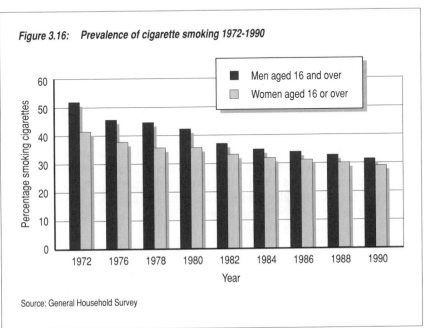

Figure 3.16:   Prevalence of cigarette smoking 1972-1990

Source: General Household Survey

Overall, approximately a third of adults smoke, a proportion which represents a substantial decline since the 1970s (Figure 3.16). Many more men used to smoke than women but the gap has narrowed considerably.

Most people start smoking when they are in their teens and then continue the habit into adult life. Substantial proportions of children have tried cigarettes or have actually started smoking on a regular basis.

To acknowledge that a huge pool of premature death, disease and disability could be eradicated if cigarette smoking became uncommon is not to underestimate the difficulties of effecting change in behaviour.

There is no single solution to the problem. Policies to reduce cigarette smoking in the population must not only recognise the addictive nature of tobacco but also the general availability of tobacco and tobacco products, the social acceptability of smoking, the pressures on people to start smoking and to continue doing so, and the commercial promotion and advertising of cigarettes. They must also find ways of providing help and support to smokers who wish to give up.

It is illegal to sell cigarettes and other tobacco products to children under the age of 16 years. Unfortunately, it is all too evident that this law is not well enforced. Children in Britain are able to buy cigarettes quite easily and there are relatively few prosecutions each year of shopkeepers for illegal sales.

The breadth of the approach which is necessary is illustrated by the measures and programmes listed in Table 3.13.

Table 3.13:   *Measures to reduce cigarette smoking in the population*

- Eliminate advertising and promotion
- Regular, innovative programmes to keep no-smoking issues constantly in the public eye
- Regular increases in duty on cigarettes
- Varied and carefully chosen warnings on cigarette packets
- No smoking in public places and workplaces
- Support and counselling services for smokers who wish to stop
- Health education for school children
- Enforcement of laws prohibiting the sale of cigarettes to young people

---

One of the most powerful channels for cigarette manufacturers to influence people and therefore to increase their sales and income as companies is through the medium of promotion and advertising. Other influences can be equally strong although not necessarily calculated to produce a specific effect. For example, the use of cigarettes by models or actors as props can glamorise smoking and reinforce its apparent desirability as a lifestyle.

Of particular concern is the extent to which cigarettes have been promoted through the sponsorship of sport and sporting events. Cigarette advertising on television is banned in Britain. The British Government also has a voluntary agreement with the tobacco industry which restricts televised coverage of tobacco sponsored events.

There is little doubt that the voluntary agreement in Britain has not been effective. Lack of Government action to legislate to outlaw tobacco sponsored sport will be increasingly difficult to defend in the face of the continuing large toll of deaths from cigarette related illnesses and the numbers of young people who continue to smoke.

Nutrition

Any consideration of the relationship between nutrition and health in an industrialised country like Britain must begin by setting the problem in an international context. In many developing countries of the World, large sections of the population are in a state of chronic malnutrition caused by the lack of adequate amounts of food. At times of war and natural disaster, as is all too evident from the widespread media coverage such events receive, situations rapidly turn to famine and large numbers of people die.

In many developing countries, protein-energy malnutrition, particularly amongst children, is present to some degree in the population all the time. In famine, or other circumstances of acute food shortage, the severe forms of protein-energy malnutrition, marismus and kwashiorkor, become common. Often there is also failure of sanitation, poor hygiene and the lowered resistance to infection (which accompanies malnutrition). This leads almost inexorably to outbreaks of communicable diseases, which then contribute to the high loss of life.

Whilst public health practitioners in the Western World grapple with a set of nutritional problems, mainly associated with dietary excess and imbalance, their counterparts in Third World countries, for example, are confronted with public health problems related to nutrition which are of an awesome magnitude.

This section is concerned with nutrition in industrialised countries, like Britain, where the dietary issues concern the balance of nutrients in the diet and whether they are present in sufficient quantities. In such countries, therefore, the issues in nutritional policy concern the measures necessary to avoid dietary deficiency diseases as well as those necessary to promote health and proper growth and development in childhood.

An expert committee advises the Department of Health on recommended daily intakes of various nutrients, including energy requirements, fat, sugars, starches, proteins, vitamins and minerals. An example is shown in Table 3.14 which sets out dietary reference values for fat intake in the population.

Table 3.14: Dietary reference values for fat as a percentage of total energy intake in the adult population

Type of fat	Recommended population average % daily energy intake
Saturated fatty acids	10
Cis-polyunsaturated fatty acids	6
Cis-monosaturated fatty acids	12
Trans fatty acids	2
Total fatty acids	30
Total fat	33

Source: Department of Health. Dietary reference values for food energy and nutrients for the United Kingdom. London: HMSO, 1991 (Reports on health and social subjects; 41).

Recommended daily intake levels of this kind are used to assess the population's nutritional status and also as a basis for targeting change to achieve particular health goals. For example, the population of Britain has shown relatively little change in recent years in the proportion of energy derived from fat. Moreover, intakes of saturated fatty acids are higher than recommended levels although the ratio of polyunsaturated to saturated fats is close to the recommended level.

The importance of diet in the causation of chronic disease has been considered earlier in this chapter as part of the discussion of risk markers for coronary heart disease and stroke. Diet may also be related to the causation of a number of other major chronic diseases, for example, some forms of cancer and hypertension. Studies of diet as a risk factor in chronic diseases are notoriously difficult to carry out and thus conclusions about causation must be drawn with great caution. In relation to cancer, there are a number of possible causal associations. Dietary fibre may reduce the risk of occurrence of cancer of the large bowel. Alcohol above safe levels is a well established risk factor for cancer of the mouth and larynx and has also been linked to the causation of breast cancer. Despite claims which have been made for the protective effect of Vitamin A in some cancers, the evidence is not clear cut. Evidence is not properly established relating to the often mooted risks of different types of dietary fat on the development of cancer at various sites. Although a controversial subject for many years, the association between high sodium intake and dietary hypertension, has led expert committees in a number of countries to recommend reductions in the amount of salt in the diet.

The Government and public health services of most industrialised countries have issued guidelines for healthy eating which are the basis of many health promotion programmes. An example is shown in Table 3.15.

Table 3.15: *Example of healthy eating guidelines to the public as part of a coronary heart disease prevention programme*

Dietary guidelines	Examples of food
Use polyunsaturated margarines and oils instead of butter, saturated fat margarines and oils, lard and suet	Sunflower margarine and oil
Avoid frying; grill or bake instead	Baked potatoes rather than chips
Reduce burgers, sausages and meat pies; choose more lean red meat, poultry and fish	Chicken and fish
Reduce cream and ice-cream. Change from whole milk to skimmed or semi-skimmed*	Skimmed and semi-skimmed milk
Restrict cakes, biscuits and chocolates; instead eat more fruit	Make cakes with polyunsaturated margarine
Go for brown rather than white; eat wholemeal and wholegrain foods	Wholemeal flour, bread and pasta. Brown rice

*Except no semi-skimmed milk below 2 years and no skimmed milk below 5 years.

Obesity is a major nutritional disorder in the industrialised world. It is an important cause of premature death and is associated with the development of a

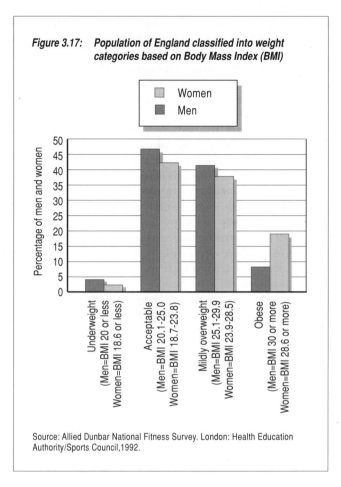

Figure 3.17: Population of England classified into weight categories based on Body Mass Index (BMI)

Source: Allied Dunbar National Fitness Survey. London: Health Education Authority/Sports Council, 1992.

number of chronic diseases, including coronary heart disease, diabetes mellitus and hypertension. Measures of obesity vary for purposes of assessing its prevalence in the population. One commonly used measure is the Body Mass Index (BMI) which is calculated by dividing the person's weight in kilograms by the square of their height expressed in metres.

This measure can be used to construct a definition of obesity and then assess the status of the population in relation to their weight (Figure 3.17).

A major element in strategies to achieve goals in nutrition and health, is to ensure that the public is well informed about the issues, the risks, and of ways of reducing them through dietary modification. There is an important role for parents in introducing their children to healthy eating alternatives and helping them to realise the importance of patterns of eating to their future health and well-being. The achievement of fundamental population change will, however, require much broader and concerted action. People's patterns of eating and their choice of food is governed by a wide range of factors, for example: family income, access to different types of food, the behaviour of other members of their social network and the powerful forces of product marketing and advertising.

For children in particular, whilst what their parents can afford and choose to give them to eat, is an important part of their early dietary experience, much of the promotion of food and food products which is directed at the younger age groups concerns potentially unhealthy eating alternatives. The mass media targeting of children, with its emphasis on sweets and chocolate, sugary soft drinks and snacks, forms a powerful current working against the interests of developing healthy eating patterns early in life.

To create a culture within Britain where healthy food choices are widely available and are adopted by a large proportion of the population poses a formidable challenge. Health services can play an important part by setting targets and gathering appropriate information about current dietary patterns. They can also take the lead in those areas where health care professionals are in a position to assess and advise people about their present food intake and provide information and assistance which will help them to make beneficial modifications. This is particularly important in the primary care setting where a relatively high proportion of the population is in regular contact with the health service. There are particular responsibilities for doctors and nurses assessing the growth and development of children to ensure that their daily nutritional requirements are being met, and to ensure that undernutrition is recognised early and corrected.

Health care professionals also have an important part to play in counselling the smaller number of people who come into contact with the hospital service as patients. It is important that the health service ensures that adequate skills and expertise in this field exist amongst their professional staff, notably that sufficient skilled dieticians are available.

Schools have a particular responsibility to introduce nutrition and health issues in the health education curriculum. They can also create catering policies which help children to develop positive attitudes towards eating for health and which will enable them to become used to healthier food.

Similarly, catering facilities in the workplace offer major opportunities to help adults to adopt and sustain nutritional behaviour conducive to health.

The food industry in all its diversity is another key element in population-based nutrition and health strategies. Industry is influenced by Government which can enjoin it at national level. It is also influenced by consumer demands and expectations. Increased labelling of food with nutritional information has been an important step forward in educating consumers about nutrition and health. A greater availability of healthier options (for example, containing less saturated fat) in processed food is still required. Similarly, such options are still in the minority amongst the choices offered by restaurants and fast food catering outlets.

The growth of vegetarianism in young people has also been important in opening up the issue of food and health to public debate (though the prime motivation behind the movement is concern for animal welfare and not health consciousness per se).

As with many other life-style related issues, the greatest challenges are with social groups within the population in which behaviour has proved intractable to change. The issue of poverty and the extent to which a limited household budget is spent on food, (particularly for its younger members) is a major concern when considering the public health problems of some parts of the population in Britain.

Infection with the human immune deficiency virus (HIV)

The World Health Organisation (WHO) has estimated that, if no effective vaccine or treatment is developed, then by the year 2000, six million people world-wide will have developed the Acquired Immune Deficiency Syndrome (AIDS). That is approximately ten times as many people as had the disease at the beginning of the 1990s. Very many more people are already infected with the Human Immune Deficiency Virus (HIV) than the number who have developed AIDS. It is estimated that the number of HIV positive people will also increase greatly, reaching 40 million world-wide by the year 2000.

The emergence of AIDS as a global threat has been spectacular. The disease was first recognised in 1981, although testing of serum taken at the time led to the realisation that it was spreading rapidly amongst some populations in the middle and late 1970s.

The nature of HIV infection

HIV belongs to the retrovirus group and, by infecting the T-lymphocyte population, gradually destroys the normal immune response mechanism. During 1981, in the United States of America, increasing numbers of cases of opportunistic infection (particularly *Pneumocystis carinii pneumonia*) and unusual tumours were reported in previously healthy homosexual or bisexual men. The presenting clinical features are often general: weight loss, fever, malaise, lymphadenopathy. The fully developed AIDS syndrome often involves opportunistic infections or patterns of malignancy infrequently seen in people with normal immune systems, although any one of a wide range of infections or malignancies can occur.

People can be HIV positive and remain asymptomatic. Whilst the precise proportion of such people who will eventually develop AIDS is not fully established, the longer follow-up studies have shown that around 50% of people will develop AIDS after ten years of infection. The first therapy to have had an impact on HIV infection and AIDS was the anti-viral drug zidovudine (AZT). It increases survival for patients with AIDS and delays the onset of symptoms and progression to AIDS in people who have HIV infection but are free of symptoms. The drug is a therapy of containment not of cure but until research yields a more effective alternative, it remains a mainstay in the treatment of infected people around the world.

Modes of transmission and risk groups

In Europe, North America and Australasia, the majority of new cases of HIV infection and AIDS up to now has been amongst homosexual men, people who inject drugs and (in the earlier phase of the epidemic) haemophiliacs who were given infected blood products. In African countries, the majority of cases of the disease has occurred amongst heterosexual people and, in these populations, considerable numbers of babies and children have become infected through transmission of the virus from their mothers who are infected.

At the beginning of the 1990s, three global epidemic patterns of HIV infection could be recognised based on a classification by the World Health Organisation

Table 3.16:   *Global epidemic patterns of human immune deficiency virus*
                (HIV) infection

Pattern	Features	Countries
I	Most virus transmission in homosexual, bisexual men and intravenous drug users	North America Western Europe Australia
	Overall population sero prevalence 1% but up to 50% in high risk groups	New Zealand Latin America
	Heterosexual transmission in the minority but increasing	
II	Male to female ratio 1:1	Sub-Saharan Africa
	Commonest transmission heterosexual	Caribbean
	Overall population seroprevalence 1% but 50% or more in prostitutes and sexually active city populations	
III	HIV infection only recently documented most cases arise from travel to or contact with cases from pattern I or II countries	Eastern Europe North Africa Middle East Asia Oceana
	Some cases from infected blood products	(excluding Australia or New Zealand)

Source: World Health Organisation.

Table 3.17:   *Modes of transmission of human immune deficiency virus (HIV)*
                infection

- Penetrative heterosexual or homosexual intercourse with an infected person
- Intravenous drug abuse (usually involving sharing of infected needles or equipment)
- Infected mother to child during pregnancy or labour or through breast feeding
- Inoculation of infected blood through a variety of potential means (including medical and dental procedures); risks to health care workers and cross-infection of patients
- Transfusion of unscreened blood or blood products

(Table 3.16), although it estimated that over 70% of HIV infections worldwide are contracted through heterosexual intercourse. The main modes of transmission of the infection are shown in Table 3.17.

The challenge of prevention

In Britain, whilst the number of cases of HIV infection arising from heterosexual transmission is still in the minority, it is rising and likely to become much more common. It is important to remember that changes in attitudes to sex and sexuality in Britain from the late 1960s onwards, led to a situation prior to the AIDS epidemic, where changes in individual behaviour increased the chances of acquiring the virus. For example, the growth of non-barrier methods of contraception came about because they were seen as a surer way of preventing pregnancy, of demonstrating sexual liberation and of enhancing sexual pleasure. Changing attitudes to relationship building, particularly amongst young people, meant that multiple sexual experiences before a stable relationship was established were increasingly seen in a positive light. The coming out movement amongst gay men was also characterised by freer sexual behaviour.

Such powerful societal trends and the individual behaviour which stems from them are difficult to modify or reverse. Yet, this is precisely what is required to halt the AIDS epidemic. For example, the transformation of the image of the condom from an unfashionable and less effective form of contraception (than the contraceptive pill) to one which is perceived as an essential and potentially life-saving component of a casual sexual encounter, is a major challenge for public health educators. Persuading people, particularly the young, to return to more stable long-lasting relationships and to cut down one night stands is equally challenging.

The importance of changing behaviour, especially in young people and in high risk groups is a major element of the global war against AIDS.

The British Government ran a major public education campaign between 1986 and 1987 (relatively early in the occurrence of the epidemic). The campaign made heavy use of the mass media: television, radio, cinema and posters. A leaflet was delivered to every household in Britain giving information about HIV infection and AIDS. A telephone information system, the National AIDS Helpline, was also established. Britain was widely praised internationally for its willingness to take an early, high profile involvement in combatting the threat of AIDS through public health education. The campaign was evaluated and found to have been extremely effective in increasing awareness about HIV infection, AIDS and the risks of transmission. Sexual behaviour amongst the population of gay men shifted with a reduction in the average number of sexual partners.

There is good evidence that young people understand the risks. There is less evidence of any major shift in behaviour on their part. Young people continue to take risks with casual or unprotected sex. A particularly telling example of the dangers for young people in these health risk-taking years is provided by an example of the results of a survey carried out in the North East of England. It shows (Table 3.18) the extent to which students would protect themselves by wearing a condom for casual sex according to their level of alcohol intake. Those who drank more were more likely to get involved in casual sex without wearing a condom. This example illustrates the way in which two behaviours in young people can produce a level of risk which could result in personal disaster, and even ultimately, death.

Table 3.18:   **Extent to which students risked casual sex without a condom according to alcohol intake**

Alcohol intake	Percentage of students risking casual sex without a condom	
	Male	Female
Non-drinker	4	4
Light drinker	9	6
Medium drinker	19	12
Heavy drinker	33	23

Source: Based on the result of a survey of 1874 students in three establishments (University, Polytechnic and Technical College) in the Tyne/Tees National Union of Students area, England.

National public education campaigns on television, radio and posters have continued into the 1990s under the auspices of the Health Education Authority, particularly to encourage condom use.

When addressing the problem of changing behaviour in young people, it is vital that national campaigns are accompanied by strong regional and local campaigns and activities. As is discussed earlier in this chapter, it is also important that initiatives taken with young people are attractive to them and are designed to be consistent with the way in which they think and view the world.

One of the problems for public education programmes for HIV infection in a country like Britain is that a number of target groups are being addressed simultaneously. Thus, the health education initiative must continue to target the sexual behaviour of gay men without leading the rest of the population to believe that HIV infection is a disease of homosexuals. Similarly, whilst heterosexual transmission is still in the minority, it is more difficult to persuade people that the threat to them is indeed real. Campaigns and programmes must also be tailored to target the behaviour, for example, of intravenous drug abusers, prostitutes, travellers to high risk areas of the world, tattooists and acupuncturists.

Public education, whilst a vital element of programmes to prevent and control HIV infection in the population, is only one part of a comprehensive range of measures which have been adopted.

Counselling, treatment and care

Other measures include ensuring that patients with symptoms or the full blown disease have access to the best specialist services and that people in risk groups or the worried well have access to locally based confidential counselling and blood testing services. The counselling service has two distinct functions. Pre-test counselling explores why the individual is asking for an HIV test, the nature and extent of their previous and present risk behaviour and the options prior to making the decision to take the test. Counselling also helps prepare the individual for coping with either a positive or a negative test result and to take the necessary steps to change risk-taking behaviour. Post-test counselling places the emphasis on helping the individual to cope with their HIV infection.

Other key elements of the overall programme include: training of staff in the care of infected people as well as in the risks of transmission during the process of patient care, clean needle exchange schemes for drug abusers, ensuring safe blood and blood products, and developing community or home-based care schemes for people with the disease (these are particularly important in high prevalence areas).

It is important that services for HIV infection and AIDS are flexible and diverse. For example, counselling services based exclusively in sexually transmitted disease clinics will not be taken up by all people who need them, some of whom will find them off-putting. A choice of contexts must therefore be provided. Increasingly health authorities and local authorities are working closely with voluntary organisations to provide non-statutory alternatives for some components of care.

Information and legislation

Information on the prevalence of HIV infection and AIDS in Britain is reported on a voluntary and confidential basis by clinicians to the national Communicable Disease Surveillance Centre in England and its counterpart in Scotland. Other information on the prevalence of HIV infection includes data from sexually transmitted disease clinics and the results of anonymous testing of the blood of patients attending hospital for other reasons (for example, antenatal clinics). Anonymised HIV surveys are also carried out on injecting drug users using voluntary saliva specimens.

The *AIDS (Control) Act* 1987 placed additional responsibilities on health authorities to report annually to the Department of Health on various aspects of the prevention, control and treatment of AIDS and to provide local statistics.

The Act was introduced to provide the Secretary of State for Health with a picture of activity underway and planned in each part of the country. The publication of a report also gives health professionals and the public in each locality an opportunity to assess the progression of the epidemic, the services which are provided and action being taken to combat the infection.

Inequalities in health

A consistent finding of public health analyses of population health needs is the poorer health status experienced by communities which are socially or economically disadvantaged. This is evident when comparisons are made between key health indicators, such as infant mortality in affluent industrialised countries compared to those in the Third World. Whilst general levels of health are much better in countries like Britain than in developing countries, differential health status within the population is marked. This phenomenon is discussed at various points in this book. The gradient in mortality between people living in the North of Britain and those in the South, the differences between social class in mortality as well as some health related behaviours, greater risk of poor outcome of pregnancy for mothers in the lower social classes and the position of triple jeopardy experienced by elderly people in one of the major ethnic minority populations are all such examples.

The observation that people in Britain who are in the lower social class groups within the population experience poorer health in relation to almost all indices of

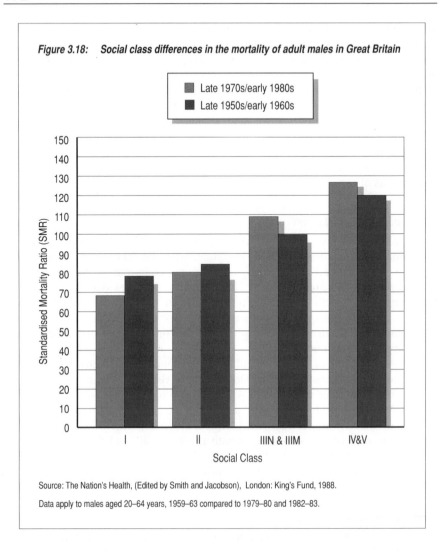

Figure 3.18:   Social class differences in the mortality of adult males in Great Britain

■ Late 1970s/early 1980s
■ Late 1950s/early 1960s

Social Class

Source: The Nation's Health, (Edited by Smith and Jacobson), London: King's Fund, 1988.

Data apply to males aged 20–64 years, 1959–63 compared to 1979–80 and 1982–83.

mortality, morbidity and disability is not a new one. The differences are very long-standing and, whilst the health of the population of Britain as a whole has improved during the present century, social class differentials have remained (Figure 3.18).

The issue was debated extensively during the 1980s. The intensity of the debate can be attributed in large measure to a report at the beginning of the decade regarded by some as highly controversial. The report of a Department of Health and Social Security *Research Working Group on Inequalities in Health*[9] better known (by the name of its Chairman Sir Douglas Black) as the *Black Report* reviewed largely routinely available information and highlighted persistent and worsening social class gradients in mortality and other indicators of ill-health. The report concluded that the cause of these inequalities in health were material deprivation and poverty and recommended solutions many of which concerned social and economic policy.

A parallel strand of work has examined the subject of inequalities in health, not in terms of national social class statistics, but at the level of local communities. An early example in Britain was the work showing the poorer health experienced by people living in inner urban areas of Teesside, England compared with their counterparts in the suburbs.

Within the Northern Region of England, differences in local communities were described in a study carried out in 1986[10] in which the population was segmented into small geographical areas encompassed by electoral ward boundaries (678 in the region as a whole). These population units were then assessed in terms of a composite measure of health which included adult mortality (standardised mortality ratios in people under 65 years), disability (permanently sick or disabled people over 16 years), babies born underweight (below 2800 grams) and four indicators of material deprivation (unemployment, car ownership, home ownership and overcrowding).

This study clearly demonstrated a strong link between material deprivation and poorer health experience. With very few exceptions, those electoral wards shown to suffer from greater material deprivation also experienced poorer health, and vice versa. The explanation for this clear association has been debated widely but remains uncertain. However, it could include housing and other environmental influences, unemployment, levels of income, lifestyle, access to services and cultural factors.

Another striking finding of this study was the extent of health inequalities observed within the region. The 678 wards were ranked by their overall health index and divided into five bands of 136 wards. If the health experience of the 136 wards with the best health record had applied to the population of 788,000 who lived in the 136 wards with the poorest health, then there would have been a saving of lives in adult life, lower levels of sickness and disability and fewer births of high-risk/low birthweight babies (Table 3.19).

Table 3.19: **Disadvantaged communities in the Northern Region: some things which would happen if those with the worst health had the experience of those with the best health**

- 1,356 fewer deaths of people under 65 each year
- 13,823 fewer people permanently sick and disabled
- 890 fewer low birthweight babies born each year

Source: Inequalities in Health in the Northern Region, 1986 by Peter Townsend, Peter Phillimore and Alastair Beattie. Published by the NRHA and the University of Bristol.

Such statistical comparisons are striking because they highlight the extent of health disadvantage experienced by some communities. The underlying causes of these differences are complex, difficult to establish clearly and undoubtedly multifactorial in nature. There is no doubt that changing these differences will only be possible over the medium to long term.

Some would argue that these are issues which can only be solved by economic, social and employment policies at national governmental level. However, the clustering of health and social disadvantage can be quite localised. Initiatives and programmes using health themes, can be targeted specifically at populations which are disadvantaged in health terms. It is vitally important, however, that such initiatives do not have a condescending orientation. The emphasis must be upon gaining a detailed understanding of the needs of the community concerned before designing programmes which are carefully attuned to its unique social, cultural and environmental characteristics. Initiatives must be participative, building upon the ideas of local people and community leaders. There must also be close collaboration between all sectors: health, local authority and voluntary, as well as industry and commerce.

The approach of community development as part of health promotion strategies has become increasingly important and is achieved with an emphasis on community

---

Figure 3.19:   *Degrees of community participation in development programmes*

Degree	Participants	Illustrative mode
High	Has control	Organisation asks commmunity to identify the problem and make key decisions on goals and means. Willing to help community at each step to accomplish goals.
	Has delegated	Organisation identifies and presents a problem to the community, defines the limits and asks community to make a series of decisions which can be embodied in a plan which it will accept.
	Plans jointly	Organisation presents tentative plan subject to change and open to change from those affected. Expect to change plan at least slightly and perhaps more questions. Prepared to modify plan only if absolutely necessary.
	Is consulted	Organisation tries to promote a plan. Seeks to develop support to facilitate acceptance or give sufficient sanction to plan so that administrative compliance can be expected.
	Receives information	Organisation makes a plan and announces it. Community is convened for informational purposes. Compliance is expected.
Low	None	Community told nothing.

Source: Brager, Specht. Community organising.
Columbia University Press, 1973

participation. Such participation is a process through which people in the community concerned can have a say or play a part in determining policies and programmes aimed at improving the population's health. Community participation is an active process which allows the people living in it to have ownership (Figure 3.19).

CONCLUSION

This chapter has described the background and the approaches used, in one of the main aspects of public health practice, the promotion of health.

Many of the health problems in a population are capable of major reduction, if not elimination, through these measures. Similarly, the promotion of health as a positive state to be attained by as many people in a population as possible is another important goal for this aspect of public health practice.

The potential for change is enormous if ways can be found to modify risk factors on a population scale and to help people adopt and sustain lifestyles which are supportive to health rather than harmful and injurious.

Much of the key to success lies in shaping the behaviour and values of children and young people. It lies in enabling them to lay the foundations for a life which will achieve the maximum of the biological span and in which most of those years will be characterised by health rather than illness, chronic disease or disability.

If these challenges can be met, as the world moves towards the next millennium, then the scale of public health achievement will be as great as the historical discoveries whose descriptions began this chapter and which transformed the health landscape of the past.

4 The National Health Service and social services

INTRODUCTION

A major landmark in the historical development of the National Health Service was the publication in January 1989 of the White Paper 'Working for Patients'. This was the result of a review of the National Health Service which was personally led by the then Prime Minister, the Right Honourable Mrs Margaret Thatcher MP, and which involved a team of Ministers, senior civil servants and advisers. The decision to undertake a fundamental review of the National Health Service after ten years in government was taken by the Prime Minister herself and appears to have been prompted by a major funding crisis which overtook the health service in the winter of 1988. Thus, the early 1990s began a period of major change in the way in which health services were to be organised, funded and delivered in Britain.

Changes were enacted in legislation which was passed by Parliament in 1990 as the National Health Service and Community Care Act. Despite this, the National Health Service moves towards the turn of the present century with a number of principles undisturbed. It remains financed largely from general tax revenue. It is virtually free of charge to the patient at the point of delivery of service. There are no qualifying conditions such as financial contribution.

This chapter describes the historical development of the National Health Service, its present structure, and the way in which it functions. The health and social services operate within a legal framework and a short description is given of the process by which law is formulated and implemented.

HISTORICAL PERSPECTIVE

The Poor Law

The development of services for the sick, aged and infirm in Britain is inextricably linked to the attitudes of society towards the poor at various points in history for it is often the case that sickness and old age are states which co-exist with poverty.

Much of the responsibility for the poor, aged and sick in medieval Britain fell on the church and on parishes, which often levied local taxes to assist them in providing relief. With the dissolution of the monasteries and religious fraternities by Henry VIII, considerable hardship was created, leaving large numbers of elderly and sick people with no means of support. Many individual items of legislation passed during the reign of Elizabeth I were rationalised in 1601 with the passage of the Elizabethan Poor Law (most commonly referred to as the 'Old Poor Law'). Under this law the 'impotent poor' (for example, the old or sick) were to be cared for in poorhouses or almshouses, whilst the able-bodied paupers were provided with work in houses of correction. Much of the responsibility for the administration of the Old Poor Law rested with individual local parishes in the form of parish overseers. Whilst tyranny undoubtedly existed, there were also many examples of caring parishes. Dissatisfaction with the Old Poor Law mounted for several reasons.

Firstly, and at the simplest level, the law was proving an increasingly costly exercise. The system of 'outdoor relief' was becoming widespread in many parishes. It proved simpler to administer payments in cash or kind to the poor, but because of the economic problems of the time, the size of the pool of such needy individuals and their families had grown. Secondly, some critics considered that the regimes in houses of correction were too comfortable for their inmates. This climate of opinion led ultimately to the establishment of a Royal Commission of Inquiry into the Poor Law and the subsequent Poor Law Amendment Act 1834 (the 'New Poor Law'). Many commentators regard this resulting legislation as being strongly aligned to the Utilitarian philosophy of Jeremy Bentham (1748–1832), and his follower Edwin Chadwick (1800–1890), the latter being intimately involved in the framing and implementation of the legislation.

It was believed that the old system of poor relief and the condition of the houses of correction might actually encourage idleness and pauperism. The New Poor Law was intended to abolish pauperism by measures based on deterrence. The system of outdoor relief for the poor was abolished. Those in need of support had to apply for it and were offered the workhouse. The workhouse regime was harsh and austere, deliberately designed to pose a very unattractive prospect for those applying for poor relief. By this central tenet of 'less eligibility' (the person receiving poor relief could not be better off than the worst-paid independent worker) it was reasoned that only those who were truly needy would accept poor relief in the form of the workhouse.

Under the New Poor Law, responsibility was taken out of the hands of individual parishes, which were grouped together as Poor Law Unions (administered by Boards of Guardians), and placed under the control of a central body headed by three Poor Law Commissioners, the aim being to introduce a uniform process of administration. Although separate provision was laid down for the sick and aged, in practice few Unions allowed themselves the expensive luxury of separate workhouses and in many mixed workhouses the able-bodied pauper rubbed shoulders with the sick, the old and infirm, children and the mentally handicapped.

Gradually, many workhouses set aside annexes or 'wards' for the care of the sick pauper. In a few, individual workhouse infirmaries were to be found and the rudiments of a domiciliary service for the sick poor were also present. Standards within such premises were, however, pitifully inadequate, with overcrowding and insanitary conditions prevailing. 'Nursing' was carried out by other inmates. Moreover, the crux of the problem was still that the law implied that poverty was a result of idleness or waywardness on the part of the individual. Florence Nightingale commented that these civilian hospitals were just as bad as, or worse than, the squalid military hospitals which she so strongly condemned in the Crimean War. Towards the end of the century, conditions had become so appalling that Parliament authorised the building of separate infirmaries with trained medical and nursing staff.

The local authority hospitals

In addition to the Poor Law medical service, the major local authorities (County and County Borough Councils) provided a separate publicly owned system of hospitals which had its origins in the isolation hospitals for infectious diseases and asylums for the mentally ill and handicapped. However, in many regions of the country in the early part of the present century, local authority hospitals were also treating other, more general illnesses. Following the transfer of the powers and responsibilities of the Poor Law to local government by a further Act of Parliament in 1929, the local authorities also took control of and administered the Poor Law infirmaries, thus creating some degree of unity. The local authority hospitals fell mainly under the jurisdiction of the Medical Officer of Health, who delegated his responsibility in each hospital to a Medical Superintendent.

Voluntary hospitals

A small number of hospitals had been provided from earliest times by ecclesiastical bodies. However, the main alternative to the publicly owned hospital system was the voluntary hospital movement, which sprang up in the middle of the eighteenth century and was run by independent organisations obtaining their finance from charitable funds and subscriptions. There was a great variation in the size and function of the voluntary hospitals, but in general they provided a standard of care which was far above that in the public sector and indeed served as a model which the latter strove to attain. Each voluntary hospital had its own committee of governors and medical care was provided by visiting physicians and surgeons who were almost always in private practice and provided their services to the voluntary hospitals free of charge.

Although the system was variable, patients who could afford to pay were often asked to do so whilst others provided themselves with some security for illness by making weekly payments to one of the hospital contributory schemes. As the involvement of the medical profession in the voluntary hospitals grew with the flourishing of teaching and research, so their function began to alter. Admission policies were selective, with an emphasis on patients with illnesses which were of a short-term or acute nature, thus ensuring a rapid turnover, or those with diseases which were of particular interest. There was little place for the elderly or chronically sick. It was this emphasis on acute medicine which was partly responsible for the extension in the last century of the State-owned hospital service to fill the gap.

The Emergency Medical Service

As part of the preparation for the anticipated receipt of military and civilian casualties during the Second World War, a hospital service was created in 1938 to be administered directly by the Ministry of Health. The number of beds in some hospitals was increased, temporary buildings were erected or premises extended, and some of the former poor law institutions were renovated or upgraded. Some centres were created with specialist facilities for example, rehabilitation, plastic surgery and neurosurgery, and the Ministry laid down what the functions of the existing hospitals should be on a regional basis.

The Emergency Medical Service is of considerable importance in the development of the health service. Although its influence was short, in the context of the long period of evolution of the service it represented a watershed for the hospital service. It resulted in the review and classification of all hospitals provided by the wide variety of agencies and brought their administration for the first time under a central authority in the shape of the Ministry of Health. This laid the foundation for the unified hospital service when the National Health Service came into being shortly after the war had ended.

Primary care

Medical services for those who did not receive care in hospital was slower to evolve. Under the Poor Law, domiciliary care or treatment by the Poor Law Medical Officer existed in some parts of the country, but the standard was very variable and care was generally very basic. Other forms of care were provided by a variety of other agencies, such as free dispensaries run on charitable lines or outpatient departments within voluntary hospitals. Other developments during the nineteenth century provided private panel systems or clubs where, by paying a retention fee, the patient could claim the services of a doctor in time of need. Friendly societies and a few industries operated similar schemes.

The National Health Insurance Act 1911 (the Lloyd George Act) was the most influential development in primary care. The scheme was directed at relieving hardship amongst working men during periods of illness. When it was introduced in 1912, it was confined to workers earning less than £160 per year and was based on contributions from the employee, the employer and the State. It entitled the insured man to choose his own general practitioner from a local panel of doctors (hence the term 'panel system') and to secure treatment (including prescribed drugs) and other consultations free of charge on demand. The exclusion of dependants' wives and children from the scheme, together with the denial of the right of insured people to receive free hospital inpatient care, meant that considerable hardship was left untouched. Moreover, a sizeable proportion of the population still paid a fee to their general practitioner for advice or treatment.

This system continued (although the eligibility was subsequently increased) until the National Health Service was established in 1948. Until then, general practitioner services were administered throughout the country by a network of insurance committees responsible for making available these services for all insured people in their locality, and representing almost half of the population.

Other local authority services

The new industrial towns, which were the products of the industrial revolution, forced the consideration of health problems on a population or community-wide basis. As a growing proportion of the population came to live in towns and work in factories so, in turn, their circumstances were characterised by scarce and over-crowded housing of a very poor standard, pollution, inadequate sanitation, a contaminated water supply and limited diet.

Such conditions were ripe for the infectious diseases to flourish, ravaging the population and taking a high toll in mortality, particularly amongst the young. The great milestones along the path to reform were the public health reports and legislation in the middle of the nineteenth century, which once again bore the mark of Edwin Chadwick, this time in the guise of public health reformer rather than implementer of the unpopular New Poor Law. The first Medical Officer of Health was appointed in Liverpool in 1847 and other local authorities soon followed suit.

These Victorian reforms led to increasing provision of pure water supply, effective sanitation, drainage and disposal of sewage and improved standards of housing. These were all factors which contributed to the reduction in mortality in the last quarter of the nineteenth century and the early twentieth century. When the National Health Service was established in 1948 public health responsibilities, including the control of the spread of infectious diseases and the environmental hazards, remained a function of local authorities.

Local authorities then turned their attention to personal health services for people in the community, a major feature of their work during the present century. The Poor Law had provided, towards the end of the last century, a form of community service (for example, for expectant mothers and children) but this was patchy and inadequate. During the first 20 years of this century, the health visitor system was developed and maternity and child-welfare clinics were opened. Thus by 1948, the local authorities not only had responsibility for a large part of the hospital service but for a whole range of community services. When the National Health Service was established they continued to be responsible for community services but lost responsibility for hospitals.

The personal social services, which were provided by the local authorities for groups like the elderly, children, the physically and mentally handicapped, also had diverse origins. In a few cases, services arose from voluntary or charitable organisations, in most others from the structure of the Poor Law with its strong orientation towards institutional care. Although local authorities subsequently assumed responsibility for certain services, it was not until the implementation of the National Assistance Act 1948 that they became responsible for providing comprehensive welfare services.

The welfare state and the National Health Service

In the summer of 1941 the Government appointed Sir William (later Lord) Beveridge (1879–1963) to chair a committee of senior civil servants charged with undertaking a survey of existing national schemes of social insurance and allied services and making recommendations. The Beveridge report, published a relatively short time later in December 1942, contained a series of sweeping proposals and recommend-ations which laid the foundation for the modern welfare state.

Beveridge based his proposals for a compulsory social security scheme on three assumptions These were that there would be a policy for the maintenance of employment, a system of children's allowances, and a comprehensive health service. The basis of the report was enacted by the post-war Labour Government and the subsequent legislation was contained in five main acts:

(1) The Family Allowances Act (1945) provided for cash allowances to the second and subsequent child.

(2) The National Insurance Act (1946) established a comprehensive contributory national insurance scheme.

(3) The National Insurance (Industrial Injuries) Act (1946) made provision for insurance against accidents, injuries and prescribed diseases due to a person's employment.

(4) The National Assistance Act (1948) finally dismantled the Poor Law, placing on local authorities the responsibility for the elderly, the handicapped and the homeless, and setting up a scheme for financial assistance on a national basis to those in need.

(5) The National Health Service Act (1946) created a comprehensive health service available to all citizens.

With the commencement of the National Health Service on 5 July 1948, the Minister for Health became statutorily responsible for providing a comprehensive health service for the population of England and Wales. All hospital property, whether it had been in the voluntary or municipal sector, came under the control of the Minister, including all but a small number of privately owned hospitals. Thus, the Minister inherited a wide array of buildings and accommodation with varying origins, traditions, functions and differing levels of upkeep and which were spread unevenly throughout the country. However, the administrative merging of these made it possible to plan a hospital service for a locality, and to rationalise the distribution of, and to make arrangements for, the training of medical, nursing and technical staff.

England was originally divided into 13 regions (four in London and the home counties and nine in the rest of the country) with regional hospital boards whose chairmen and members were appointed by the Minister. A further region, Wessex, was created later to make a total of 14. These regional boards appointed hospital management committees to be responsible for the day-to-day running of individual hospitals or groups of hospitals. Teaching hospitals had separate arrangements, being administered by Boards of Governors appointed by the Minister and responsible directly to him rather than the regional hospital boards.

The National Health Service also provided general medical, general dental, ophthalmic and pharmaceutical services on a contractual basis with local Executive Councils. Thus, with the advent of the National Health Service, primary medical care was also provided free and as a right for all who wished to request it.

Aside from therapeutic services which were based in hospitals or general practice, the National Health Service laid down a range of other services concerned with the health of the population which were delivered mainly by major local authorities (Counties and County Boroughs). This was the only part of the new service which had specific responsibility for the prevention of disease. However, little detail was specified giving considerable scope for innovation by individual local authorities. The authorities discharged their functions through Health Committees whose chief officer was the Medical Officer of Health. In addition to the general responsibility for developing a preventive function, local authorities were charged with providing a range of supportive services. These included a wide variety of 'community' services (such as health visitors, home nurses, domiciliary midwives and home helps) to provide care, support and advice to people in their own homes; a responsibility for the control of infectious diseases including immunisation and vaccination; the care of expectant mothers, infants and young children; the provision of an ambulance service and the provision of health centres.

The last of these, health centres were seen as a major role for the local authorities at the time but were very slow to get off the ground. As early as 1920 the Dawson Report had recommended that local authorities provide, equip and maintain health centres where groups of doctors and other health care staff could work together. By 1966 only 28 purpose built group practice premises, housing about 200 general practitioners, had been established.

The first experiments with local authority nursing staff attached to practices occurred in the late 1950s and early 1960s. General practice at this time was experiencing problems. The perception that general practitioners were failed hospital doctors was commonly held. The general practitioner's income was wholly dependent on the number of patients registered with them, and they received no assistance from the Government towards the provision of adequate premises or supporting staff. In consequence morale amongst general practitioners was low. Many United Kingdom graduates emigrated to North America.

In 1966, as a result of The Charter for the Family Doctor Service, a new contract for general practitioners introduced major change. A three part payment system of basic practice allowances, capitation fees and item-of-service payments was supplemented by group practice allowances and incentives for doctors to work in under-doctored areas. Partial reimbursement of the salary costs of practice clerical and nursing staff was instituted, and funds were made available for the building or upgrading of premises.

These steps encouraged a trend towards group practices, the employment of ancillary staff, the imaginative development of premises and an expansion in the range of services offered to patients. Attached district nurses and health visitors became commonplace and practices progressively sought to accommodate these staff in their premises. These positive developments were accompanied by the expansion of vocational training for general practitioners, which became mandatory in 1982, and the establishment of academic departments of general practice in the medical schools.

The unified health service

Between 1948 and 1973 the health service was organised in a so-called 'tripartite' fashion whose three components were:

- The hospital service (administered by Regional Hospital Boards and a network of hospital management committees at a local level) and teaching hospitals (administered by Boards of Governors);
- The family practitioner services (with contracts held by Executive Councils);
- The local authority health services (which operated within the sphere of local government administration to provide public health services in the form of infectious diseases and environmental hazard control, preventive services and community based services).

In 1974, a major administrative reorganisation of the National Health Service took place. Its aim was to provide a better, more sensitive and co-ordinated public service. Before 1974, it had never been the responsibility, nor had it been within the jurisdiction of any single named authority, to provide a comprehensive health service for the population of a given area. As a result it had not been easy to balance needs and priorities rationally and to plan and provide an integrated service within the resources available. From 1974, local authority health services were brought within the National Health Service along with hospital services. The service was organised geographically around 14 regional health authorities and below them area health authorities.

A further restructuring took place in 1982. The 1982 restructuring attempted to solve further problems by removing one administrative tier (area health authorities) and devolving from the centre the responsibility for providing the service within available resources. New district health authorities were created and were left to decide on the type of organisational structure most suited to local needs. Before the impact of this 1982 reorganisation could be fully realised, further major changes in the organisation of the service were stimulated by a National Health Service Management Inquiry in 1983. The most noticeable consequence of this, the 'Griffiths Report', was the introduction for the first time, of general managers at various levels within the health service.

The National Health Service and Community Care Act 1990 followed the White Paper 'Working for Patients', the end product of a review of the National Health Service. This review had been prompted by unwelcome publicity in the winter of 1988 which had focused on two perceived shortcomings:

(i) Incidents of hospitals closing beds, deferring or redirecting admissions or sending doctors on extended leave to limit workload in order to stay within budget, despite continued real increases in health service funding.

(ii) The existence of 'perverse incentives', whereby extra workload in the most efficient, effective and sought after hospitals was not matched by extra funding, and these hospitals were the first to have to limit their services.

These National Health Service reforms, arguably the most radical since 1948 despite the absence of any formal structural reorganisation, introduced a new approach to funding and regulating the delivery of hospital care. The proposals ended the conflicting roles of district health authorities (DHAs) in which operational involvement in health care provision (in local hospitals) within their geographical boundaries was coupled with serving the needs of the population. The proposals also ended the system of funding which offered no incentive to hospitals to treat more patients, improve quality, or to provide a wider range of services.

The main features of the 1990 reforms are summarised in this section of the chapter and considered in more detail in the one which follows. The principal thrust of the reforms was to separate responsibility for purchasing health care from its provision. District health authorities and general practice fundholders became service purchasers, funded according to the health needs of their population. Hospitals and other provider organisations were free to concentrate on improving the quality, effectiveness and efficiency of health care in order to win service contracts, the means of regulating service delivery between purchasers and providers.

National Health Service Trusts whether hospitals or other providers of services have their own Trust Boards directly accountable to the Secretary of State and significant freedom in the way they can employ staff and invest in capital infrastructure. Trusts are dependent upon contracts with purchasers for most of their income, keeping services provided in line with the requirements of the populations they serve.

Fundholding General Practices have their own budgets to cover some hospital and community services, prescribing and practice staff. At present the scheme is restricted to practices with more than 7,000 patients. The hospital element covers most outpatient referrals, investigations and a limited range of elective procedures. However, general practice fundholding has been demonstrably successful in stimulating improvements and innovation from hospitals, resulting in more effective services appropriate to the needs and demands of patients.

Changed Health Authority membership replaced large and cumbersome Authorities with streamlined 'boards' based on a more business-like model capable of a sharper and quicker focus on priorities. Additionally, for the first time, chief officers were also board members.

New funding arrangements clarified markedly the previously confused relationship between populations, service workload and resources. For the first time, central funding could be allocated on the basis of population size weighted for level of need, to purchasers. From there, funding now flows through service contracts to providers according to the amount of work that they are contracted to do (this is often referred to as 'money following the patient'). This arrangement not only paved the way to removing most of the previous considerable disparities between the resources available to different populations, it also potentially abolished the perverse incentive whereby the hardest working hospitals were the first to use up their fixed allocation and be obliged to cap workloads.

These changes are described in more detail in the next section. Aside from 'Working for Patients' the legislation which led to the 1990 health service reforms also incorporated the main principles of two other White Papers 'Caring for People' and 'Promoting Better Health'. The former set out proposals for the reorganisation of community care and the latter introduced changes to the general practitioners' contracts. The reorganisation of community care which was created by these changes is described later in the chapter.

After a period of 25 years of relative stability, the 1990 General Practitioner contract brought about a major shift in emphasis in the following areas:

- health promotion
- systematic chronic disease management
- consumer responsiveness
- preventive care targets
- population surveillance.

To meet the challenges posed by the new contract most practices employed more staff, particularly practice nurses and practice managers, and a large majority became computerised. Practice income on average increased. The 1990 contract demonstrated that, with the appropriate financial incentives, practices could respond and develop their services rapidly. Improved performance in achieving targets for immunisation and cervical smear screening based on practice populations occurred.

The next section of the chapter deals with the structure and function of the present health service in more detail. The present arrangements reflect changes brought about by the 1990 health service reforms.

THE PRESENT STRUCTURE AND FUNCTIONS OF THE NATIONAL HEALTH SERVICE

The introduction of health care markets (Figure 4.1) was one of the fundamental pillars of the White Paper 'Working for Patients'. The proposals and subsequent legislation contained a number of key ingredients: the creation of an environment of competition amongst providers of service with the aim of bringing down costs and raising quality; greater choice for, and more emphasis on, consumers of health services; greater accountability of professionals and funding mechanisms which rewarded services sought after by patients and referring general practitioners.

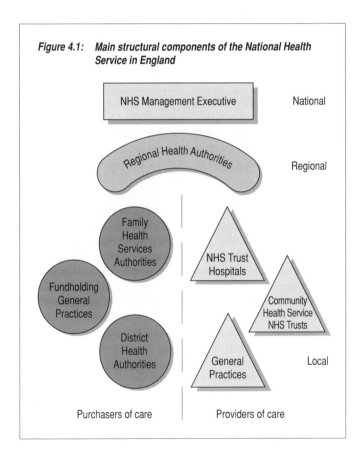

Figure 4.1: *Main structural components of the National Health Service in England*

The reforms introduced the prospect of a new degree of clarity in several key respects:

(i) The purpose and aims of each part of the National Health Service at district health authority level and below were designated and differentiated, and core roles defined.

(ii) The funding of health care was simplified through purchasers according to resident population weighted for need, and providers according to the workload, type and quality of service actually delivered.

(iii) The quality, volume and costs of services were explicitly specified through contracts.

This new environment released four significant forces for improvement driving the National Health Service towards higher standards and better quality of care. Firstly, service purchasers used their knowledge of services, their ability to compare potential providers and the leverage of service contracts to foster higher specifications of patient care. Secondly, the inherent competition between providers stimulated them to develop new and improved services to offer to purchasers. Thirdly, contracts offered a quite new form of explicitness, providing a direct mechanism to foster quality. Finally, the reforms also put in place at hospital level quality improvement and development systems, including medical audit.

Whilst there is considerable scope for local decision-making in the provision of health care to the people of Britain, services are delivered within a clear national framework which is underpinned by legislation. This places responsibility for securing the appropriate services in response to the population's needs in the hands of statutorily defined health authorities and also provides a clear chain of accountability to the Secretary of State for Health and hence to Parliament.

In most other sectors in which individual consumers seek a service or goods, they do so through the exercise of choice, in many situations backed by purchasing power. This process encourages the providers of the service or goods to maintain standards and contain costs and the consumer generally benefits.

Allowing such a process to take place in the health care field has a number of serious drawbacks. Most importantly, it cannot guarantee that a hospital or other provider will exist which maintains a service that is difficult or expensive to deliver, and thus there is a risk that at least part of the population's needs cannot be met. Secondly, because of the highly technical nature of most medical care, consumers are not always in a position to judge for themselves what represents a high quality of service and therefore to make the most appropriate choice when they need help. Thirdly, in the National Health Service, the general practitioner is often acting on the patient's behalf so that the customer-service interface is quite complex.

However, to raise standards and levels of cost effectiveness without the competitiveness of a market for health care has proved difficult in the National Health Service over the years. Whilst the inherently high standards of professionalism in the service, the altruism of staff, the setting of fixed budgetary limits, and performance related contracts for managers have all helped to push the service in this direction, the system of organisation of the health service has not in the past had the momentum to provide major consumer-orientated changes quickly and spontaneously.

The health service now in existence in Britain is not a free market. It is probably best described as a managed market in which the perceived benefits of competition and choice have been introduced, whilst aiming to ensure comprehensive coverage of the community's needs and equality of access to services.

The strategic direction and management of the health service is carried out at national and regional level. At more local level, however, the first stage in the provision of care is that the health and health care needs of populations should be properly assessed, with services increasingly secured to meet those needs through a series of service agreements or contracts, between a purchaser of care and a hospital or other provider of services.

The provision of a comprehensive health service clearly goes far beyond the high profile of hospital-based specialist services which only meet a narrow range of health needs. Critical elements of the British health care system thus include the infrastructure of primary care and community services at local level, as well as other mechanisms directed towards improving the health of the population, through the promotion of health.

The next two sections of the chapter set out in more detail the main structural and managerial elements through which the health service is organised and the processes through which health care is secured and provided.

The Department of Health

The Secretary of State for Health is accountable to Parliament for the National Health Service in England, whilst the Department of Health has a number of major functions, including the management of the National Health Service and the Personal Social Services. The Department of Health is staffed by senior and junior civil servants, professional staff (including the Chief Medical Officer and the Chief Nursing Officer), technical and scientific staff and health service managers.

Although ultimate accountability for the National Health Service at national level rests with the Secretary of State for Health, he or she is assisted by four ministerial colleagues: a Minister for Health and three Junior Health Ministers, also called Parliamentary Under Secretaries for Health, (two in the House of Commons and one in the House of Lords).

National Health Service Policy Board

Whilst the Secretary of State for Health determines policy for the National Health Service, as well as on health matters more generally, he or she receives advice from a range of sources including senior civil servants, external advisers and expert committees. His or her main source of formal advice on policy for the National Health Service comes from a Committee called the *National Health Service Policy Board* which he or she chairs.

In the early 1990s, the Policy Board included amongst its members the Minister for Health, both Parliamentary Under Secretaries for Health, the Chief Executive of the National Health Service, the First Permanent Secretary in the Department of Health (its most senior civil servant), a number of senior industrialists, a senior clinician, Regional Health Authority Chairmen, the Chief Medical Officer and the Chief Nursing Officer. Because most of the members of the Policy Board are appointed in a personal (rather than a representative) capacity, its membership can change from time to time.

In addition to advising Ministers on strategy and policy in the National Health Service, the Policy Board also sets objectives for the National Health Service Management Executive (see below for a description of its role) and monitors the performance of the Executive.

The Secretary of State and other Health Ministers also meet on a regular basis with Regional Health Authority Chairmen and this represents another important route of advice and views from the service on national policies which are being considered or implemented.

National Health Service Management Executive

The day-to-day management of the National Health Service at national level is in the hands of the Chief Executive of the National Health Service, who is supported by a team of other senior managers (or 'directors' as they are usually called). The size of this group of senior managers and areas of individual responsibility will often change to reflect prevailing priorities in the National Health Service or career progression of the individuals concerned. At any one time, for example, the team is likely to include a Director of Finance, a Director of Human Resources, a Medical Director, a Director of Nursing and a Director of Research and Development, as well as Directors covering other areas of responsibility.

This team of directors, is formed as a Management Board, the National Health Service Management Executive (NHSME), under the leadership and chairmanship of the Chief Executive.

The NHSME set three strategic goals for the first half of the 1990s and identified a number of ways in which these goals would be achieved. These goals are set out below in order to give an impression of the Executive's role and orientation:

Strategic goals

- To ensure, through the National Health Service and within available resources, significant improvements in the health of the population through the delivery of services providing health promotion, prevention and diagnosis of illness, and high quality cure, care and rehabilitation.
- To ensure that these services are provided effectively, efficiently and economically, in response to identified needs and with regard to the wishes of the patients.
- To ensure that the National Health Service provides the structure and support for its staff satisfactorily to carry out their jobs and develop their careers.

The NHSME has its primary managerial relationship with regional health authorities (see below for a description of their role). The Chief Executive of the National Health Service meets regularly with the general managers of regional health authorities to discuss the implementation of policy as well as to review progress and developments within the service. In addition to formal meetings, there are a great many informal contacts between the Chief Executive, other Directors of the NHSME, senior managers, civil servants and their counterparts in regional health authorities, as well as in National Health Service Trusts, district health authorities and family health services authorities (see below for descriptions of their roles).

In addition, the NHSME and Department of Health staff will often be in contact with staff at operational level (whether managers, doctors, nurses or other professional staff) through site visits to see at first hand and to learn about service developments and problems.

The management of the health service at national level is also characterised by a great deal of team work involving staff of all disciplines. On any one day, Government buildings will contain a substantial number of meetings involving managers from national, regional or local level as well as doctors, nurses and other professional staff. Such meetings will vary in their purpose, format and content but will range from single *ad hoc* events to discuss a particular issue, through working parties considering service programmes, to more permanent advisory committees.

This is an important and democratic part of the management of the service and ensures that there is commitment to national policies and programmes by those working in the field and that action initiated by the NHSME is informed by the knowledge and expertise of those closer to the operational service level.

Health authorities

Below the Department of Health, the next organisational and managerial level of the health service consists of health authorities.

The National Health Service and Community Care Act 1990 created three types of statutory health authority: regional health authorities (RHAs); district health authorities (DHAs); and family health services authorities (FHSAs). Although, strictly speaking, these bodies did not exist in Law until the new Act came into force in the Summer of 1990, RHAs and DHAs had been a part of the service prior to this and Family Practitioner Committees (FPCs) had been the predecessors of the FHSAs.

Regional Health Authorities

The Health Service in England is divided geographically into 14 health regions, each managed by a regional health authority (RHA).

RHAs are strategic bodies which do not themselves deliver services directly. They are responsible for ensuring that the health care needs of their regions' populations are met through the provision of a range of high quality services and that there is efficient and effective use of the resources which are available for the regions' health care.

They ensure this largely by working closely with, and ensuring the good performance of, DHAs and FHSAs. RHAs have less direct involvement with hospitals and other providers of care and little in their day-to-day management and performance. However, RHAs may have contact with managers of hospitals and senior medical staff working within them on a range of issues such as the development of particular programmes (for example, medical audit); the assessment or encouragement of new service developments (for example, transplantation services) and in trouble-shooting situations (for example, where particular hospital services are threatened by low take up by purchasers or where there are severe financial pressures which threaten to jeopardise services).

RHAs are staffed by a team comprising managers, senior professional and technical staff often with appropriate support staff. The size of this team varies according to the Authority concerned.

Each RHA will organise its core management structure differently, but each has a team of senior managers headed by the Regional General Manager with groups of staff accountable to him or her. Although the precise number, titles, and responsibilities of the senior managers (or directors) vary, all RHAs have a Director of Public Health and a Director of Finance. The other Directors and the staff grouped under them in the organisation may be defined in professional terms (for example, Director of Personnel) or in functional terms (for example, Director of Business Planning).

The functions of a RHA can be broadly specified as follows:

- Setting strategic direction for health and health care in the region and ensuring commitment at all levels in the service to achieving agreed goals and objectives.
- Allocating resources in such a way that, as far as possible, they will achieve maximum health improvement and maximum health care benefit and ensuring financial stability of all health care organisations for which the RHA is accountable.
- Assessing health need and health status on a region-wide basis and ensuring that service response and other activities in the region effectively meet need and improve health status.
- Monitoring and regulating the purchasing and provision of health care in the region to ensure that local populations have access to a choice of services which are of high quality.

The RHA itself is a Board headed by a non-executive Chairman with other non-executive members (all are appointed by the Secretary of State for Health). The RHA membership also comprises a General Manager (its Chief Executive), and other Executive members (who are also senior managers of the Authority).

District health authorities

In the health care market created by the 1990 health service reforms district health authorities (DHAs) became one of the principal purchasers of care. This marked a fundamental change in their role. The DHA's primary functions now are in relation to health needs assessment, determining how these needs will be met, and placing contracts with hospitals and other providers to secure the services required by their local population. These hospitals may be within the district's own boundary or within the geographical area encompassed by another DHA. Whereas the DHA had previously been very much involved with the operational management of its local hospitals, the Act created a system whereby responsibility for the purchasing of service would be separated from responsibility for its provision. In this way, DHAs (as purchasers of care) have been encouraged to look more widely to obtain the most appropriate services for their populations at the best price, and not automatically to place contracts with local providers.

The creation of an environment in which DHAs concentrate on the purchasing function and have no managerial interest in a hospital or community services unit within their boundaries became much easier where the local providers opted to become National Health Service Trusts.

The principal functions of a DHA can be summarised as:

- The assessment of the health needs and health care of its local population.
- Deciding upon priorities for meeting those needs in the light of regional and national strategic guidelines.
- The placing of contracts to secure high quality services for meeting the prioritised needs of the population in a way which gives good value for money.
- Promoting health and preventing disease, disability and premature death.
- The monitoring and evaluation of the impact of these processes on quality of care and the health of the population.

Like RHAs, DHAs are staffed by a team of managerial and professional staff, each of whom is ultimately accountable to the authority's District General Manager (or Chief Executive).

Individual DHAs have taken different approaches to the organisation of their core staffing structure but in most the Director of Public Health (and his or her department) will play the major role in relation to health needs assessment and in advising on aspects of the contracting process, particularly in relation to clinical content and standards of care. Other senior managers and professional staff within the DHA will usually take the lead in other areas of work such as negotiating and placing contracts for services, in resource allocation and financial management and in monitoring and assessing the impact of the district's policies.

In carrying out these functions, DHAs maintain close working relationships with FHSAs (see below) and local general practitioners. They seek their views on the services provided and on issues which affect the provision of care, such as likely patterns of referral of patients to hospital. They must also have strong mechanisms for taking account of the views and wishes of service users.

The DHA Board has a membership structure similar to that of the RHA. It comprises a non-executive Chairman (appointed by the Secretary of State) and non-executive members (appointed by the regional health authority). These members are joined by executive members (who are also senior managers of the authority). As with the RHA, the latter group must include the Chief Executive and a Director of Finance.

Family Health Services Authorities

Of the three new kinds of health authorities created by the National Health Service and Community Care Act 1990, family health services authorities (FHSAs) have seen the greatest change to their responsibilities. Prior to the Act as Family Practitioner Committees (FPCs) they were responsible for contracting with general medical practitioners, general dental practitioners, ophthalmic opticians and community pharmacists. These various practitioners were, and continue to be, paid on a so-called *independent contractor* basis. Family Practitioner Committees had responsibility for maintaining lists of these contractors and taking responsibility for their remuneration. FHSAs have now taken over these responsibilities.

FHSAs have also taken over many of the other functions of the Family Practitioner Committees, for example, appraisal of doctors' surgery premises; arranging for improvements to premises; reimbursing doctors for the employment of practice staff and the investigation of complaints. However, FHSAs also have a range of new responsibilities in relation to gathering information to help in the assessment of the health needs of the local population; formulating policies and plans for the development of primary care services; setting and monitoring prescribing budgets for individual general practitioners; monitoring and administering the budgets of fundholding general practitioners; providing information to patients and seeking user views of primary care services and, very importantly, monitoring the performance of general practitioners in relation to their contract and the preventive targets (such as immunisation and vaccination and cervical cancer screening).

This major change of emphasis in the management of primary care services and the central role of FHSAs in this process has sometimes led to comparisons between them and the old Family Practitioner Committees, in which the latter are described as having been 'pay and rations' bodies.

This is a rather unkind and unfair description of the Family Practitioner Committees and undervalues much of the excellent work which they carried out. Nevertheless, however inappropriate the phrase, it does throw into relief the distinction between a body whose main focus was on the payment of doctors and other professional staff as independent contractors and one which takes an additional wider role in relation to primary care service development.

The Chairman of the FHSA (appointed by the Secretary of State) is a non-Executive. There are other non-Executive Members (appointed by the Regional Health Authority), who include those from health care professional backgrounds as well as lay people. The General Manager (or Chief Executive) is a member of the FHSA but there are no other Executive Members (a situation which contrasts with RHA and DHA membership).

Joint working between DHAs and FHSAs

In many parts of the country DHAs and FHSAs work very closely together. Patterns of joint working vary but it is not uncommon to have consortia type arrangements where a single management team serves both authorities. In addition to reducing managerial costs, this has the advantage of integrating the function of primary and secondary care purchasing so that care can be viewed on a whole population basis.

Fund-holding General Practices

The National Health Service and Community Care Act 1990 created a new service entity called the Fundholding Practice. This is a mechanism which allows the larger general practices to be allocated their own budgets for the purchase of certain services on behalf of their patients.

The fund covers four areas: hospital services for outpatient referrals, investigation and a defined list of elective procedures; prescribing of drugs; certain community health services and employment of practice staff. Fundholders are entitled to redeploy the fund across the budget headings and this has allowed them, for example, to employ a physiotherapist in the practice rather than contract for the service from a hospital. Equally, any savings from the fund may be used for anything that improves the care of the practice's patients.

Hospital services are purchased through contracts between fundholding practices and the hospital concerned. For those hospital services not covered by the fund and for non-fundholding general practices the purchaser is the district health authority.

General practices which are large enough (practice population 7000) can apply for fundholding status to the regional health authority which decides on whether to approve the application. The key criterion in evaluating proposals by general practices to become fund-holders is the practice's capacity to manage the fund effectively and efficiently.

The regional health authority concerned is required to determine the size of the fund to be offered to each of the practices granted fundholding status.

Providers of care

District health authorities and fundholding practices negotiate contracts for services with hospitals and other providers to secure the volume, range and quality of service which they require.

There are a number of different types of provider of care in the internal health market which comprises the health service.

National Health Service Trusts

National Health Service Trusts are a service entity which had not previously existed, created by the National Health Service and Community Care Act 1990. The purpose of the Trust concept is to create considerable managerial freedom and autonomy for hospitals, community units and other providers of care or services (for example, ambulance services) whilst retaining them under the overall organisational umbrella of the National Health Service.

The managerial team of a National Health Service Trust is headed by a Chief Executive with a Board of Directors which comprises a non-executive Chairman (appointed by the Secretary of State), together with executive and non-executive directors (the latter appointed by the regional health authority and the Secretary of State for Health).

National Health Service Trusts have a number of freedoms which are not available to other service providers within the National Health Service. They are free to determine separate terms and conditions of service and levels of remuner-ation for their staff; they can borrow money (for example, for buildings and equipment) from commercial sources; they are able to retain surplus revenue for investment or expenditure, for example, on buildings or equipment; and within certain restrictions, they are permitted to buy and sell land, buildings or other assets.

National Health Service Trust hospitals will enter into contracts with district health authorities, fundholding practices and other purchasers of care, to provide defined services. Usually, the district health authority within whose boundary the National Health Service Trust Hospital is situated will be the largest purchaser of the Trust's services, but the Trust hospital will often have contracts with other district health authorities within the region, certainly with fundholding practices and perhaps also with private health care organisations.

National Health Service Trusts, particularly those which are hospitals, have a responsibility to maintain a balance of services for patients. It would not usually be appropriate for a Trust hospital, which provided a range of specialist services typical of a general hospital, to narrow its provision down to a smaller number of more profitable services, especially if this caused major difficulties in accessibility to care for the local population.

The Secretary of State for Health retains reserve powers to intervene in a Trust's affairs in the rare circumstances where it may be necessary.

Directly managed Units

National Health Service hospitals and other National Health Service providers of services which have not applied for and been granted Trust status are referred to as directly managed units (DMUs). In most cases, managerial responsibility is to district health authorities but this relationship is an arms length one as far as most operational matters are concerned.

DMUs do not have the freedoms which National Health Service Trusts have. For example, they cannot retain or invest financial surpluses, they cannot borrow money, they do not own their own assets (such as buildings and equipment).

Private and voluntary hospitals

The majority of hospitals and other providers of services in the British health service are within the framework of the National Health Service (either as Trusts or DMUs) but an increasing proportion of care and services is provided by hospitals managed by private or voluntary organisations. However, this still represents only a small proportion of all the care and services available.

District health authorities and fundholding general practices may purchase care, through contracts, from providers in the private and voluntary sector, though the principal purchasers of private health care are still the patients themselves either paying directly or through medical insurance plans.

Structure of the NHS in Wales, Scotland and Northern Ireland

There are differences in Wales, Scotland and Northern Ireland in the administrative structure of the Service, although the main principles are the same as in England.

KEY FUNCTIONAL PROCESSES OF HEALTH DELIVERY

The overall purpose of health services in Britain is to provide advice, assessment and treatment for patients, and to enhance the quality of life for those with special and long-term care needs (for example, the elderly, the mentally disordered, the physically handicapped and those with chronic diseases). There is also a responsibility to deliver services efficiently and, where appropriate, to address problems of inequity (Figure 4.2).

The process begins with the formulation of strategic goals and aims at national, regional and local level and ends with a process through which purchasers of care come together with providers of care in a number of stages (Figure 4.3).

The first stage involves the purchasers of care, principally district health authorities, carrying out a comprehensive needs assessment for their resident population. From this starting point, district health authorities will draw up a statement of their purchasing intentions. This statement will reflect the priorities which the district health authority has assigned to different areas of service and will serve as a plan of how the authority will deploy its resources for the forthcoming financial year, the volume of services which will be purchased, and specifications in relation to quality of service requirements. Using the statement of purchasing intentions, district health authorities seek to establish contracts with hospitals and other providers of care for a particular level, quality and cost of service. Once the service is being delivered the district health authority will ensure that it is monitored and the basis and timing of the monitoring arrangements are something which is agreed between purchaser and provider at the time that the contract is agreed.

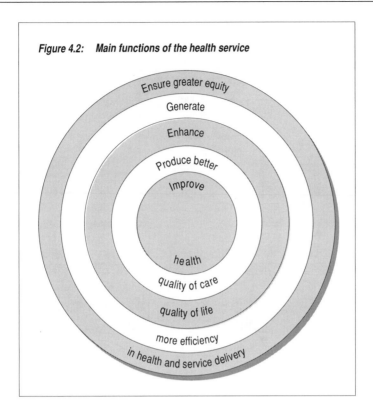

Figure 4.2:   Main functions of the health service

Ensure greater equity
Generate
Enhance
Produce better
Improve
health
quality of care
quality of life
more efficiency
in health and service delivery

Whilst the major purchaser of care remains the district health authority, fundholding practices and other purchasers will also go through these stages, albeit on a smaller scale, in securing services for the populations for which they are responsible. These stages which the purchaser goes through are referred to as business planning.

A hospital or other provider of health care will also have to undertake business planning. It will have to make an assessment of the health care it is likely to be able to provide or asked to provide. On this basis, it will produce a business plan setting out the range of services which it intends to provide, its income from contracts placed by purchasers and the resources it requires to meet these contractual commitments.

Setting policy and strategy

The direction for the improvement of health and development of health care through the activities of the health service is set at a number of levels. National policy is formulated by Ministers and the National Health Service Management Executive drawing widely on expert advice and information. One of the most difficult issues is how to set priorities. Although in theory, a number of areas of policy will have particular emphasis and importance, the reality is that the health service has to cope with multiple priorities and ensure progress on almost all of them. This is in contrast to the approach taken in private sector business where

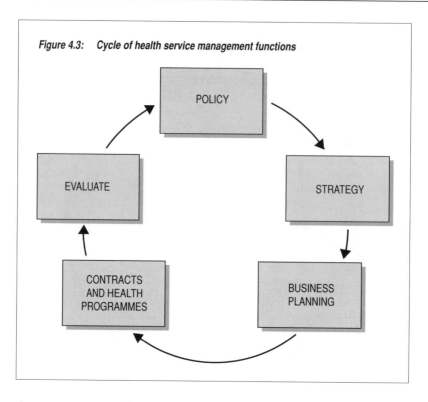

Figure 4.3:   Cycle of health service management functions

good management practice would see a company concentrating on a relatively small number of clearly expressed goals.

In the health service, the flow of new ideas, information, policy guidance and new initiatives is constant and one of the major challenges is to channel this stream into manageable courses to inform and stimulate health care development.

The range of potential inputs to this planning process is very diverse and encompasses information arising from health needs assessment, developments in provision, policy and strategy as well as wider influences such as the availability of resources, demographic and social change (Figure 4.4). There is a need to evaluate information some of which is quite technical. It is important, for example, to draw in the research and development perspective to ensure that a proper evaluation is undertaken of new technologies and interventions which are claimed to be beneficial to patients or to the population. Policy and strategy set at national level is developed and extended within regional health strategies and then implemented at local level through the process of contracting and through the establishment of health programmes.

Business planning

Business planning is a management process common to all organisations within the health service. It is often the process through which strategy is turned into action; it is the bridge between setting strategy and negotiating and agreeing service contracts. It is a continuous process rather than a discrete exercise.

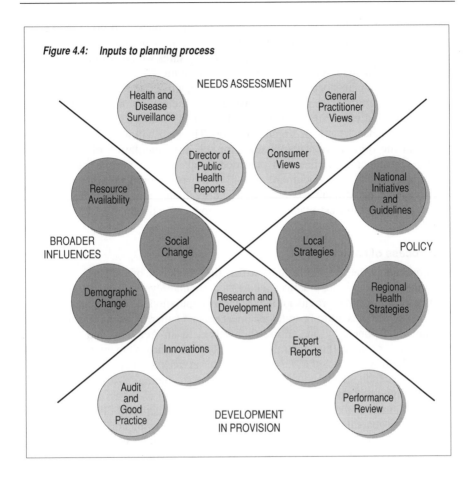

Figure 4.4: Inputs to planning process

The Boards of health authorities and National Health Service Trusts set objectives and goals for the organisation, identify likely available resources, assess the organisation's strengths and weaknesses as well as opportunities for, and threats to, growth and development (commonly known as SWOT analysis).

Contributions to the business planning process also come from the operational level of service. These involve identifying options for change in management and operational practices and in investment requirements. They also involve evaluating current service levels, comparing the performance of other purchasers and providers, and expressing the aspirations and requirements of the different functions within the organisation. In the case of hospitals, these will be the clinical services, the operational support services such as catering, and portering as well as the general management functions.

The crux of business planning is the bringing together of these two processes and producing a business plan which sets the direction for the coming year. The National Health Service is no different from any commercial business environment in that it is not possible to plan accurately or exactly what will happen in the year ahead. The business plan must therefore consider the implications of all likely situations which may arise during the course of the year. Financial planning is a key element of the business plan. The costs of action plans and programmes can usually be forecast with a reasonable degree of accuracy but the organisation also needs to make provision for potential financial pressures which cannot be foreseen. This is called risk assessment and contingency planning.

The business plan document is a series of objectives and goals supported by specific programmes or action plans as the means to achieve them. The programmes and plans are prioritised and matched to likely available resources. Precise timescales are set for implementation. The plan will also identify the lead person in the organisation responsible for the implementation of each action. However, producing the business plan document is not the end of the business planning process. The document provides the benchmark against which the organisation's performance is measured and evaluated and this review must be continuous if the business planning process is to be effective.

The process of contracting

The contract is the means through which the purchaser of care (district health authority or fund holding practice) secures a particular level and quality of services from hospitals or other providers of care for its population.

Patients who present to hospital as emergencies, either through referral by their general practitioner, by presenting themselves to an Accident and Emergency department, or after calling an ambulance, may require any element of the possible range of help which hospital-based specialist services are capable of providing. This may include specialist opinion, investigation, therapy with drugs or other measures including operative intervention.

The majority of the non-emergency demand will arise from clinical workload generated by general practitioners referring patients following consultations.

Thus, depending on the clinical specialty concerned, a relatively large proportion of the elective work of the hospital service will involve providing specialist assessment or an opinion (usually on an outpatient basis) on patients referred by a general practitioner. Such patients may require further investigation or treatment by hospital-based specialist services but many will be referred back to their general practitioner with advice on further management of their problem.

A group of patients, in addition to baseline investigation, will require more complex or advanced forms of investigation before their problem is defined. They may require further specialist intervention to resolve or alleviate theirproblem (provided either on an inpatient or outpatient basis) or they may again be referred back to the care of their general practitioner with advice only on treatment.

A further group of patients at any one time will have their problem defined in terms of a need for intervention by specialist services, either in the form of an operation, another type of procedure or some kind of non-operative treatment. Some will have the condition or treatment monitored, others will have further specialist interventions, either in response to changes in their health or at pre-determined times as part of their overall clinical management plan.

It is not possible within this diversity of clinical problems which patients may have and the consequent variation in care requirements and resource consumption, to predict accurately (in advance) the numbers which will require particular programmes of care.

Contracts are therefore concerned with covering eventualities and they can be framed to do so in a number of ways ranging from a broad catch-all approach to a more specific basis for some groups of patients or some treatments.

Types of contract

There are three broad types of contract for clinical services. The first and most general is the block contract in which a purchaser agrees with a hospital or other provider of care that a payment will be made to enable patients to have access to a defined range of services. Specifications may be made about the quality of service but the block contract is not based on an agreed volume of work to be undertaken. This type of contract has the advantage of simplicity and tends to be used where information systems are weak and monitoring of the volume of work is difficult or in situations where predicting the volume of work is problematic (accident and emergency is an example of such a service). The disadvantages are (for the purchaser) that it is difficult to ensure that maximum value for money is being obtained and (for the provider) that the numbers of cases presenting for treatment in the contract may exceed expectation and available resources.

The second type of contract is more specific and is called the cost and volume contract. In this type of contract, the purchaser agrees with the provider that a particular volume of work will be dealt with and the two parties fix a price. Quality criteria will also be included. This type of contract has advantages over the block contract in enabling a greater degree of certainty on the part of the purchaser (in what amount of work will be carried out) and the provider (in what amount of work will need to be coped with). Sometimes, cost and volume contracts contain a clause agreeing that additional work will be carried out at marginal cost.

The third type of contract is the cost per case contract and is the most specific of the three. In this type, the agreement between purchaser and provider is based upon the concept of a payment for the cost of each case. The cost per case contract has the particular advantage for the purchaser in enabling it to obtain the best price for the category of care. However, this type of contract is not so widely applicable because it can only be used effectively where the category of care can be well specified. It is particularly well suited to treatments which are provided in a number of specialist centres and where the volume of cases which the District Health Authority has within its population is relatively small (an operation such as coronary artery by-pass graft would be a good example). The cost per case agreement also tends to be used for isolated cases where patients are treated outside their district of residence and their home district health authority is subsequently invoiced.

Contracts are set following discussion and negotiation between purchaser and provider and should be seen in the context of continuing contact between the two. Contracting is a process, not an event.

When placing contracts with providers, district health authorities will reflect the referral patterns and preferences of general practitioners within the district and will ensure contracts cover all predictable patient referral flows. However, the district health authority is unable to predict where all residents will require access to services. For example, a resident of any district may be on holiday in another part of the country and require hospital treatment, and refer him or herself to the nearest hospital. This is called an Extra Contractual Referral (ECR). A second example of an ECR is where a general practitioner refers a patient for a specialised treatment which is only available in one or a few particular hospitals. It is unlikely that the health authority will have a contract for such a service if the referrals are very few and irregular. For ECRs, the hospital administering the treatment charges the health authority in which the patient lives on a cost per case basis. In setting their financial plans for the year, district health authorities make a provision for expenditure on ECRs.

Health programmes

Not all developments in health care can be achieved through the contracting process. This applies particularly to the improvement of health where for example the aim might be to reduce mortality from coronary heart disease or stroke or to reduce cigarette smoking amongst teenagers. Here, health authorities will wish to design health programmes to achieve the desired change. Such programmes may involve health education campaigns through local media, counselling of high risk individuals or working with non-health service bodies to create more opportunities for healthier leisure pursuits. Approaches to the promotion of health are described in detail in chapter 3.

Evaluation and monitoring

The process of evaluation and monitoring of health services should be a continuous one. The basis for it is something which should be agreed before implementing service contracts or health programmes. The lessons learned from the evaluation process can be used to inform the next year's decisions about service development and investment of resources.

The process of law making

Although a considerable proportion of English law is case-law (sometimes called Common Law) which has been derived by setting precedents in court cases, as far as the health and social services are concerned, the powers for providing services are derived almost entirely from Acts of Parliament – Statute Law. The process of law making is complex and only a brief outline is described in order to provide a basic understanding of the procedure.

An underlying principle of modern British democracy is to seek to obtain wide agreement on proposed legislative changes. It is often the practice nowadays to promote wide discussions on a major social issue before introducing it to Parliament. There are several methods for achieving this.

The appropriate Minister may issue a discussion paper in the form of a 'Green Paper' or consultative document, in which he invites comments within a specified period of time. The next step may be a 'White Paper' which makes firm proposals for changing the law, having taken into account the results of the consultative process. The firm proposals may be in a Parliamentary Bill. For example, two Green papers, a consultative document and a White Paper preceded the National Health Service Reorganisation of 1974, whilst three White Papers preceded the 1990 Act. Alternatively, the Minister may appoint a Committee or, if the issue is of sufficient importance, a Royal Commission to collect information, interview witnesses, sift evidence and produce a report with recommendations. On the basis of such reports, the Minister may accept some or all of the recommendations and again set out an outline of proposed changes to legislation as a White Paper. This sequence of events occurred, for example, when the Report of the Committee on the Allied Personal Social Services (The Seebohm Committee) was followed by the Local Authority Social Services Act 1970.

When the Government's final proposals are ready, they are put into a Bill which is introduced to Parliament with a copy to all Members. This is referred to as its first reading. The second reading of the Bill involves discussion of the main points and, if approved, it is referred to a committee of Members of Parliament which considers the Bill clause by clause (as each paragraph is termed). This takes place either in a committee room or as a 'Committee of the whole House' in the House of Commons Chamber. The Bill is then returned with any amendments for a further debate in which amendments can still be proposed. This is referred to as the Report stage. After a third reading it passes to the House of Lords for a similar procedure before it is finally submitted to the Queen for Royal Assent.

An individual Member of Parliament may introduce a Bill – a Private Member's Bill. An example in the field of social legislation is the Chronically Sick and Disabled Persons Act of 1970, which was introduced by Mr Alfred Morris MP. Less commonly, Bills can be introduced first in the House of Lords.

After receiving the Royal Assent, the Bill becomes an Act and the paragraphs that were previously still clauses are now referred to as sections. It is customary for the Act itself to be concerned only with broad principles. Powers are given to an appropriate government Minister to make regulations and orders (subordinate regulations) dealing with the detail. It is important to realise that these regulations carry the same force in law as if they were part of the Act from which they are derived. However, Ministers can only make law in this way within limits laid down by the original Act. Regulations are subject to Parliamentary procedure, but this is much quicker and simpler than the elaborate and lengthy procedure that most Bills go through on their way to becoming Acts.

Thus, a flexible means of law making is available to meet changing and unforeseen circumstances. In addition, the Minister may issue circulars or memoranda on the subject of the Act. These are not legally binding, but in practice are usually implemented by health and local government authorities. Some legislation, particularly in relation to local authorities, makes powers available but does not make it a duty to implement them. The term 'permissive' legislation is used in this context.

QUALITY OF HEALTH CARE

In a modern, consumer-oriented society one of the cornerstones of the process of supplying goods and services is an emphasis on quality. In turn, one of the principal stimuli in a market economy for improving quality and raising standards, is competition amongst suppliers and providers to produce a better product or service as economically as possible, and which meets the expressed needs or wishes of the purchaser.

The health care sector has not been immune from this emphasis on quality, though it is perhaps fair to say that in the past there has been a less formal and comprehensive approach to quality assessment and improvement within it. There are a number of possible reasons for this. There is an inherent belief in some quarters, that standards of professional training and practice are so high that they guarantee that the practitioner delivering the service will do so at a uniformly high quality. Undoubtedly, it is also the case that the complexity of defining and measuring quality in the health care field is much greater than in many other sectors (for example, industry) and this has also been an impediment to developing a stronger quality ethos in health service provision. The approach to assessing and improving quality can be potentially very threatening to professional staff, such as doctors and nurses, particularly if it is felt that health service managers may also wish to become involved in discussions about the quality of the services they provide.

Finally, the high standing which the health service (as a public service) has had in the hearts and minds of the British people and the fact that it has been provided free at the point of delivery also contribute to the previous lack of emphasis on quality.

This section of the chapter describes some of the key themes underlying the approach to quality in health care and gives an account of the main mechanisms through which quality of care can be influenced.

Concepts and definitions of quality

The development of conceptual frameworks to define quality of health care has spurned a major literature on the subject in biomedical and health services journals, particularly over the last three decades.

One of the most important and widely respected classifications of quality in health care is that originally propounded by the North American Avedis Donabedian[1] in which there are three approaches.

Structure

One approach to assessing the quality of health care is to examine the amount and nature of facilities and staff available to it. Examples of such *structural* measures would be: hospital beds per thousand population, and the number of senior doctors per thousand population.

The structural aspects of quality in health care are often used in making comparisons between health services in different parts of a country or in international comparisons. Thus, variation may be found between services in the number of surgeons per head of population or in the number of ophthalmology out-patient clinics available to different populations.

Such differences in the structural aspects of health care quality can be useful in initiating discussions about the adequacy of health care facilities available to different populations. They can also be valuable in stimulating change or improvement where, for example, levels of staff or facilities are very low compared to those which are agreed as being required to operate an effective service.

The main problem with relying on the structural approach to assess how 'good' or 'bad' a health service is, is the fact that there is seldom adequate evidence to demonstrate what levels of facilities or staff are required to produce good results for particular types of patient care. It by no means follows, for example, that one service with a higher number of surgeons per head of population than a neighbouring service will yield better results for hernia repair operations (low in-hospital complication rates and low long-term recurrence rates).

Thus, whilst structural measures are still an important aspect of assessing the quality of health care, they are of limited value when taken alone and are best regarded as only one part of an overall concept which also embraces process and outcome measures.

Process

A second attribute of quality is concerned with what is done for and to a patient, or group of patients, and how well it is done. Assessment of the quality of care based on the process approach to quality can be wide ranging. For example, the evaluation of a programme for control of high blood pressure (hypertension) might be assessed by establishing how adequately the population at risk of developing hypertension had been identified, how thoroughly diagnostic criteria had been determined, how valid and accurate were the blood pressure readings which were taken, how other associated medical conditions were detected and managed, whether agreed treatment protocols were being followed, whether patients were complying with treatment regimes, what proportion of patients who had been diagnosed as hypertensive had their blood pressure stabilised at agreed levels, how often patients were followed-up and how adequate were these subsequent clinical assessments.

All these are examples of processes of care which can be used as a basis for assessing aspects of the quality of clinical services given to hypertensive patients. In practice, assessing quality in this way requires establishing agreed standards of good practice in the process of care concerned against which the actual service can be compared and hence assessed. Whilst the process approach adds much greater depth to the assessment of quality than the structural approach, it cannot be viewed in isolation from it nor from the third attribute, outcome measurement.

Outcome

The final attribute of quality in the Donabedian triad is concerned with the outcome of the health care episode for the patient. Does she or he get better? Are there any clinical complications? Is he or she satisfied with the care delivered? Does he or she survive the illness or disease occurrence? Outcome is the final arbiter of the quality of care provided. There are numerous possible approaches to defining outcomes of health care or of a health service's activity.

One approach which is often quoted and easily remembered is based on the *five D's: death, disease, disability, discomfort and dissatisfaction*. Thus, for example, assessment of the outcome of care for a man admitted to hospital as an emergency for treatment of a ruptured aortic aneurysm might be in terms of whether he survived (*death*); whether the aneurysm was technically well corrected surgically (*disease*): whether he returned to 'normal' physical, psychological and social functioning after discharge from hospital (*disability*); whether he remained free of residual pain (*discomfort*); and whether the interpersonal as well as the technical aspects of the nursing and medical care and the environment in which it was provided were pleasing to him (*dissatisfaction*).

This and similar classifications of outcomes are probably best used for illustrative purposes because most are either too simplistic or too detailed to be generally applicable. The most important issue in considering outcome as an aspect of health care quality is to remember that there is a *population* and a patient care *dimension*.

The practical application of outcome assessment of the quality of health services, whether at the population or at individual patient care level, is still in its infancy. Partly, this is because of the virtual absence of routinely available data through which outcome can be assessed. This situation is rapidly changing as greater emphasis is being placed on the importance of the outcome dimension in assessing the quality of care.

The Donabedian classification has been dealt with at length because it remains the most enduring and widely respected conceptual approach through which the quality of health care can be defined and assessed. It is important, however, to remember that these concepts are closely inter-related as well as dynamic. Determining the way in which health facilities (*structural*) are used (*processes*) to produce the end result of care for the patient (*outcome*) is the real route to improving the quality of care.

It is important also to remember that health care has different attributes upon which judgements about quality can be made. The health service professional's definition of high quality care would probably rely heavily on *technical* considerations (for example, how well the therapeutic or investigational aspects of the care were delivered). On the other hand, many patients would place a high or low value on the care they receive based on the interpersonal or amenity attributes of their care (for example, kindness, courtesy, explanation, information giving and standards of lighting, heating, food, toilet and washing facilities).

All are important quality considerations and it cannot be assumed that high quality in one attribute automatically means high quality in the others. For example, a surgeon may be excellent in terms of communication and empathy with his patients but obtain less satisfactory surgical results than a colleague who is a masterly technical surgeon but treats his patients like a 'slab of meat'.

Finally, an attribute of health care quality which is particularly important from the public health perspective is the care received by the community embracing such quality issues as access to, and equity of, care provided to the population.

Methods for improving quality

A number of mechanisms within the National Health Service are directed towards improving the quality of health care provided and some of these are described in this section.

Quality improvement through contracts for services

In a health care system, such as the National Health Service, in which there is a framework of contracting for clinical (and other) services in an internal market, there are at least three major forces acting to influence the quality of care provided.

- The first is the tendency for the purchasers of service to place contracts based upon experience. Thus, for example, patients' poor experience of an obstetric service (such as lack of attentiveness of staff or a high perinatal complication rate) should lead the purchaser of services (whether a district health authority or fund-holding practice) to negotiate improvements in the quality of service from the provider concerned. If this does not then take place, the purchaser has the ultimate sanction of switching the contract to another hospital which is able to provide the quality of service required.

- The second is the tendency for the provider of service to compete based upon quality. As far as the hospitals (or other providers of services) are concerned, developing new ideas and offering new services or improved ways of delivering an existing service will give a competitive edge, the opportunity to win more contracts and therefore a powerful incentive in terms of income for the hospital. This is a process which should usually lead to the raising of standards and higher quality of care.
- The third is what is specified in the contract: the opportunity for purchasers to make explicit, publicly in their contracts, requirements for the quality of service to be provided is a further stimulus for improving quality.

The overall impact of these various elements in any particular locality will have a major effect on the quality of care provided.

Whilst the emphasis in purchasing and provision of health care should be that quality comes first, it should not be forgotten that cost is also very important. Hospitals and other providers of care must demonstrate and provide high quality service, though not by increasing costs so as to make them uncompetitive on pricing. In turn, district health authorities will wish to procure the highest quality services across a broad range, whilst working within a constrained budget. There are always trade-offs between quality and cost, but it is important to recognise that there are also trade-offs between different elements of quality for example, between local access and waiting times.

Quality clauses in contracts represent an increasingly important route through which district health authorities and fund-holding general practices see themselves achieving a higher standard of care for their patients who require hospital services.

Medical audit

Medical audit is the approach through which doctors critically examine their own and each other's practice, so that the lessons learned from such a scrutiny can be used to make improvements in professional practice, and hence the quality of care.

The term medical audit is largely a British one, and, in other countries it is more common for the process to be described as peer review. Medical audit or peer review is not a new phenomenon, examples of it having been practised can be found much earlier in this century, and in even more distant medical history. However, the early 1990s saw medical audit being formally introduced as part of the contracts of all senior medical staff in the National Health Service and as an integral part of postgraduate medical training programmes.

The stimulus for this was the National Health Service Review White Paper 'Working for Patients'. Indeed, one whole Working Paper[2] was devoted to the subject of medical audit.

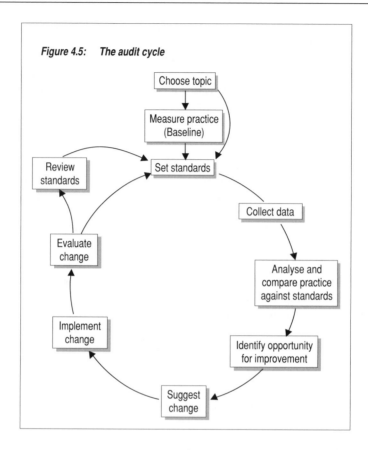

Figure 4.5:   The audit cycle

In this Working Paper, medical audit was defined as:

'The systematic, critical analysis of medical care, including the procedures used for diagnosis and treatment. It also concerns the use of resources and the resulting outcome and quality of life for the patient.'

It is vital that any medical audit programme is methodologically sound, such that appropriate conclusions can be reached and hence appropriate action planned and undertaken. If this is not the case, then the time and effort involved will have been wasted. Valid medical audit techniques must be in place to allow the audit to take place continuously as part of the day-to-day work of a clinical team.

The process through which effective medical audit is conducted is by progress around the audit cycle (see Figure 4.5). A key component of the cycle is the setting of standards and comparing current practice against these standards. The setting of standards is something for all members of the clinical team to agree upon but should be undertaken using the best available medical evidence and knowledge.

There are four main medical audit techniques or methods in common use.

Critical incident review. This is a common type of audit where members of the clinical team review and discuss adverse outcomes such as case fatalities or complications. This so-called 'death and disaster' meeting is a time honoured and valuable part of clinical practice and postgraduate education. It is valuable as part of a systematic medical audit programme but discussion of individual cases cannot itself lead to progression around the audit cycle. However, such an approach may identify opportunity for more formalised development of standards, protocols or guidelines against which practice may be compared using a population of patients. This then allows for collation of aggregated data with the opportunity for cyclical audit.

Random case note reviews. Individual case note review, within a peer group discussion, has value but again there is a risk of subjectivity and limited application directly to the audit cycle. Such individual case note review is most valuable if comparison is made against already agreed standards of practice (such as the practice of clinical record keeping).

Critical event monitoring. This approach builds upon critical incident discussion but collates information over time so as to generate aggregated data in the form, for example, of rates such as wound infection rates, return to operating theatre rates. There is enhanced opportunity for cyclical audit.

Criterion based review. This is probably the most effective of the medical audit approaches. It involves developing explicit standards which are agreed by consensus in relation to diagnosis, treatment, investigation and/or presenting complaints with comparison of how patients in the service have been dealt with against these standards. Aggregated data are collected and analysed, opportunities for improvement identified, change instituted and data collected to demonstrate whether improvement has occurred.

To carry out medical audit properly requires an infrastructure and a process to build in the results to identify service improvements.

Confidential Enquiry into Perioperative Deaths

Although the majority of medical audit activity is carried out as an integral part of clinical work at hospital level, there are examples of medical audit initiatives on a regional or a national scale.

One such initiative is the Confidential Enquiry into Perioperative Deaths (CEPOD)[3] which was first established on a pilot basis in three health regions and was later extended more widely. The approach of CEPOD was based broadly on the longstanding Confidential Enquiry into Maternal Mortality (see chapter 6 for a fuller description of this) which has used a peer review mechanism to identify avoidable factors in maternal deaths during pregnancy and labour.

The first pilot studies of CEPOD used a similar system of confidential reports by peers in the surgical and anaesthetic specialties on the circumstances of deaths which occurred amongst hospital patients within 30 days of a surgical or anaesthetic procedure.

The results of the pilot studies showed firstly, that a very low number of perioperative deaths occurred in the pilot regions and, secondly, that death was attributable to 'avoidable' surgical or anaesthetic factors in a small proportion of all perioperative deaths.

However, amongst the deaths which were deemed 'avoidable' a number of important findings were made. These included issues about inadequate time and attention being given to rescucitating patients or dealing with intercurrent medical conditions before they were operated upon; instances of lack of adequate supervision of junior surgeons and anaesthetists by consultants; and situations where surgeons who were generalists were operating on patients with conditions which would have been better dealt with by a surgeon with specialist skills in the field concerned.

The results of the CEPOD studies are only made available in aggregated and anonymised form. Thus no individual doctor or patient can be identified. This is an essential pre-requisite of any peer review based upon voluntary notification of cases and participation, if the continuing cooperation of the professionals concerned is to be achieved.

An initiative like CEPOD produces improvement in the quality of care in two main ways. Firstly, the knowledge of those involved that they are participating in a peer review process may in itself raise standards by making them more aware, and self-critical, of their practice. Secondly, the formal report of the results of a major peer review exercise of this kind, containing analyses and recommendations, is a means through which the profession can amend· existing practices. Where necessary, change can take place in the organisation of clinical care. Training programmes can be established to address the issues raised. Following the conclusion of the first CEPOD study, the system was extended to a National Enquiry in which the methodology was strengthened in a number of respects.

Total Quality Management (TQM)

The experience of the commercial sector, both industrial and service, can inform strategies for quality improvement and quality management in health care. This wider quality debate is most clearly apparent in the recent history of North American and Japanese manufacturing industry. It is not so long since the Japanese were renowned for producing cheap, poor quality merchandise, and American industry predominated in such areas as camera production, stereo and hi-fi equipment manufacture. Today, the Japanese have gained a major share of the North American and, indeed, world markets in consumer goods. They now produce and export merchandise which competes with alternatives on quality and not simply price.

The reason for this dramatic turnaround in the competitiveness and market position of Japanese industry is widely recognised as being grounded in the adoption of relatively simple theories of quality improvement. Ironically, the theorists who have been credited with stimulating this process in Japan are American, particularly W Edwards Deming[4] and Joseph M Juran[5].

The basic postulates of their theories which underpin the school of Total Quality Management (TQM), are relatively simple but provide an interesting contrast to the approach to improving quality of care taken by medical audit. Both TQM and medical audit are charged with the purpose of producing quality improvement but perhaps the major difference between the approaches is inherent within the different emphasis that they place on the two elements of the phrase *quality improvement*.

Medical audit tends to be concerned more with the definition of quality, with the setting of standards, and with measurement of performance against such standards. TQM is more concerned with the vision of continuous improvement, being less concerned with definitions and standards and more focused on the processes and systems necessary to stimulate improvements. As such, TQM recognises the dynamic nature of quality improvement to a greater extent than traditional approaches to medical audit. It is less concerned with identification and sanction of outliers and more with the improvement of the whole. Its influence is aimed at the whole population rather than the tail of a distribution, a concept that should be comfortable for those with knowledge of the principles of epidemiology and public health. For the same reason, this approach recognises the multidisciplinary nature of quality improvement.

Professionally led medical audit can often become an isolated, ring fenced activity focusing on physician performance and hence discouraging synthesis into a corporate view of quality. The techniques employed for quality improvement from this model tend to focus on influencing and changing individual physician behaviour. This carries with it the danger of developing what has been termed the *bad apple* approach[6]. This concentrates on the outlier and potentially engenders fear and distrust, stimulates defensive attitudes and practices on the one hand, and risks development of complacency and satisfaction on the part of the majority, rather than instilling the desire and culture for continuous quality improvement.

In the short-term, it is likely that medical audit activity will continue to be seen as separate from other quality perspectives. In the longer-term, however, it is likely that the fragmented view of quality will be synthesised into a more corporate view of quality of health care in the National Health Service which is shared by management and all the caring professions and which enhances and focuses upon consumer perceptions and experience.

In the industrial field and in the service industries, the TQM approach is based on the philosophy that by continually improving the processes of production (or the delivery of service) expensive consequences such as scrapping defective products, expenditure on warranty agreements and re-manufacturing will be avoided. By concentrating on quality productivity will improve.

The traditional approach to quality control in industry was initially based upon the concept of inspection to detect defects. This has a number of disadvantages. Firstly, and most importantly, it does not gain commitment of the whole workforce to improving quality. Instead the issue is seen as the concern of a separate quality department or inspector. This instills in the workforce a feeling that they are not being trusted and, even worse, creates the situation in which they will only achieve a high standard of work when being watched or inspected. Secondly, when the process of manufacture is not properly designed, and the raw material inadequate, then no amount of inspection will remedy the problem. This approach inspects out poor quality, rather than building in good quality to the systems of management and production.

The TQM approach seeks to reduce the importance of inspection as a quality tool and instead to involve the whole workforce, using to the full, their knowledge and expertise of the process of manufacture constantly to improve it so that the defects, errors and poor products are eliminated.

The overall benefit for a company which is engaged effectively in TQM is success of its business. Reduction in errors and defects not only increases quality, it reduces costs (from remanufacture, replacement goods, inspection), improves profitability and, by satisfying customers, attracts more of the market share.

Whilst a key element of TQM is reducing unnecessary variation in the production process, another is the emphasis on the customer and his or her wishes and expectations. This customer ethos extends not just to the external customer but also to internal customers within the organisation. Indeed, in TQM terms, the very definition of quality of the product or service relies heavily on the customer's views of what constitute good or bad quality.

The potential applications of TQM to the health care field are not yet fully apparent such that large numbers of practical examples cannot yet be cited. However, perhaps one example at this stage will illustrate the potential benefits of quality improvement to a health service. A complication of hospital care, particularly in the elderly, is that of pressure (or 'bed') sores.

In this example, good quality care would be a hospital inpatient stay for an elderly person in which he or she was free of pressure sores. An approach in which all nurses on the ward discussed, planned and reviewed the process of nursing care so that pressure sores were eliminated would have advantages over an approach in which a matronly figure inspected patients for evidence of pressure sores for which individual nurses could then be blamed for failing in their duty.

The former, TQM-based, approach would reduce or eliminate pressure sores (improve quality of care), reduce costs (length of stay reduced, no need for skin grafts or other treatment), increase productivity (by enabling other patients to be admitted and treated), and improve market share (district health authorities would be more likely to place contracts with a hospital with a reputation for a low incidence of pressure sores).

Thus, there are parallels between TQM in the business sector and in health care. In this example, the health service's aim of eliminating pressure sores could be seen as analogous to a Japanese electronic company in which concentration on improving the processes of production of television sets led to products in line with customer requirements (improved quality), reduced costs (fewer defects resulting in re-work, scrapping, payment of warranty agreements), increased productivity (less workforce time devoted to re-manufacture or correcting defects), increased market share (more satisfied customers).

The introduction of TQM is not simply a matter of exposing and adopting the techniques, it requires major organisation-wide change in terms of the culture and orientation. It places major responsibilities on senior management to create the kind of participative environment in which all members of the organisation are valued, their skills and efforts rewarded and an environment in which there is a recognition that employees generally want to do their best and should be comprehensively and actively involved in the process of quality improvement.

Patient empowerment

In the past, concern with quality has largely focused on improving standards of diagnostic and treatment techniques delivered by doctors and other health care professionals. This perspective on quality improvement is still very important but increasingly attention is being given to seeking and acting upon the views and expectations of users and potential users of health services. In a message to the United States Congress in 1962, President John F Kennedy identified four basic rights of consumers (Table 4.1). These rights embody fundamental principles which

Table 4.1:   ***Basic rights of consumers***

- The right to be informed
- The right to be heard
- The right to choose
- The right to safety

Source: President John F Kennedy. Message to the United States Congress, 1962.

if applied to health services would constitute a powerful commitment to users of services. In Britain, the Patient's Charter is the health service element of the Government's Citizen's Charter, an initiative introduced to raise standards and ensure greater accountability in the delivery of public services.

The Patient's Charter[7] sets out a range of rights and standards for all those using health services. These include maximum waiting times both for diagnosis and treatment as well as a range of other guarantees and entitlements.

Genuine empowerment of patients as consumers of health care requires a cultural shift in the way in which services are traditionally delivered. It involves not only listening and talking to patients about the care which they receive, but also genuinely taking their views and opinions into account when designing services. It also means enabling them to make informed choices and becoming partners with health professionals in the care provided.

Complaints

The number of formal complaints made by patients is relatively small in relation to the total episodes of care provided by the health service. Though this undoubtedly represents a generally high level of satisfaction with the public health care system in Britain, there is some evidence that people who wish to complain do not do so either because they do not know how or because they believe that it would be pointless to do so.

Complaints made by patients about their care represent an important opportunity to learn lessons about possible service failures, which can then be translated into improvements in service quality. An important factor in judging the quality of a health service should be how quickly and effectively complaints are resolved. Patients will wish to see their concerns taken seriously, their complaint investigated, a clear explanation given, and follow-up action taken.

People who are unhappy about the clinical care they receive in National Health Service hospitals face several options for expressing their dissatisfaction. They can raise their concerns informally with the health professional concerned to have them settled by discussion and explanation; they can make a complaint formally to the hospital or health authority management, when it will be dealt with using the Hospital or Family Health Services Complaints Procedure. Alternatively they can take their complaint to law.

Hospital complaints procedure

Virtually all written complaints to health authorities concern the hospital service, but the same procedure also applies to community services outside hospital (but not primary care which has a separate machinery).

There are about 12,000 written complaints made to the hospital service annually by patients, former patients or by relatives or friends of patients. The investigation of complaints of a non-clinical nature, (for example, those relating to nursing or administrative matters) is co-ordinated by the district health authority or hospital manager and all members of staff involved are fully informed of any allegation and given an opportunity to reply. They are advised of their right to seek advice of their professional associations before commenting. A reply to the complaint is sent by the manager of the district health authority or hospital following agreement with the senior staff concerned. Should a complaint of this nature fail to be resolved at local level, it can ultimately be referred to the Health Service Commissioner (Ombudsman) provided that the complainant is not considering action through the courts.

Complaints relating to the exercise of clinical judgement by hospital medical and dental staff are dealt with in three stages under the clinical complaints procedure. Although a complaint may be made direct to the consultant in charge of the patient, to a health authority, to a hospital, or one of its officers, it is the responsibility of the consultant in charge of the patient to investigate the clinical aspects of a complaint, usually after seeing the complainant and discussing the matters which have given rise to his or her anxieties. The formal reply is normally sent by the hospital manager after the clinical matters are agreed with the consultant concerned. Sometimes the consultant may send a written reply direct to the complainant dealing with the clinical aspects.

The second stage is reached if the complainant is still dissatisfied. The Regional Director of Public Health is informed and, after further discussion with the consultant concerned, may consider it valuable to have a further talk with the complainant. If this fails or it is thought there is no useful purpose in further meetings, then the third stage of the procedure is put into effect. The Regional Director of Public Health then, after discussion with the consultant, seeks the names of two independent consultants from the Joint Consultants Committee of the British Medical Association nationally. These independent consultants will be in active practice in the appropriate specialty and at least one, and usually both, would be from outside the region concerned. They will conduct an Independent Professional Review. This involves a visit to the hospital concerned to discuss the case with the consultant against whom the complaint was lodged, and any other staff involved, and there will be access to the clinical records. The independent consultants also discuss the complaint at first hand with the complainant, who may be accompanied by relatives or friends (complainants, especially at this stage, are encouraged to seek help and advice from their local Community Health Council). They then make their independent report in confidence to the Regional Director of Public Health who advises the local manager, who in turn writes formally to the complainant on behalf of the hospital or health authority.

The third stage procedure involving independent professional review is intended for complaints of a substantial nature involving clinical judgement, but not those which would appear to be the subject of action through the courts or by the more formal procedure of the health authority.

Whilst this procedure allows a thorough and searching investigation of a serious complaint, it has a number of disadvantages. Firstly, it is often very lengthy. From the time of the initial complaint to the receipt of the result of the Independent

Professional Review by the complainant it will take several months and often longer. Secondly, a complaints system in which doctors investigate other doctors, no matter how impartial in practice, is not one which will enjoy the confidence of the complainant as to its genuine independence.

Moreover, the production of the report by the independent consultants following the Independent Professional Review, marks the conclusion of the clinical complaints procedure and there is no mechanism under which the complainant can contest the findings of the report should he or she disagree with them. However, if a complainant is dissatisfied with the administrative handling of his or her complaint by a health authority, then he or she may refer the matter to the Health Service Commissioner.

There is little doubt that poor communication is a main and recurring theme in complaints made about health care. This situation can only be remedied by greater emphasis on high standards of communication by all health professionals (which in some cases will require changes of attitude as well as increased awareness of the problem) and inclusion of the teaching of communication skills to those in training.

Many of the more serious complaints involve patients who have died. Practical experience of dealing with complainants suggests that better and more sensitive bereavement counselling at the time of death could resolve matters which subsequently become manifest as complaints. Complaints of a more serious nature which are considered to be unsuitable for action by the health authority's officers are dealt with by more formal means which may involve setting up a committee of inquiry.

Family health services complaints procedure

Complaints made by the public to the family health services authority (FHSA) concerning the family practitioner service (medical, dental, pharmaceutical and ophthalmic) can be made orally or in writing. The time limit for receipt of complaints varies for the profession involved.

Complaints made against a general medical or other practitioner can be dealt with informally through a process of conciliation or formally through a so-called 'Service Committee'.

Many complaints made to the FHSA are resolved informally, sometimes with the help of a lay conciliator appointed by the authority who may interview both the complainant and the practitioner as part of the process of resolving the complaint.

Complainants who remain dissatisfied after the informal procedure can have their complaint dealt with by formal investigation (Service Committee). Certain types of complaint are dealt with by the formal investigation in the first place. Under this procedure, the Chairman of the Service Committee first considers the complaint and may seek further information. He or she may consider that there are no grounds for thinking that the practitioner has breached terms of service and may report to the FHSA accordingly. Alternatively, the decision may be taken to progress the complaint within the Service Committee, often with a hearing at which the complainant, the practitioner and (possibly) witnesses may attend. A complainant may be assisted in presenting his or her case to a Service Committee (a Community Health Council officer will often assist).

In all cases involving a Service Committee investigation of a complaint, the complainant and the practitioner are sent a copy of the report. Complainants have a right of appeal to the Secretary of State for Health.

The Service Committee comprises professional and lay people. Essentially the procedure deals with alleged breaches of terms of service (or contract) by practitioners. Inevitably many hearings of Service Committees within FHSAs do stray into issues of clinical judgement since this may be necessary in order to decide whether a breach of terms of service has occurred.

Complaints made about practitioners contracted to FHSAs usually fall into one of three main groups: technical; financial and those related to service delivery. The last of these may be further sub-divided into those concerned with organisation of care or the process of delivery of care.

Examples of technical breaches would include prescribing on the National Health Service prescription form (FP10) drugs or appliances that should not be prescribed; failure to notify the FHSA about surgery times or prolonged absence; failure to make satisfactory deputising arrangements and failure to issue medical certificates.

Allegations about financial breaches of terms of service commonly relate to improper acceptance of fees for certificates that should be provided free at the point of delivery under the terms of service, or services for which patients registered under the National Health Service should not be charged. Questions relating to false claims for payment may also be investigated under the Service Committee procedures and in extreme circumstances may be referred for investigation by the police and charges brought.

Examples of breaches of terms of service relating to defects in the organisation of the delivery of care would include messages, such as a request to visit, failing to reach the doctor; failure to refer to hospital or specialist services because arrangements are not made, or a positive test result being mislaid or not acted upon.

A number of breaches occur as a result of deficiences in the process of the delivery of care. The commonest of these is failure to visit a patient at home. Whilst general practitioners do not have a contractual obligation to visit any patient at home at their request, they do have to visit if the patient's medical condition warrants this. Allegations about failure to visit usually succeed because the doctor, by not visiting the patient, has failed to put himself or herself in a position to make an adequate clinical judgement about the patient's medical condition.

The other main group of complaints that usually succeed do so on the basis of the doctor failing to provide appropriate or necessary medical services, usually meaning urgent referral or admission to hospital. The doctor found in breach will have failed to put himself or herself in a position to recognise significant symptoms of signs, or, having recognised them, failed to act expeditiously on them.

The greatest number of complaints made to FHSAs about family practitioner services relate to issues of attitude or behaviour of professional staff. The Terms of Service do not govern such issues and cannot be investigated under the Service Committee procedure. FHSAs make use of informal processes to address and resolve them.

In cases where a breach of terms of service is deemed to have occurred, a number of options are open to the FHSA:

- Warn the doctor to comply more closely with his or her terms of service in the future but take no further action.
- Make a financial withholding of payments due to the doctor.
- Refer the doctor to the National Health Service Tribunal for consideration of continuing fitness to practice. This would be an option normally required in circumstances of repeated breaches of sufficient magnitude to call into question the effect on patient safety if the doctor remained on the NHS medical list. The Tribunal cannot disqualify the doctor from practising outside the NHS.
- Refer the doctor to the General Medical Council (GMC). In severe cases of professional misconduct or incompetence the GMC may suspend or disqualify the doctor from practising. This would include both NHS and non-NHS practice.
- Use a combination of these actions.

Health service commissioner (Ombudsman)

An independent Health Service Commissioner (Ombudsman) is appointed by Parliament. This official has powers to investigate complaints from members of the public who consider that they have suffered injustice as a result of a failure in a service provided by a health authority or a hospital, or failure to offer a service it has a duty to provide, or other examples of maladministration. He or she reports directly to Parliament.

There are, however, a number of circumstances in which the Commissioner is precluded from carrying out an investigation. Examples of these are purely clinical matters, professional services provided by doctors and others, staff appointments and if the aggrieved person has taken proceedings to a court of law.

A member of the public must always complain first to the responsible health service organisation before referring the matter to the Commissioner. Many complaints relate to waiting time for hospital treatment, lack of communication from health professionals to patients and relatives, failures in services, poor handling of complaints themselves or the administration or management of health services. The Health Service Commissioner produces an annual report in which he comments on the issues which have been reported to him and which he has investigated. He also produces regular anonymised reports of selected investigations.

Courts

A patient has recourse to the courts of law where he or she may allege clinical negligence. Settlements are often made out of court and this is the main route of complaint through which he or she can obtain financial retribution. This is an increasingly common route for complainants in Britain, and is a major feature of medical practice in the United States of America where patients are much more litigation-minded and doctors are inclined to plan their clinical management in a way which is least likely to lead to litigation, even if it may not be the best approach to a particular clinical problem (so called 'defensive medicine').

Community Health Councils

Community Health Councils (CHCs) represent the views of the consumers to health authorities and, although not directly involved with individual complaints, act as the official watchdog for the local community, inevitably receiving adverse comments. They have no duty to investigate complaints but will usually advise a complainant about which procedure to follow and may attend with him or her at the hearings of complaints.

Each Council is made up of members with a particular interest in the health services. Half are appointed by the local authorities, one-third by voluntary organisations and one-sixth by the RHA. Although no upper or lower limit for membership is set, a total of 18–24 members would normally ensure an appropriate representation of local interest.

There is a CHC for the area covered by each district health authority (a few have two) and its basic job is to represent the interests of the public in each health district. Councils have right of access to public information, have the right to visit hospitals and other institutions and have access to health authorities, in particular, to the senior officers managing services.

District health authorities are expected to consult CHCs when making plans for service developments, particularly where proposals involve important changes affecting the public (for example, the closure of a hospital or change of use of facilities). The district health authority meets formally with its Community Health Council at least once a year. In addition, less formal meetings take place between the authority's members and officers and the CHC's representatives. CHCs publish annual reports and the district health authorities are required to publish replies to reports, stating action taken on specific issues contained in them.

Health Advisory Service

This service was formed following an unfavourable report on conditions in a mental hospital in Wales in 1969. A description of it is included at this point in the chapter to illustrate another way in which professional standards are reviewed and improved.

The Health Advisory Service focuses on a number of service areas in particular: mental health problems, the elderly, the elderly mentally ill, children and adolescents with mental health problems as well as drug and alcohol misuse. It carries out its function through a Director and a small number of full-time staff. However, extensive use is made of senior professional and managerial staff (from within the health service) who work on a temporary or part-time basis to assist the Health Advisory Service with particular initiatives. Such initiatives may be in the form of thematic reviews of a particular issue (for example, the quality of child and adolescent psychiatry services), an advisory role to health authorities on the development of a particular service (for example, day care for the elderly) or a trouble-shooting function (for example, where there are problems or concerns about standards of care in a unit for the mentally ill).

The Audit Commission

The Audit Commission is a body which has overall responsibility for the external financial audit of all local authorities as well as the National Health Service in England and Wales.

Part of its role involves ensuring the best use of the public funds which are allocated to the authorities concerned. In addition to examining the way in which

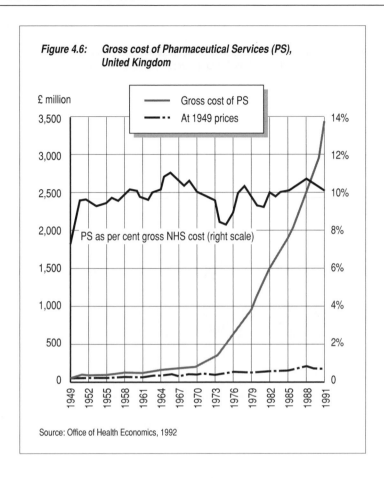

Figure 4.6:   Gross cost of Pharmaceutical Services (PS),
               United Kingdom

Source: Office of Health Economics, 1992

funds are used within individual authorities, the Commission also undertakes regular reviews of specific subjects and makes recommendations which particularly focus on value for money issues. Say, for example, the Audit Commission has examined the use of acute hospital beds, day case surgery, and community care. The usual method of conducting these reviews is for the Commission's staff to study services in a number of parts of the country and draw up a report based on its findings. Health authorities are then encouraged to examine the implications for their local services in the light of the Commission's report and implement changes as necessary.

PRESCRIBING AND THE USE OF MEDICINES

Prescribing of medicines is one of the main interventions used in the delivery of health care. Medicine usage accounts for a substantial proportion of the health service's budget each year (Figure 4.6).

A range of data are available to enable trends in general practice prescribing to be examined. They are provided by the Prescription Pricing Authority which

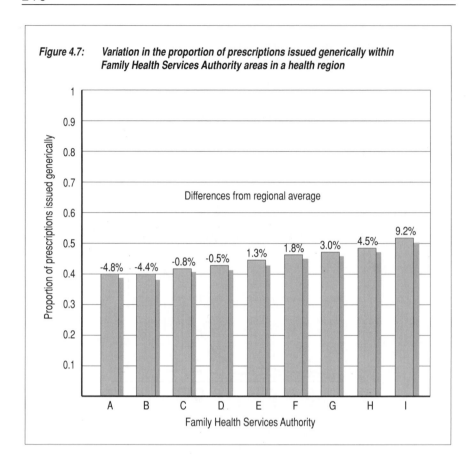

Figure 4.7:   Variation in the proportion of prescriptions issued generically within Family Health Services Authority areas in a health region

analyses prescriptions written by general practitioners. Analysis of such data allows comparisons of medicine usage between general practices and family health services authorities in a number of key respects, for example, the number of prescriptions written, the net ingredient cost and the therapeutic class of drug used. The presentation and discussion of such comparative data allows the quality of prescribing as well as the use of resources to be explored which ultimately potentially benefits patient care (Figure 4.7). Similar data are not routinely collected nationally to allow prescribing and medicine usage in hospitals to be examined. However, most hospitals now have computer-based systems for issuing drugs to wards and clinics and these enable patterns of medicine usage to be examined at a local level.

The National Health Service and Community Care Act 1990 introduced new arrangements for the monitoring and management of medicine usage in primary care through the Indicative Prescribing Scheme. Under this scheme, each general practice must set an indicative prescribing amount which is a non-cash limited estimate of each practice's annual prescribing needs. The scheme enables targets to be set for more rational prescribing and enhances opportunities for greater efficiency in the use of resources.

The control of medicines

With the increase of new pharmaceutical products in recent years there has been growing concern about the safety and side-effects of medicines.

The legal basis for monitoring and control of therapies for both human and animal use is the Medicines Act 1968, which brought together a number of previous pieces of legislation. Since the Act originally came into force regulations, orders and information leaflets have been issued by government departments on various aspects of the control of medicines.

Under the Act responsibility for control of medicines is vested in the 'Licensing Authority' which is, in effect, the Secretary of State for Health, acting on behalf of all United Kingdom Health Ministers. The controls have a wide variety of aspects. A licensing system governs the development, marketing, manufacture, import and wholesale distribution of 'medicinal products'. Criteria are laid down for what constitutes a medicinal product and powers exist to extend the definition. This has already been carried out for many substances, for example, in relation to surgical suture material, dental fillings and contact lenses. The licensing system also covers the issue of new medicinal products for the purposes of conducting clinical trials to evaluate a new therapy in human beings. Medical and dental practitioners are exempt from the licensing procedure in so far as they still have freedom to prescribe unlicensed products for individual patients. The question will hardly ever arise since the majority of practitioners will be prescribing medicinal products which ultimately derive from a manufacturer or supplier which will itself hold a licence under the regulations. However a doctor or dentist may import a medicinal product without licence provided that it is to treat a specific patient and not to build up a stock for general usage. He or she may also manufacture (make up) an unlicensed medicine for an individual patient and maintain a small stock. The use of unlicensed products is rare in general practice, but much more frequent in hospital medicine because of clinical trials and other specialised patient needs.

Aside from licensing, other aspects of control include registration of pharmacies, promotion and advertising (both to the medical profession and the public), post-marketing safety surveillance, and labelling of packages and containers. The Medicines Act makes no provision for regulating the price of medicines or their availability under the National Health Service. The licensing process is concerned solely with quality, safety, efficacy and it does not take into account factors such as the clinical need for the new medicine or relative efficacy between drugs with similar safety profiles. Indeed, consideration of these issues as part of the licensing process would be unlawful under European Community directives on medicines licensing. Instead, the Secretary of State for Health controls prices through the Pharmaceutical Price Regulation Scheme (PPRS) which is a voluntary agreement between the Government and the major pharmaceutical companies operating in the United Kingdom. In addition, the availability of and reimbursement for, medicines prescribed in the National Health Service is regulated by the National Health Service Act 1977. The Secretary of State for Health administers this control machinery through the Medicines Control Agency (MCA) of the Department of Health which is staffed by doctors, pharmacists, scientists, lawyers as well as administrative and clerical staff.

The Medicines Control Agency's main functions include:

- Direct involvement with all aspects of licensing, both of medicinal products and of manufacturing and wholesale facilities.
- Providing an inspectorate to make sure that the Act is enforced.
- Monitoring and reporting adverse reactions to medicinal products (together with the Committee on the Safety of Medicines).
- International liaison, particularly through the World Health Organisation and the European Community.

The Act allowed for the establishment of a Medicines Commission. Members from the relevant professions are appointed by the Secretary of State for Health and advise him or her in relation to the execution of the Act. Upon the recommendation of this Commission, the Secretary of State has established a range of expert committees to provide advisory functions on specific topics (for example, the Committee on Safety of Medicines, CSM). Many of these standing committees have themselves established expert subcommittees to deal with individual aspects of their overall responsibility, for example, the CSM's subcommittees on safety and efficacy and on pharmacovigilance.

A particularly important role of the Committee on Safety of Medicines and the Medicines Control Agency is to involve members of the medical profession directly in the process of detecting untoward reactions from drugs. This is undertaken through the 'yellow card' system, whereby individual medical practitioners can report, in strict confidence, a suspected adverse reaction in an individual patient. The Committee on Safety of Medicines maintains a confidential register of such information that it has obtained from this and other sources. This database contains more than 300,000 adverse drug reaction reports and constitutes a major source of information on drug safety. Anonymised analyses from the register are available to health professionals on request.

In response to drug safety information received through yellow cards or from other sources, the Licensing Authority has powers to revoke a product licence or to suspend the licence for a period of three months. When such regulatory action has been taken, it becomes unlawful for anyone to promote the use of that medicine (although its use by a practitioner in individual patients is still legally permissible). Alternatively, the product licence may be varied and the manufacturer required to issue new data sheets with revised dosage, contraindications, or precautions. An example of the value of this system of reporting is provided by the events which led (in August 1982) to the suspension of the anti-inflammatory drug Opren (benoxaprofen). The Committee on Safety of Medicines had received more than 3500 reports of adverse reactions to the drug, including 61 deaths, mainly in the elderly, when the suspension of the product licence was made (initially for three months) under the terms of the Medicines Act, 1968. More recently, the anticholinergic drug, Terodiline, was voluntarily withdrawn from the market by its manufacturer, after the United Kingdom yellow card system had revealed an association with serious cardiac arrhythmias.

Information and quality in prescribing

The doctor actually carrying out the prescribing, whether based in hospital or in general practice, has a number of channels through which to learn about the efficacy of various alternative therapies, and their potential hazards and side-effects:

(a) *From pharmaceutical companies:* either directly from medical representatives of the companies concerned, via advertising in medical journals or by advertising literature mailed to him.

As this is the major source by which medical practitioners acquire information about medical products and because of the large sums of money at stake in the drug industry, there has been concern about the potential for pharmaceutical companies to make unjustified or misleading claims about the efficacy of their products. Control on standards in advertising to the professions is maintained through regulations issued in accordance with the Medicines Act 1968. Aside from these safeguards, the system of data sheets is also an attempt to prevent biased information about a product being put across to a practitioner. It is a legal requirement that within the preceding 15 months before any advertisement or promotion (either written or oral) of a product is undertaken, a standard data sheet must be sent to the practitioner setting out objectively full details about the product. In addition to this, a Data Sheet Compendium is published by the Association of the British Pharmaceutical Industry (ABPI) and mailed free of charge to all medical practitioners and pharmacists. It contains data sheets from many of the products on the market, so that details of dosage, route of administration, contra-indication, markings, side-effects and other details are available in one volume. The ABPI also operates a voluntary code of conduct which covers promotion of medicines by its member companies. Breaches of the code are investigated by the ABPI's Code of Practice Committee, to which health professionals can refer complaints. Another publication which contains brief data on many drugs and is produced by a commercial organisation and sent regularly to doctors is the Monthly Index of Medical Specialties (MIMS). This also contains advertising material.

(b) *Drug Information Service:* most health authorities provide a hospital-based service staffed by pharmacists with special expertise to maintain and provide information on drugs and medicines from a number of different perspectives including indications, relative merits, efficacy, side-effects, safety and costs. This impartial advice or information is open to all medical practitioners, pharmacists and other relevant professionals working within the district.

(c) *British National Formulary (BNF)*: this is produced by the medical and pharmaceutical professions and is brought up-to-date and sent without charge to doctors and pharmacists within the National Health Service every six months. It is orientated towards the treatment of specific disorders and thus provides an impartial opinion on indications for, and the relative merits of, various alternative therapies.

(d) *The medical literature:* articles in the medical journals will report clinical trials of new or existing therapies for particular conditions, as well as reporting potential side-effects. Some more specialised journals deal specifically with prescribing.

(e) *Postgraduate education or training:* in the course of study for postgraduate examinations or through attendances at lectures and seminars many practitioners will keep abreast of recent developments in therapeutics.

There is increasing emphasis on seeking ways to improve the quality and cost-effectiveness of prescribing through education programmes, publications, drug information services and audit of drug therapy. Audit may be performed on a 'macro' scale, through drug utilisation review (DUR) in which patterns of prescribing and outcomes of drug therapy are studied in populations. DUR was pioneered in Scandinavia and the United States of America, and is now developing rapidly in the United Kingdom and the remainder of Europe.

A complementary approach is the review of drug therapy for effectiveness, safety, cost-utility and patient convenience in individual patients. This is increasingly seen as an integral component of the clinical audit process at patient, practice or hospital level.

Safety

Before a drug receives a product licence the Licensing Authority must be satisfied that it is safe in relation to its intended use. This is a relative judgement. For example, a new anticancer drug or an antiviral agent for use in AIDS would be permitted to exhibit more frequent or serious toxicities than a new addition to the penicillin group of antibiotics. Information on safety of new drugs is generated through a range of animal studies including carcinogenicity, mutagenicity and reproductive toxicity in several species. Appropriate standards of chemical and pharmaceutical quality must also be achieved. After appropriate animal testing, new drugs are introduced into clinical use through a continuous process of clinical development that is conventionally divided into four phases. Phase 1 studies constitute first use in man, where the clinical pharmacology of the drug is invest- igated in small numbers of healthy volunteers or patients. Phase 2 studies comprise clinical investigation for efficacy and safety in larger numbers of patients, typically 200–300. Phase 3 studies are formal randomised clinical trials on a substantive scale, in up to more than 1,000 patients. Phase 4 studies, also known as post-licens- ing studies or post-marketing surveillance (PMS) consist of further surveillance, particularly for safety, in large populations after the drug has been launched.

Adverse reactions to drugs can be broadly sub-divided into two groups. Type A (augmented) reactions are exaggerated responses to the drug's normal pharmaco- logical reaction, for example, bradycardia with beta-blocking drugs. They are common, predictable, usually dose-related, and rarely fatal. Type B (bizarre) reactions are unrelated to the drug's normal actions, usually not dose-related, and uncommon. However, they are often serious and may carry a high mortality, for example, hepatorenal syndrome caused by benoxaprofen, or oculomucocutaneous syndrome caused by practolol. Much effort in adverse reactions monitoring and post-marketing surveillance is therefore directed at identifying and avoiding Type B reactions.

RESOURCES FOR THE HEALTH SERVICE

The health service in Britain represents a major area of Government expenditure. This section of the chapter describes how the finances of the health service are determined and deployed. In addition to financial resources, there are three other major elements of the health services resources, its staff, its estate and its information.

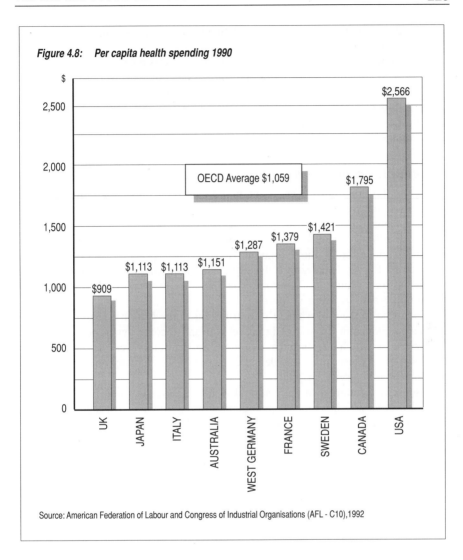

Figure 4.8: Per capita health spending 1990

OECD Average $1,059

UK	$909	
JAPAN	$1,113	
ITALY	$1,113	
AUSTRALIA	$1,151	
WEST GERMANY	$1,287	
FRANCE	$1,379	
SWEDEN	$1,421	
CANADA	$1,795	
USA	$2,566	

Source: American Federation of Labour and Congress of Industrial Organisations (AFL - C10),1992

Financial resources

Trends in health service expenditure

In its first full year of operation, the National Health Service cost approximately £10 per head of population but by the early 1990s, it had increased to over £500 per head. Over the same period the proportion of the Gross Domestic Product (GDP) dedicated to health care increased from 4% to over 5.7%. Spending on health care varies greatly between different countries of the world (Figure 4.8).

The extent to which spending on health services changes over time is determined by a number of factors including demographic changes (for example, the proportion of elderly people in the population will have a major effect on expenditure because they are an age group with a high level of need for services), advances in medical technology, inflation within the economy and inflation within the health service system (determined by pay rises to health service workers and rising drug and equipment costs).

It is important to remember that the health service is a cash limited service so that any increasing need for expenditure has to be contained within the available resources. In effect this means that priorities have to be determined between different types of service and at times this can cause great difficulty and public concern, especially in situations where individual patients are seen to be disadvantaged by not having the services they require.

Allocation of funds to the National Health Service at national level

Each year, the Government decides upon the size of the allocation of money to the National Health Service and other public expenditure programmes (for example, Defence, Education, Transport, Social Security).

This decision is made between Ministers of the various Departments of State and the Chancellor of the Exchequer as part of a process called the Public Expenditure Survey (PES) and is usually made public in the Chancellor's Autumn Statement to the House of Commons. The PES allocations cover the financial year which runs from 1 April to 31 March.

In addition to the Government's contribution to the National Health Service, it also receives income from cost improvement and income generation schemes in the service for which targets and assumptions are set. It receives income from other sources such as prescription and dental charges and fees paid by private patients in National Health Service hospitals.

Resources committed to the National Health Service fall into two broad categories: *revenue* which is money spent on day-to-day running costs such as medical and non-medical staff, drugs and other consumables and *capital* which describes money spent on items such as buildings or equipment. On this basis, the allocations are made by the National Health Service Management Executive within the Department of Health to lower tiers of the service in the following main categories.

Revenue for hospital, community health and primary care services. Revenue is allocated to each regional health authority (and to special health authorities) in England to cover the cost of the purchasing of hospital, community health and primary care services for patients as well as to fund the management and other costs of securing a comprehensive range of health care.

The size of each regional health authority's share of this national allocation is determined on the basis of the region's population size adjusted by age profile, local standardised mortality ratios and in the Thames regions some geographical weightings in and around London.

Capital allocations. The main purpose of the capital allocation is to fund hospital building or development programmes within the regions. Each region will have a capital programme designed to replace, modernise and repair its existing stock of hospitals and equipment. These capital programmes have a long time span because the stages between planning a new hospital development to becoming fully operational can be many years and a reasonable degree of financial certainty is required if these plans are to be properly made.

Allocation of funds to operational service level

The allocation received by regional health authorities from the Department of Health forms the basis of the onward transmission of funds to operational levels of the Service. Regional health authorities make their allocations in a number of broad categories which are described in this section.

District Health Authority allocations. District health authorities need funds at the beginning of each financial year to enable them to purchase services for their populations.

These funds are allocated by the regional health authority to its constituent district health authorities on the basis of a *weighted capitation* calculation. The basis of the allocation is per head of population with adjustments being made for factors such as age and mortality (as a proxy for morbidity) which will affect the need and demand for health services. Regions have some discretion in determining their own sub-regional allocation formula but these must be broadly on the same basis as the national formula for allocations by the Department of Health to RHAs.

General practice fundholder allocations. Regional health authorities allocate funds to general practice fundholders to purchase hospital services, community services, drugs and to fund practice staff.

Family Health Services Authorities allocations. Family health services expenditure is largely on services provided by its contractors (general medical and dental practitioners, ophthalmic opticians, pharmacists) and is not cash limited. This means that the funding requirements of family doctors, dentists and other contractors will be met even if they exceed forecast levels although there is an expectation that they will remain within financial balance. Expenditure on general medical services (GMS) which covers practice staff and premises and family health services authority management costs is cash limited.

Human resources

The most important asset of a service industry like the health service, is the people it employs (Table 4.2). Either directly, or indirectly, they are the means through which the patients or consumers of health services receive the help they need.

The health service has traditionally employed a wide range of professional staff. Doctors, nurses, physiotherapists, clinical psychologists, occupational therapists are examples but there are many others. In addition, there are many groups of staff which perform specialist technical jobs: for example, medical physicists and information technologists. During the 1980s and early 1990s, there was much greater emphasis on general management posts and management posts in relation to specialist functions such as finance and personnel. Finally, a further group of staff essential to the efficient and effective running of the service is the very wide range of personnel providing an infrastructure of support to other levels of the service, for example: drivers, porters, catering staff, ward clerks, records officers, medical secretaries, engineers, laboratory technicians, public relations officers.

Table 4.2:   **National Health Service directly employed staff by main group, England 1990**

Staff group	Number	Percentage
Nursing and Midwifery	463,790	48.9
Administrative and Clerical (including management)	155,720	16.4
Ancillary	132,650	14.0
Medical and Dental	58,120	6.2
Professional, Scientific and Technical	53,290	5.6
Professions allied to Medicine	45,600	4.8
Ambulance	18,890	2.0
Maintenance	16,040	1.7
Works	3,910	0.4
Total	948,010	100

Medical staff

There are three main categories of doctors employed within the health service. They are those working in specialist areas of clinical practice (mainly within hospitals or in the community); those who are general practitioners; and those who are working within the field of public health medicine.

A career in hospital medicine is the first choice of about half the graduates of British Medical Schools. Most young men or women embarking on such a career will have, as their ultimate goal, a consultant post in one of the clinical specialties. Before they reach this point, all will have completed a structured programme of training.

The distribution of medical posts within the various training grades is controlled on a national basis to ensure, firstly, that there are sufficient doctors available to fill posts at different levels and, secondly, to create sufficient opportunities for progression to their substantive career post (for example, consultant in the hospital service).

A key feature of British medical education is the emphasis on postgraduate and continuing medical education for qualified doctors to carry on from the undergraduate teaching they receive while medical students.

This approach is supported by a specific organisational infrastructure for postgraduate and continuing medical education in each region. In each, there is a Postgraduate Dean (sometimes called Director of Postgraduate Medical Education) who is responsible for establishing overall educational objectives and ensuring that they are achieved. Similar Postgraduate Deans cover dental postgraduate training.

For the hospital service, the Regional Postgraduate Dean is supported by a network of Clinical Tutors for each local service, who are part-time appointees and almost invariably members of the consultant staff in the hospital concerned. Clinical Tutors are responsible for organising local education programmes in line with the overall objectives set by the Regional Postgraduate Dean. They hold budgets and are responsible for manning the Postgraduate Centre (which is a feature of most large hospitals).

The Regional Postgraduate Dean's professional support is different for the general practice side of the service. Here, there is a specific Regional Adviser for

General Practice who is accountable to the Postgraduate Dean and who works through an infrastructure of Associate Advisers (or General Practice Clinical Tutors) who are responsible for organising and implementing training programmes at local practice level. The different structure of postgraduate education and training for general practice, with the essential feature of vocational training schemes means that there is a more extensive network of general practitioners with designated organisational roles at local level (for example, Vocational Training Scheme Organisers and Trainers in individual practices).

The Regional Postgraduate Dean is a joint appointee between the regional health authority and its corresponding university. He or she holds and manages the budget for postgraduate medical and dental education in the region, has administrative support provided to discharge this role and is advised by a Regional Medical and Dental Education Committee. Another essential ingredient to the organisation of postgraduate medical education is maintaining high standards in its delivery. The Royal Colleges have an important role in this respect. The Colleges (and Faculties) discharge their role in a wide variety of ways but particularly in terms of formulating training programmes for their specialty or clinical discipline and inspecting posts to grant them recognition for training purposes. Each Royal College or Faculty has one or more Regional Advisers who advise the College nationally, as well as advising the Regional Postgraduate Dean and the regional health authority, on training matters for their specialty.

Public Health Medicine

In addition to doctors working in hospital and in general practice, the medical workforce of the National Health Service also comprises public health doctors. The specialty of public health medicine (formerly called 'community medicine') is entered as part of a structured programme of postgraduate medical training. Training involves in-service and academic components. Trainees sit a two part examination leading to Membership of the Faculty of Public Health Medicine of the Royal College of Physicians of the United Kingdom.

A number of consultant-level posts exist for doctors who have satisfactorily completed training in public health medicine. Directors of Public Health are the senior public health doctors of district and regional authorities in England (the titles of health authorities and of the senior public health doctors differ in Scotland and Northern Ireland). They form part of the health authority's senior management team and head a department of public health medicine within the authority.

There are also posts of Consultants in Public Health Medicine. They, too, are based within health authority departments of public health. Some public health doctors specialise in communicable disease control and where this is the case they may be appointed to posts as Consultants in Communicable Disease Control (see also chapter 9). Other public health doctors work within academic institutions such as medical schools where they major on teaching and research and usually have honorary contracts with health authorities to undertake public health duties within the National Health Service.

Within the health service, the role of departments of public health and the doctors who staff them differs from place to place. However, in the majority the work will encompass health needs assessment in the population, disease surveillance and control, the design of health promotion programmes and advising the health authority on a wide range of health policy and public health matters. Each Director of Public Health is required to produce an Annual Report on the Health of the Population in his or her locality. Such reports vary in format but will usually draw attention to the main health problems and issues as well as making recommendations for action.

The estate

A major element of the resources of the health service is its estate: the buildings, land, plant and equipment from which services are delivered. The management of the resources which make up the estate is a complex and wide-ranging process. It involves the deployment of existing capital assets to meet service needs and strategic decisions about new investments. The planning and building of new hospitals is itself a complex process and includes the establishment of an initial business case, detailed planning and design, acquiring land, procurement, construction and commissioning.

Management of the estate also involves maintenance and renewal of building machinery and equipment. It involves ensuring that rigorous safety standards are met and, increasingly it involves addressing environmental issues (such as energy consumption and waste management).

Information

The fourth element of the health services resources, information, is considered in chapter 1.

SERVICES PROVIDED BY LOCAL GOVERNMENT

Local authority services, particularly education, environmental health, housing and personal social services, have an important bearing on the NHS.

Organisation of local government

The population of each county and district elects representatives (councillors) to the Parliamentary Franchise (virtually everyone over the age of 18 can vote). The full Council of a local authority (either county or district) consists of all elected councillors and acts as a corporate body with responsibility for providing services in a locality. It elects a chairman, who in some authorities is known as the 'Mayor'. In order to discharge its functions the Council defines its duties and divides into service-orientated committees, each of which elects a chairman. It is a statutory requirement to establish committees for education, social services and the police. Aside from these it is for each Council to decide which other committees it thinks necessary.

The structure of local government in England and Wales is a complex one. Since major re-organisation in 1974, most areas have two main tiers of local government, District and County Councils, between which the designated functions of local government are divided. Thus in these areas, County Councils have responsibility for issues such as education, social services and policing while the districts manage such services as Housing and Environmental Health.

The exceptions to this arrangement are the metropolitan areas where so called 'unitary' authorities exist which contain the functions of both District and County Authorities.

In 1991 the Government announced the formation of a Local Government Commission which was charged with devising a new configuration for local government in England and Wales. Whilst it was charged with looking at the most appropriate configuration in each area, Ministers made it clear that the concept of unitary authorities would be expected to be recommended for most areas on the grounds of reducing duplication and improving communication. The likely result of the Commission's work will be dramatically to re-model the face of local government as it exists today.

Within both County and unitary authorities, a number of Chief Officers are appointed to head departments and provide the services for which they are responsible. In local government the chief officer is a manager of all staff in his or her department, irrespective of their discipline. Local authorities are free by statute to determine the numbers and categories of staff they appoint to carry out their functions, although they must appoint a Chief Education Officer, a Director of Social Services and a Chief Constable (if these officers are appropriate to the duties of the Council). The chief officer of the department is then responsible to a committee of elected members. The Director of Social Services for example is responsible to the Social Services Committee.

Council and Committee meetings are required by law to allow the public and press access to council affairs. To ensure co-ordination between departments, most authorities form their chief officers into corporate management teams under the chairmanship of a Chief Executive officer.

This management team considers matters concerning the authority as a whole, not just individual departments and usually reports to a major committee which has responsibility for policy and resources.

Local government derives its powers to provide services from Statute Law. Legislation can be either mandatory (making it a duty) or permissive (giving powers which can be used at discretion). Even the mandatory legislation is written in general terms so that there is scope for interpretation tailored to local needs. The result is a wide variation in the quality and quantity of services provided by different authorities throughout the country.

Local authorities are empowered to raise money from a local tax to finance their annual expenditure, but this has in recent years amounted to an ever smaller proportion of local government's financial requirements (in the early 1990s around one quarter of their expenditure). The rest comes from central government through a system known as the revenue support grant. It is calculated using a complex formula (the 'Standard Spending Assessment') which takes into account various factors, including population characteristics (proportion of children, old people and number receiving services). Central government has the potential to reduce the grant if it finds that a local authority acts in defiance of some important policy matter or that a local authority has not been effective and efficient in its provision of services. While the use of these default powers is rare, it is also possible for central government to control local government expenditure by capping the level of local taxation. During the late 1980s and early 1990s these 'charge capping' powers were used with ever-increasing frequency.

Organisation of social services departments

The Local Authority Social Services Act 1970 required local authorities to establish social services departments. Much of this legislative basis arose from the Report of the Committee on Local Authority and Allied Personal Social Services, chaired by Sir Frederic (later Lord) Seebohm, which presented its recommendations in 1968. This report made wide-ranging proposals, suggesting that social services should be family-orientated and community-based and that more needed to be done for the under fives, elderly people, those with physical and mental disabilities and the 'neglected flotsam and jetsam of society'. People, it considered, should be treated as individuals rather than categorised into groups based on age or type. It also concluded that the service in general should be better organised. Thus, the 1970 Act incorporated the recommendations in the Report to integrate the many social work functions and establish social services departments. Welfare and children's departments, parts of the health departments of local governments as well as social workers in hospitals came under a unified administrative structure. Social workers in education and housing departments were not included, neither were probation officers.

The National Health Service and Community Care Act 1990 and the Children Act 1989 together set out a new agenda for Social Services Departments in the 1990s. The main responsibilities of social services departments are to provide protection for children in need, and to meet broader social care needs by arranging the provision of residential, day and domiciliary care services and respite care. A new emphasis was placed on developing a policy of care in the community. This requires social services departments to enable people who have problems associated with ageing, disability or mental health to live in their own homes wherever feasible and sensible. Social services departments are able, unlike health authorities, to charge clients for the services they receive and they are also empowered to assess an individual's ability to pay. These charges vary from authority to authority as they are, at least in part, dependent upon local decision.

The services provided by social services departments to individual groups in society who are potentially vulnerable: people with physical and learning disabilities, older people, children in need and the families of all these groups are described in detail elsewhere, but an overview of the structure and function of a social services department is given here. It should be remembered that there is variation amongst individual local authorities in the way in which these services have been organised and indeed in the actual services which are provided.

Legally, the Director of Social Services is the Chief officer of the department. The post is held by a person with managerial experience as befits an executive of an organisation with a budget of millions of pounds. Until recently this person was also invariably qualified as a social worker. While this is still normally the case, a trend has been established in recent years to place greater emphasis on the managerial as opposed to the social work attributes of the candidates for such posts.

Consequently an increasing number of Directors are not holders of social work professional qualifications.

Traditionally structured departments often have a Deputy Director and a third tier of Assistant Directors who have responsibility for functional divisions. There is a considerable variation in the way in which these divisions are defined and financed in different localities. However, typical divisions might be given separate responsibility for residential and day care, domiciliary support services (for example, home help service, meals on wheels), administration and training, finance and research. As social services departments work responded to the implications of the final stage of the implementation of the NHS and Community Care Act in 1993, such structures became modified to reflect an increasing separation of direct service provision from assessment and the commissioning of care services.

Organisational structures of social services are not uniform around the country. For example there has been effective merging of Housing and Social Services Departments in several of the London Boroughs. More radical still, some unitary authorities have sought to restructure on the basis of an abolition of the departmental structure (though as mentioned above certain designated Directors are legally required) and its replacement with a series of functionally based sections (for example, an 'Assessment' section which would be the point of entry for all local authority services such as housing, social services, education). Given this increasing diversity, coupled with the re-definition of local authorities structure and functions resulting from the Local Government Commission, no 'typical' structure of a social services department can currently be described.

At a lower level in the organisation, the day-to-day provision of care to people in the community has traditionally been carried out on a geographical basis through 'local teams' of social workers and support staff who are the main route through which problems are first channelled. These teams vary in remit depending on the structure of the department with many being geared to the needs of one particular 'client group' (for example, children and families, mental illness, physical handicap, learning disabilities). Often two or three teams are combined to form an area organisation controlled by a manager with a title such as area director or sector manager.

Care in the community

The community care component of legislation introduced in the early 1990s set out six key objectives for service delivery:

- To promote the development of domiciliary, day and respite services to enable people to live in their own homes wherever feasible and sensible.
- To ensure that service providers make practical support for carers a high priority.
- To make proper assessment of need and good case management the cornerstone of high quality care.
- To promote the development of a flourishing independent sector alongside good quality public services.
- To clarify the responsibilities of agencies and so make it easier to hold them to account for their performance.
- To secure better value for taxpayers' money by introducing a new funding structure for social care.

The changes required to deliver these key objectives were phased in from April 1991 to April 1993.

By April 1991, local authorities had to have in place:

- Revised complaints procedures.
- Inspection units.
- New social care services for people with mental health problems.
- New arrangements with voluntary organisations for social care for people with drug and alcohol problems.

The revised complaints procedures were required to provide an effective means of enabling actual or potential service users (or their representatives) to complain about the quality or type of service provided by the social services department. They therefore had to give clear information to all relevant people about how to complain, and had to provide an independent appeal or review mechanism. Complaints procedures had to set out a timescale within which a department would guarantee to resolve a complaint, and had to reflect the need for confidentiality and impartiality at all stages.

Ever since the enactment of the 1984 Registered Homes Act, social services departments have been responsible for inspecting and registering residential care provided by the independent (ie, private and voluntary) sectors. Under the 1990 Act their role was widened. Inspection units were required to be set up at arms-length to the main departmental service management function and be accountable for ensuring the quality of care provided in public, private and voluntary residential care. They were also expected to support and assist in the general development of quality assurance programmes within the department. Social services departments were required to collaborate effectively with district health authorities in the development of inspection and quality control. District health authorities retained responsibility for the registration and inspection of nursing homes. The two authorities were recommended to develop a joint strategy for inspection and quality control, working together wherever possible. In a few areas this process of collaboration between district health authority and social services department inspection units has led to a single joint inspection unit being formed to combine the functions of the social services department in respect of residential care providers (of all types) and the district health authority in respect of independent sector nursing homes.

New social care services for people with mental health problems were encouraged by the provision of a specific grant from central government. Local authorities had to make a 30% contribution to the expenditure and nationally, in the first year of implementation, a total £30 million could be spent on these new social care services. A condition of receiving the money was that district health authorities and social services departments agreed spending plans locally, so that new services could be developed to complement existing ones.

Additional funding was made available to local authorities to pay voluntary organisations to provide social care services for people with drug and alcohol problems. Again, the grant could only be paid if a 30% contribution from local authorities was raised and inter-authority agreement reached.

Community Care Plans

By April 1992, and annually thereafter, district health authorities, local authorities and family health services authorities had to produce Community Care Plans. The remit of these plans was to "state clearly authorities' strategic objectives for meeting their populations' community care needs". Wherever possible, these were expected to be a single plan published by the three authorities. Where a single plan could not be produced, the three authorities had to ensure that the separate agencies plans were based on local joint planning agreements. The purpose of community care plans is to set out strategic objectives and priorities for community care. These must be based on an assessment of local need, and on an account of resource assumptions. A key feature of the plans is that they are required to be public documents and it is necessary that there is a wide process of consultation with other agencies, users and carers during the preparation of the plan. The process of community care planning is a key method through which health and local authorities are becoming joint commissioners of services on behalf of their populations, rather than main providers of health and social care.

New mechanisms and funding arrangements

1993 was the implementation date for the most far-reaching changes laid out in the White Paper 'Caring for People'. By that date, the following procedures had to be in place:

- Assessment systems for all clients who approach the SSD for support.
- Payment and charging mechanisms for SSD services.
- Contracting arrangements.
- Management information and budgeting systems.

Several of these derived from the need for social services departments to be organisationally and managerially prepared for a major transfer of funds from the Income Support system administered by the Department of Social Security (DSS) to the local authority. This transfer (some £399 million in 1993/94 alone) was at the heart of the "Community Care" reforms. Under the pre-1993 system, the budget for Income Support payments to pay for residential and nursing home care provided by the non-statutory sector was not cash limited and not well related to the needs of the individual for such care. As a result of this funding structure, a massive expansion in residential and nursing care occurred during the 1980s (with the budget rising from £10m in 1979 to £1000m in 1989) regardless of whether the people concerned could more appropriately be cared for in their own homes. In order to ensure a needs-led approach, from 1993, people entering residential or nursing home care with public financial support have been funded by the social services department rather than through the Income Support system. This funding is only available after a full assessment of the individual's need for such care (as opposed to alternatives such as increased domiciliary support) has been undertaken. Thus, a single unified budget for the purchase of social care was created and managed through local authorities.

The legislation requires assessment to be developed and seen as a function in its own right, separate from services which are arranged as a consequence of assessment. It must be based on the needs-led principle, and users and carers have to be actively involved in individual assessment. Authorities are required to take positive steps to ensure that people with communication difficulties can participate fully in the assessment process. Full information about appropriate services must be available, so that users can exercise choice in developing a plan of care. The outcome of the assessment process is to secure the most cost-effective package of services to meet assessed need. This package must be set out in an individual care plan, which is then a key tool in monitoring the effectiveness of services. NHS professionals are required to collaborate with the social services department on individual assessments when an individual's health care needs are relevant to deciding which social care services are required.

Payment and charging mechanisms for social services department services involve a means-testing system. Whilst social services departments have always had the power to charge for services, many had opted not to do so, and others had charged a flat rate, irrespective of income, so as to avoid the need to means-test. Once the unified social care budget was in place, however, an assessment of ability to pay became essential.

Contracting arrangements for social care were conceived on a similar basis to those introduced as part of the 1990 reforms of the National Health Service. Contracting required a division between the purchasing and the providing strands of the organisation of social care for the first time. Unlike the National Health Service however, where contracting is predominantly at population needs level, contracting for social care is mainly based upon the purchase of care packages for individuals.

Care management and budgeting systems are a key means by which to ensure effective delivery of the individual care plan. Care managers are a new type of professional whose remit is to act as brokers across the statutory and independent sectors. They are not directly involved in service delivery, nor in managing services which they arrange. They are expected to take on responsibility for purchasing some or all of the services set out in the individual care plan and, to do this task, manage a devolved budget. The devolution of budgets to the level of care managers represented a significant change in the previous practice of social services departments, and was designed to bring decision making closer to users and their families.

Taken together, the changes for community care which were set out in the National Health Service and Community Care Act 1990 represented a major change in the organisation and delivery of health and social care services in the community. The development of the needs led approach; the focus on the needs of carers as well as clients; the separation of purchaser and provider functions and the requirement for statutory agencies to work more closely with each other as well as with private and voluntary bodies were all key elements in developing a new system designed to meet the emerging challenges of the late 1990s and beyond.

The duties of social workers

Social work is a young profession with its roots in the post Second World War welfare state. Whether working in the community ('field'); hospital or in settings such as education or in the courts, the social worker will receive referrals either directly from, or indirectly about, a member of the public ('client'). Referrals will normally be requests for social care or support in some form. In a minority of cases, they will be queries about the need for child protection.

The social worker will make an appraisal of the problem which will involve an assessment of the clients and usually also their home environment, family relationships and network of social contacts. The process of assessment may involve asking for and receiving reports on the client from other agencies (for example, general practitioner, hospital consultant, or probation officer). There will be filter mechanisms in place to ensure that social workers only receive problems of a severity warranting professional assessment with more straightforward requests for assistance being dealt with by either administrative or vocationally trained staff.

The ultimate aim of the social worker is to assess need and then ensure that the client receives the most appropriate type of services to meet, most effectively, his or her particular needs. This may mean referral for a service provided by the social services department itself (for example, a residential home for a frail elderly person; the provision of a home help for a physically handicapped person or arranging for a day-nursery place for the child of a one parent family) or another local authority service (for example, the housing department). It may mean bringing the problem to the attention of another agency entirely. A voluntary organisation, for example, may provide a service which is particularly appropriate for the client's needs. Liaison with the health service may be more formal in the case of the hospital social worker, but as in community care, health service professionals and social workers liaise on a regular basis over particular patients' or clients' needs. The advent of care management as a result of the Community Care reforms described in the previous section augments this traditional role in assessing need and arranging services by allowing the social worker to establish contractual relationships with the various providers of elements of the care package. This process enables the individual to receive effective services and the local authorities to be sure of value for its money.

Social workers are supervised in these processes of assessment of need, choice of the most appropriate response and (if acting as a care manager) the purchasing of the resulting care package by a first line manager (usually titled Team Leader). Traditionally, social workers may decide that, aside from referral to specific services, the client and her or his family would benefit from a structured analysis of their problem via a helping process known as 'casework'. The advent of care management with its separation of assessment from service provision will not normally preclude the social worker engaging in such work with clients, although if long-term counselling is required, this is likely to be the subject of a specific referral.

Throughout the 1980s, an increasing proportion of social work time was taken up with child protection work. The Children Act 1989 radically changed child care law and practice, and was developed partly as a response to dramatically increased awareness of child protection issues and the need for clarification of the rights of both children and parents. At a time of reduced expenditure in social services departments, most have had to introduce priority lists, so that some clients are put on a waiting list before assessment. Child protection work is always a high priority, and lower priority has consequently often been accorded to the more general types of support to frail and vulnerable people. The Community Care reforms require publication via Community Care Plans of eligibility criteria for services in order to make clear the priorities of the social services department and their relation to the assessed social care needs of the population.

The role of hospital social workers is slightly different from their colleagues in the community. In addition to dealing with specific problems concerned with clients or their families which are referred to them, they will have a number of continuing responsibilities in connection with the process of hospitalisation. This will vary considerably according to the type of hospital in which the social work service is being provided. In many settings, a major role will be facilitating the process of discharge. This may, for example, involve the assessment of the patient's capacity and home circumstances and arranging for such domiciliary support services as might be required. In a psychiatric or mental handicap hospital, social workers will often be part of a multidisciplinary team which reviews current inpatients in case-conference or discussion. They will also have a special responsibility, in connection with the admission and possible compulsory detention of patients under sections of the Mental Health Act. It is a requirement of the Department of Health nationally that discharge procedures for every psychiatric patient are agreed at local level with the relevant social services department (the so-called 'Care Programme Approach'). In an obstetric unit the function may entail providing advice on entitlement to benefits or intended adoptions.

The range of services which social workers may provide for clients is shown in Table 4.3.

Table 4.3: Some services provided by social workers to clients

- Assessment of need
- A means of providing access to resources
- Therapeutic and supportive function
- Advice and information - counselling
- Helping clients to make decisions
- Statutory functions (court work and compulsory admission)
- Obtaining new resources
- Promoting the needs of children and inarticulate adults to other agencies
- Child protection

CONCLUSIONS

The basic principles of the National Health Service have remained intact since it was introduced after the Second World War. This is despite a number of major reorganisations which have changed its structure and management. Also when viewed internationally, it is generally acknowledged as a relatively efficient system of delivering health care to the population. Changes which will occur up to the end of the twentieth century and beyond are likely to include: a further growth in diagnostic and treatment technology, further ageing of the population, a greater emphasis on the promotion of health, a change in the role which the hospital will play in the health care system, and rising consumer expectations. It will be important for the National Health Service to adapt to and meet these challenges as they occur.

5 Physical disability

INTRODUCTION

Many disease processes are wide-ranging in their impact. In some, the result is disability, a state in which the individual may experience loss or limitation of physical function; reduced opportunities in social functioning; economic hardship or disadvantage, negative attitudes and prejudice. Aside from disease, disability can arise through other causes, such as fetal abnormalities and accidents.

Disability is an important issue for public health for a number of reasons. Firstly, the proportion of people who develop disability could be reduced with more effective health promotion measures aimed at eliminating the underlying causes. For example, a greater number of serious fetal abnormalities could be identified through improved detection programmes in the antenatal period. Secondly, the effective use of treatment and rehabilitation services directed at restoring function in people who are already ill or injured can reduce residual disability. For example, an active multi-professional approach to the clinical recognition, treatment and rehabilitation of people with stroke helps to prevent long-term major disability in some of those affected. Thirdly, people with disability represent an important group within the population with special needs. It is a responsibility of those planning and providing services to ensure that the needs of people with disability are clearly identified and that an appropriate and personalised response is made to them. To undertake this task properly poses enormous challenges. It is not simply a question of making adjustments in the delivery of health services. The needs of people with disability are very wide-ranging and addressing them requires approaches in areas such as: building and environmental design, transport, employment, education, communications, and leisure.

Perhaps the greatest challenge is to create an infrastructure of help, support and care which enables people with disability to be fully integrated within society as well as creating a climate in which they are recognised and respected as individuals, with commensurate rights and entitlements. This chapter deals with the nature and causes of physical disability as well as the needs of people who are so affected and the range of responses which can be made to them.

THE MEANING OF DISABILITY

Whilst many classifications and definitions of disability have been formulated, the most widely accepted is that adopted by the World Health Organisation in the early 1980s[1].

In this a sequence is recognised:

disease or disorder → *impairment* → *disability* → *handicap*

Progress through the sequence is not necessary or inevitable but each of the terms has been given a particular meaning which is helpful in exploring the concepts both for individual need and for population needs assessment.

Impairment

Disturbance of the normal structure or functioning of the body, which may be temporary or permanent.

A state of impairment represents a deviation from normal bodily function or status, irrespective of whether it arose from injury, disease or congenital malformation. It is concerned with parts or systems of the body that do not work.

Disability

Loss of, or restriction in, functional ability or activity as a result of impairment.

A disability represents a limitation in tasks or activities, either physical, social or psychological, arising from the impairment. Disability is about things people cannot do.

Handicap

A disadvantage for a given individual, resulting from an impairment or a disability that limits or prevents his or her fulfilment of a role that would be expected (depending on age, sex, social and cultural factors) for a group of which that individual is a member.

Handicap is very dependent on the structure and attitudes of the society in which the individual exists; handicap therefore is a relative concept.

Practical implications

The applicability of these concepts depends very much on the underlying cause of the disability, the characteristics of the individuals and the community or society in which they live. Even for particular causes of disability, people can vary greatly in the impact which the disease process has upon them. For example, a person with diabetes mellitus, by definition, is impaired since there is a disturbance to normal functioning of one organ of the body. For many diabetic people, careful self-regulation of their disease through urine glucose monitoring, diet, exercise and insulin injection will mean that they are not disabled: there is no loss or restriction of functional ability or activity because of their impairment. On the other hand, a diabetic person whose disease has progressed or been badly controlled may have complications of the illness (for example, blindness, poor circulation to the limbs) which will seriously interfere with his or her ability to function. Diabetic people will be handicapped if, for example, they are unable because of their disease to follow a particular occupation or career which would otherwise have been open to them.

Numerous other examples can illustrate the way in which the components of disablement are manifest. A person with red/green colour blindness has an impairment but is unlikely to have a disability if there is no restriction of activities. However, their choice of occupation could be restricted. For example, normal colour vision is required for driving trains. This would give rise to a handicap or disadvantage. A young woman who has been rendered paraplegic in a road accident and is confined to a wheelchair will be impaired, disabled and also handicapped.

Stigma

Of even greater importance than a conceptual framework when considering the needs of people with disability are the ways in which disability is perceived by society and its individual members, the way in which people with disability themselves are affected by these attitudes and the extent to which they cope with them. The stigma of disablement is very deep seated in contemporary, western society. Whilst the degree of tolerance towards it is much greater than in the past (when people with disability were often punished or outcast from communities) there is no doubt that, even in modern Britain, stereotypic assumptions abound. Many disabled people are treated and regarded as different. Many able-bodied people harbour feelings of discomfort and even revulsion when coming into contact with disabled people.

As a result of the way in which people with disability may be treated by other members of society, they themselves may develop feelings of frustration, resentment and serious loss of self-esteem. These and similar feelings may be major barriers to people with disability coping with and overcoming their problems.

Terminology used in the chapter

Having described this formal classification of impairment, disability and handicap, in the remainder of the chapter, to permit ease of communication, the terms 'people with disability', 'disabled people' and 'disablement' are used interchangeably and in an everyday sense, rather than the technical one described above.

THE ASSESSMENT OF NEED

There are no comprehensive data available to describe the size of the problem of disability and its nature at local population level. This is for a number of reasons. Firstly, most information systems are derived from contact with hospital services, whilst many people with disability will be living in the community and will not necessarily be receiving care from hospital-based services. Secondly, the needs of disabled people have not in the past been a high priority for service providers. Therefore, building up accurate information on the numbers of those disabled and on their needs has not been a concern. Thirdly, for information on disability to be of any value, it must encompass some of the definitional issues which were discussed in the previous section. Gathering valid data on this basis is extremely complex in practice.

Causes of disability

The major underlying causes of disability (Figure 5.1) are consistent across a number of surveys. In examining population need locally, some insights into the size of the problem of disability can be derived by estimating the number of people with conditions such as stroke. This disease-based approach does not provide information on the full range of disability nor does it yield data on levels of incapacity amongst disabled people, the most important issue when assessing need and planning service responses. Some information is available from the national sample survey, the General Household Survey which asks questions about long-term incapacity. Disability registers maintained by local authorities under the Chronically Sick and Disabled Person's Act 1970 yield data of variable quality and are only of very limited use for local needs assessment.

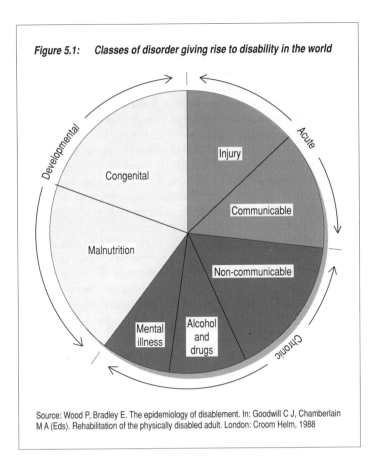

Figure 5.1:   Classes of disorder giving rise to disability in the world

Source: Wood P, Bradley E. The epidemiology of disablement. In: Goodwill C J, Chamberlain M A (Eds). Rehabilitation of the physically disabled adult. London: Croom Helm, 1988

Pattern in the population

The most comprehensive information on the numbers of people with disability and the nature of their problem comes from a series of national surveys undertaken during the 1980s. Originally commissioned by the Government in 1984, the Office of Population Censuses and Surveys (OPCS) carried out four separate surveys between 1985 and 1988.

They covered adults in private households, adults in communal establishments, children in private households and children in communal establishments. The surveys were far more comprehensive than those undertaken previously because they included all types of disability and not just those of a physical origin.

A ten point scale of overall severity of disability was developed by the OPCS Team. Category 1 represented the least severe end of the scale and category 10 represented the most severe end. A person in category 1, for example, might be someone who has difficulty hearing a normal voice even without any background noise, whereas someone in category 10 might be someone suffering from severely impaired mobility in the aftermath of a stroke.

The survey estimated that there were 6.2 million adults in Britain with one or more disabilities. Of these 422,000 (7%) lived in some kind of communal establishment. Some 360,000 children in Britain had disabilities of which only 5.6 thousand (2%) were living in communal establishments. In all, 14.2% of the adult population living in private households had at least one disability.

Figure 5.2 shows the estimated number of disabled adults living in private households and communal establishments in Britain. The largest numbers were in the least severe categories and the lowest numbers were in the most severe categories. The numbers increased with age overall and in each severity category. Disabled adults were generally older than the rest of the population (Figure 5.3).

In the population as a whole, locomotor disorders were the most commonly cited cause of disability. Also mentioned frequently were hearing and visual problems and difficulties with personal care (Figure 5.4). For those living in communal establishments mental disabilities, particularly dementia, were mentioned most often followed by disorders of the musculo-skeletal system and nervous system.

Only a minority of disabled adults under pensionable age was found to be in work compared to the general population (Figure 5.5) and those who were in employment had lower earnings (Figure 5.6) compared to other people.

These major national surveys were very important in describing the size and nature of the problem of disability in the population. Increasingly, it will be necessary to gather similar data at a more local population level if the needs of disabled people are to be properly assessed and then addressed by those planning and providing services.

Visual and hearing disabilities

People with sensory disabilities are a group with special needs within the disabled population. The two principal categories are people with blindness and those with deafness. There are various definitions of blindness and deafness in use depending on the context.

The National Assistance Act 1948 defines blindness as "that a person should be so blind as to be unable to perform any work for which eyesight is essential". There is no statutory definition of partial sight. However, in practice this category refers to those who, although not blind within the meaning of the Act, are substantially and permanently handicapped by defective vision caused by congenital defect, illness or injury.

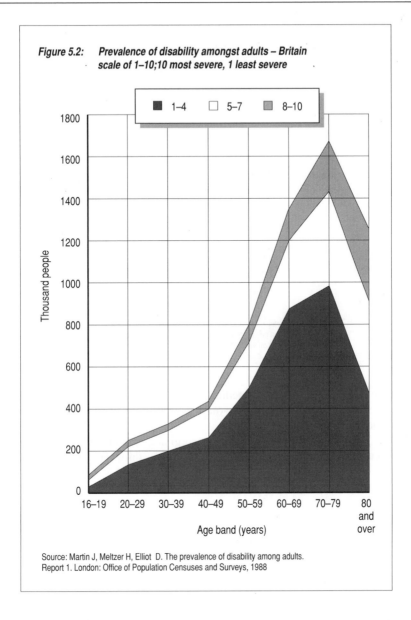

Figure 5.2: Prevalence of disability amongst adults – Britain
scale of 1–10;10 most severe, 1 least severe

Source: Martin J, Meltzer H, Elliot D. The prevalence of disability among adults.
Report 1. London: Office of Population Censuses and Surveys, 1988

A register of blind and partially sighted people is held and maintained in most localities of Britain although participation is voluntary. The information recorded is made available to care agencies, thus enabling the registered person to gain access to services more easily. A person is placed on the register following an examination by a medical practitioner with experience in ophthalmology (usually a consultant ophthalmologist). Absolute standards are not laid down but usually someone with visual acuity less than 3/60 for both eyes on the Snellen chart would be regarded as suitable for registration as blind. Alternatively better visual acuity but impaired fields of vision could also lead to someone being registered as blind. Similarly,

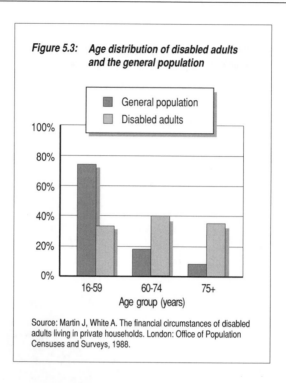

Figure 5.3: Age distribution of disabled adults and the general population

Source: Martin J, White A. The financial circumstances of disabled adults living in private households. London: Office of Population Censuses and Surveys, 1988.

there is no definition of partial sightedness but visual acuity between 3/60 and 6/60 for both eyes or field impairment would usually qualify a person as partially sighted for registration purposes.

It has been calculated that the blind register can underestimate the true prevalence of blindness in a population by up to a third. However, the data do provide a broad indication of the size of the problem and its causes. Information shown in Tables 5.1 and 5.2 is taken from an area where the level of ascertainment

Table 5.1: *Rates of blind registration in Leicestershire, England per 100,000 population by age and sex*

Age group (years)	Male	Female
0 – 4	13.3	7.7
5 – 14	0.0	1.8
15 – 29	2.9	1.9
30 – 44	4.4	5.7
45 – 64	5.4	7.6
65 – 74	48.5	91.4
75 and over	405.7	474.8
All ages	24.2	48.0

Source: Thompson J R, Du L, Rosenthal A R. Recent trends in the registration of blindness and partial sight in Leicestershire. British Journal of Ophthalmology 1989; 73: 95–9.

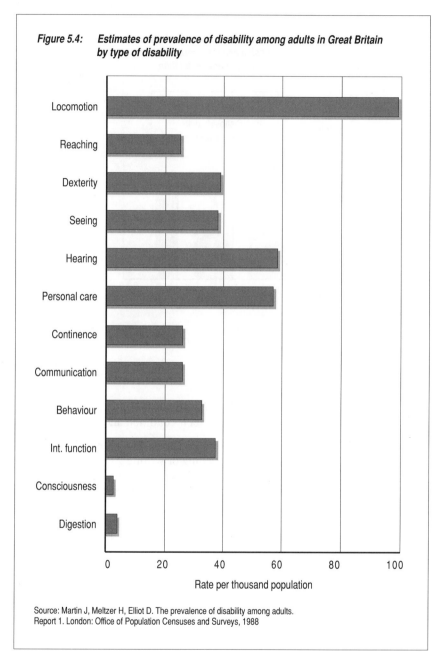

Figure 5.4: *Estimates of prevalence of disability among adults in Great Britain by type of disability*

Source: Martin J, Meltzer H, Elliot D. The prevalence of disability among adults.
Report 1. London: Office of Population Censuses and Surveys, 1988

of the blind register is relatively high. Registration of partial sightedness is much less complete. Specifically conducted population-based surveys are the best way of estimating the size of the problem of blindness and partial sightedness but they should not be lightly entered into because they require considerable skill and resources to be undertaken properly.

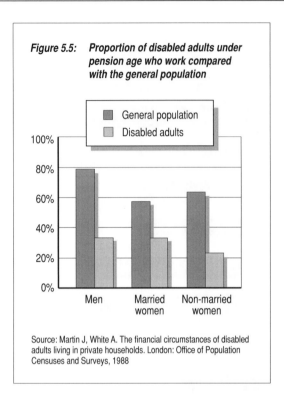

Figure 5.5:   *Proportion of disabled adults under pension age who work compared with the general population*

Source: Martin J, White A. The financial circumstances of disabled adults living in private households. London: Office of Population Censuses and Surveys, 1988

People who suffer from a disabling hearing loss to the extent that they require help from services are usually categorised on their condition and needs as follows.

(a) *Deaf without speech*: Those with no useful hearing and whose normal method of communication is by signs, finger-spelling or writing.

(b) *Deaf with speech*: Those who (even with a hearing aid) have little of no useful hearing but whose normal method of communication is by speech and lip-reading.

(c) *Hard of hearing*: Those who (with or without a hearing aid) have some useful hearing and whose normal method of communication is by speech, listening and lip-reading.

Table 5.2:   Cause of blindness registration (percentages) in people aged 65 years and over

Cause of Blindness	Percentage
Senile macular degeneration	47
Cataract	20
Glaucoma	12
Diabetic retinopathy	2
Others	19

Source: Thompson J R, Du L, Rosenthal A R. Recent trends in the registration of blindness and partial sight in Leicestershire. British Journal of Ophthalmology 1989; 73: 95–9.

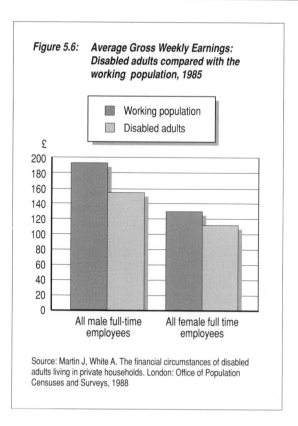

Figure 5.6:   *Average Gross Weekly Earnings:*
              Disabled adults compared with the
              working population, 1985

Source: Martin J, White A. The financial circumstances of disabled adults living in private households. London: Office of Population Censuses and Surveys, 1988

The first two categories usually apply to those who are deaf at birth or became so when very young and require specialised help. There is a register for deaf people. Participation in registration is voluntary and is not a prerequisite for help or services. The register is maintained by the Social Services department under the National Assistance Act 1948.

When considering the level and range of services required for people with hearing impairment, population health needs assessment must consider a number of perspectives (Table 5.3).

The prevalence of hearing loss in the adult population of Britain is not available from routine data sources but can be derived from well designed surveys (Figure 5.7). Hearing impairment is strongly age-related.

Table 5.3:   Needs assessment in relation to services for the hearing impaired:
              factors to be taken into account

- Size of the population with particular degrees of hearing impairment.
- Demographic composition of the hearing impaired sub-population.
- Distribution of type of hearing impairment (middle ear vs cochlear).
- Nature of disability and handicap experienced by hearing impaired people.

Source: Derived from Davis A, Thornton R. The impact of hearing impairment: some epidemiological evidence. Proceedings of 14th Danavox symposium. Presbyacusis and other age-related aspects. Ed JH Jensen, 1990.

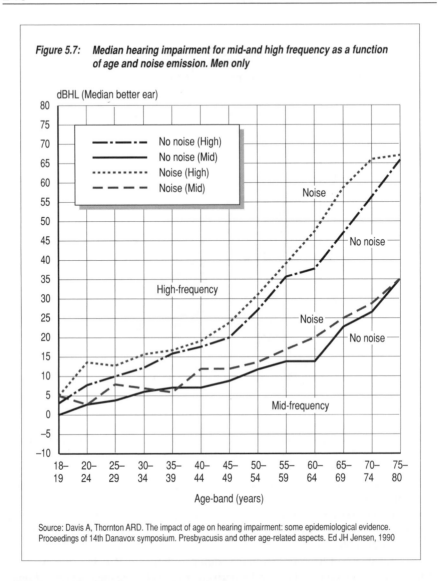

Figure 5.7:   Median hearing impairment for mid-and high frequency as a function of age and noise emission. Men only

Source: Davis A, Thornton ARD. The impact of age on hearing impairment: some epidemiological evidence. Proceedings of 14th Danavox symposium. Presbyacusis and other age-related aspects. Ed JH Jensen, 1990

SERVICES FOR PEOPLE WITH DISABILITY

At the end of the nineteenth century School Boards were required to ensure that all blind and deaf children under their jurisdiction received suitable elementary education. Earlier in the present century, education authorities were given additional powers to provide special education for epileptic and mentally handicapped children and this was made obligatory in 1914. During the latter half of the nineteenth century, a number of voluntary societies were founded which were concerned with the welfare of particular groups of handicapped people such as those who were blind, deaf and crippled. The Workman's Compensation Act 1897 and the National Insurance Act 1911 began to make some material provision for the sick and people injured in industrial accidents.

In the second decade of this century, the importance of after care for tuberculosis was demonstrated. The first village settlement for people with tuberculosis was established (the Bourne Colony), later transferred to the village of Papworth in Cambridgeshire. At a time when people with tuberculosis were barred from most normal occupations, this settlement provided a special environment in which tuberculosis patients could work and live normally with their families under medical supervision.

During World War I, rehabilitation regimes including physiotherapy, hydro-therapy, remedial exercises and occupational therapy were organised for ortho-paedic cases. Meanwhile, the work of St Dunstan's Hospital for blinded soldiers and sailors showed how experts with a medical approach could train disabled people to acquire self-reliance and compensatory skills.

The large number of military and civilian casualties sustained during World War II brought about rapid innovations in rehabilitation methods and in special schemes for disabled people. Under the Emergency Medical Service, a large number of hospitals were taken over by the Ministry of Health for the care of war casualties and evacuated civilian patients. The improved resources together with a commit-ment towards war casualties stimulated a progressive attitude. The range of occu-pations for which disabled men were trained greatly widened to include, for example skilled engineering work. Rehabilitation methods similar in principle to those used in orthopaedic practice, were applied to other categories of sick and injured people. Furthermore, an increasing emphasis was placed on the involve-ment of patients in their own treatment through techniques such as group exercise and remedial games.

The development of services for the rehabilitation of people with spinal injuries, although a specialised field, has also done much to stimulate improvements in rehabilitation services generally.

As with other groups with special needs the emphasis in providing help, support and care for people with physical disability must lie in comprehensive needs assessment by all relevant agencies working together. To meet the large range of health, social and other needs of people with a disability, requires well-coordinated and managed services and a personalised approach in organising the care and support required. The health service is only one of the agencies involved in providing such care. Local authority Social Services departments have the lead role in the new Community Care legislation, fully implemented in April 1993.

Medical and rehabilitation services

A cornerstone of the health services' response to the problem of disability is the provision of high quality rehabilitation services. In the past, such services have grown up around war time medicine: notably the Second World War and the Vietnam War. Survivors of serious injury often had considerable residual disability and their function was often considerably improved by targeted intensive rehabilitation programmes.

In Britain, though there have been some centres of excellence for rehabilitation medicine, the majority of local services have had to make do with general, rather than special expertise. This is rapidly changing. It is now recognised that an organised, team-based approach to rehabilitation is an essential feature of local services for people with disability. Not only has there been a growth in rehabilitation as a specialty of medical practice, but there has also been increased recognition of the value of therapy services. The continuing growth of voluntary and charitable organisations and of the disabled persons movement have also been important forces for change. It was the advent of the disabled persons independent living movement in the United States of America that was a major force in the development of rehabilitation and disability services in that country.

Rehabilitation services have a number of functions. Firstly, they must undertake a full assessment of the disabled person, ideally in their home or other place of residence. This will enable functional capacity to be assessed and the scope for restoration of lost functions and acquisition of new skills to be identified. It will also identify the need for special equipment to be supplied or for adaptation to the person's day-to-day living environment. Secondly, rehabilitation services will set out to establish a clear care plan, agreed with the person concerned and their informal carers (if any). Thirdly, the service will set in hand measures and services to deliver the care plan. The circumstances vary greatly. In some cases, rehabilitation will begin following an acute hospital admission for example, because of stroke or traumatic injury. In other cases, rehabilitation services may be offered to someone who has had a long-standing problem, for example, multiple sclerosis, but has never previously had help of this sort.

It is important to recognise that people with disability often have long-term care needs which will continue to benefit from rehabilitation services and the notion of rehabilitation as a single course of therapy is increasingly outmoded. This means that rehabilitation services will not be exclusively provided on a hospital site but will be delivered on a community-basis. Local rehabilitation teams are multiprofessional, using skills such as physiotherapy, occupational and speech therapy in addition to those of medicine and nursing.

Within the National Health Service, there are increasing numbers of consultant posts in Disability Medicine or Rehabilitation Medicine which are filled by people with specialist training. In addition to being core members of local rehabilitation teams, such consultants perform a liaison and specialist advisory role with consultants in other disciplines (for example, neurology, geriatric medicine, orthopaedics, rheumatology) where conditions giving rise to disability are commonly seen amongst their patient population.

Whilst many hospitalised patients will be able to receive help from the rehabilitation team and still remain within the service which is treating their underlying problem, some designated hospital inpatient facilities are required specifically for the treatment of people with disability. In some parts of the country, these facilities are provided in a rehabilitation unit to which patients (for example those with strokes or injuries) can be transferred for intensive rehabilitation prior to discharge and their re-integration within the community. In addition to this type of facility, most localities will need inpatient beds to care for more severely disabled people in a hospital environment. This particularly applies to the younger physically disabled, a group who have traditionally been victims of the lack of a co-ordinated approach to care.

Specialist facilities are also required for the rehabilitation of people with acute traumatic injury of the spinal cord and people who have sustained head injuries. The physical, psychological, social and financial consequences of both of these types of disability are profound and justify the specific attention of services to ensure high standards of care for the groups of patients concerned.

It is also important to ensure that services specifically address the needs of young adults so that the transition from childhood to adulthood is as smooth as possible. The Disabled Persons Act 1986 has acted as a stimulus in many areas for the development of advisory services for the disabled young school leaver.

Many people with disability require specialist medical, surgical and nursing treatment to deal with locomotor and bladder problems. Close liaison is needed between the rehabilitation team and the hospital services concerned to ensure that the nature and timing of any intervention is the most appropriate.

Disabled living centres

A major focus of local services for people with disability is the Disabled Living Centre. Such centres act as a resource and information facility and provide a wide range of aids, appliances and equipment to help people with disability. Centres will undertake assessment of people to judge what sort of aids and equipment are most appropriate to their needs and will also provide advice and supervision on their use in the home environment. In some cases, this will involve home visiting by the Centre's staff. Most Disabled Living Centres provide many additional services. Typically they will give information and advice to people with disability and their families on issues such as health and social services, employment, benefits and entitlements, and sports and leisure opportunities. Their advisory function in relation to benefits may extend to an advocacy role and to representing people with disability at tribunals and hearings. They will also often serve as an educational resource to pass on expertise about caring for people with disability. Many Centres are funded from charitable sources but additional funding is usually also provided by health and local authorities. Many disabled people live relatively isolated, 'one-off' lives. A local Disabled Living Centre can provide continuity of support, advice and help to empower and enable those with disability to have access to the complex range of services which are available.

Some specialist services

Whilst services such as those provided by the Disabled Living Centre are intended to be accessible to all people with disability in a particular locality, the nature of some people's disabilities will mean that they have needs which can only be met by more specialised services. The nature of such services has developed in different ways around the country either in response to a particular need, or because of local initiatives, or as a result of the enthusiasm and commitment of certain individuals or organisations. Nevertheless, there are some specialist services which are more generally available. These may be based at Disabled Living Centres or delivered from other locations.

Continence services

Many people with disability experience a degree of urinary incontinence. This subject is discussed more fully in the chapter on elderly people but much of the core service is the same. Because the embarrassment and stigma of incontinence of urine or faeces is particularly great, an important function of continence services is to promote awareness of the problem as well as to provide practical help and support. Continence services are usually run by a continence adviser, invariably with a nursing background, who assesses the extent of the person's problem and advises on the most appropriate continence and toileting aids.

Stoma care services

A stoma is an artificial opening to the outside of the body from one of the internal organs. The more common types of stoma are created after bowel surgery for diseases such as cancer of the bowel, ulcerative colitis and Crohn's disease. A stoma may also be created involving the urinary tract. People who have a stoma have special needs for advice, counselling and practical support. Although this may be provided by the hospital surgical service which created the stoma, increasingly, specialist services using trained stoma care nurses or therapists provide pre-operative counselling, after care and continuing support to patients.

Pressure sore services

Pressure sores are a particular hazard for people with disability. Their consequences can be serious and their treatment is potentially very costly. They are preventable. Many pressure sores develop amongst people who are hospitalised, particularly the elderly. The avoidance of pressure sores in this group relies upon high quality nursing care. Similarly, for people who are confined to bed in their own homes, skilled nursing care in the community will reduce the occurrence of pressure sores. For people with disability who are in wheelchairs or whose mobility is seriously restricted, it is important that they receive advice and counselling from expert staff on the measures they need to take (regular shifting of position, weight distribution cushions, special mattresses) to avoid developing a pressure sore.

Counselling services

The psychological consequences of disability are, for most affected people, profound. Counselling and psychological intervention can provide, therefore, an important and much valued element of core services for disabled people.

Sexuality is just as important a facet of life for disabled people as for the able-bodied. A person with disability will often be handicapped sexually and this may have far-reaching effects on his or her self esteem and psychological state. Many people with disability will not realise that they can gain sexual fulfilment. Therefore, it is very important that this domain of disability and handicap is not regarded as a need to which services respond as an after thought. There are very strong arguments for a counsellor being a core member of the professional team of every local disability service.

Driving assessment services

The dominant feature of many disabilities is restriction of physical mobility with its potential to limit social contacts and produce difficulty in coping with aspects of independent living such as shopping, leisure, or visiting places of entertainment. For many people with disability, a car or other means of personal transport will be one of the most important features of their lives. Disability arising from a wide range of causes will affect people's ability to drive (for example, stroke, epilepsy, muscular dystrophy, amputation, rheumatoid arthritis). A person's fitness to drive must be taken into account by the Driving and Vehicle Licensing Centre (DVLC) based in Swansea whose staff (making use of medical advisers) will decide whether the disability could constitute a danger when driving. Medical reports and assessments will usually be required from the person's local doctor.

A disabled driver has three main needs. Firstly, to be fully assessed. Secondly, to be advised on the type of car most suited to his or her needs (with adaptations and modifications where appropriate). Thirdly, to receive advice on how to finance the purchase.

There are a number of assessment centres for disabled drivers around the country which provide these services. It is important that local disability services have good links with them so that they can ensure disabled people have access to the centres, even though they may live some distance away.

Prosthetics and orthotics

A prosthesis is a device which replaces a missing part. For example, the fitting of an artificial limb to a person who has lost all or part of their limb due to amputation because of trauma, vascular disease or cancer.

There are many other types of prostheses and they are becoming increasingly sophisticated as a result of advances in modern science and technology as well as higher expectations of people themselves.

The fitting of prostheses is one which *par excellence* requires a service based upon an ethos of high quality and patient-centred care. In the case of an artificial limb, the scope of the service should involve pre-operative counselling, the operation itself, the assessment and fitting of the prosthesis, gait training, after-care and support. Such an approach requires general practitioners, surgeons, physiotherapists, occupational therapists, other members of the rehabilitation team and prosthetic fitters, engineers and suppliers working closely together. Increasingly, for example, it is recognised that the quality of a surgical amputation is a vital determining feature of a successful prosthesis for the patient. The idea that amputations should be left for the most junior member of the surgical team to gain experience is being re-thought. It is a growing practice for amputations to be performed by senior surgeons who undertake larger numbers of such operations and who work closely with the prosthetic and rehabilitation teams.

An orthosis is an appliance or piece of equipment which is attached to the body to enhance function. Orthoses can range from splints or collars applied to support an arthritic joint to calliper-type devices used to assist movement where muscles are weak or paralysed, to devices which support or redistribute weight (for example, special footwear). The orthosis is usually arranged following a prescription by a consultant. Orthotics has a long tradition in the health service but there has been concern that this important service for people with disability has not been well integrated with other aspects of their care. This has in part come about because a high proportion of orthoses have come from private firms whose orthotist (the person who usually undertakes the assessment) is also the supplier on behalf of the company concerned. The potential for a conflict of interest in such a dual role is obvious, even though it may not be manifest. Moreover, whilst many devices are cosmetically unappealing and are not well liked by patients, there have not been major changes in their features over the years. Greater attention is now being given to issues of assessment, manufacture and supply of orthoses together with ways of ensuring that a high quality product is made available to the patient, whilst at the same time ensuring value for money.

Wheelchair and special seating services

Wheelchairs are an important aid to mobility for people with disability. The majority are prescribed and supplied at local level with the assessment being provided by staff of the Disabled Living Centre or from another local service base. Some disabled people will require a more specialised chair and, in such cases, assessment and supply may have to be arranged at a centre dealing with special problems and serving a wider population. A wide range of wheelchairs (non-powered and powered) are available both for indoor and outdoor use. The wheelchair service is also responsible for assessing and providing special seating for disabled people with major postural problems.

Communication aids

Difficulties with speech and communication are an important consequence of some causes of disability. For this reason, a speech therapist should also be a member of the team providing core rehabilitation services for people with disability at local level. In addition to speech therapy services, some people can greatly benefit from a mechanical aid to communication. Each person should receive careful individual assessment to determine which of the many possible aids to communication are best suited to their needs. These range from simple voice amplifiers, to devices controlled by non-affected parts of the body (for example, eyeball, finger, chin, toe) which will link up to electronic typewriters, computers, or to the more complex communication and environmental controls systems (such as the Possum system).

Technical aids and medical physics services

The supply of technical aids specifically tailored to an individual's needs is an essential part of disability services. The Medical Physics department of a hospital will be the usual route through which such services are delivered.

Aids for sensory disabilities

It is important to ensure that people with sensory disabilities such as visual and auditory impairment have had a proper clinical assessment. They must also have access to medical and surgical treatment where they can potentially benefit from it. Having said this, a proportion of blind or deaf people will not have a problem which is amenable to specific intervention. The approach is then to ensure that they receive aids and equipment to minimise the degree of disability and handicap caused by their condition. In the case of the deaf, this can mean the fitting of a hearing aid, or other devices to assist amplification of sound, aids to the home (such as lights on telephones and door bells), and vibration devices for the profoundly deaf.

Similarly, the range of aids and equipment for blind people is now quite large. Longer term measures used in the rehabilitation of blind people include teaching them to read Braille and Moon and touch typing. Some of these services are more appropriate for the younger blind rather than very elderly people. The Wireless for the Blind Fund can arrange for any registered blind person in need of a radio to have one. Free membership is available to blind people for the Braille National Library for the Blind and for the Royal National Institute for the Blind which also has a large talking book library.

Braille dials can be fitted to most gas and electric cookers. Clocks and watches are available with special markings and embossed playing cards, chess, dominoes, draughts and other games are obtainable.

A number of occupations have traditionally become well established for blind people. There are several two to three year courses for piano tuners, most of whom set up their own businesses. Training courses are also available for blind people who wish to take up audio and shorthand typing and switchboard operating. Physiotherapy is also popular with blind people and many have successful careers in teaching, social work and the law, as well as in newer areas of employment, such as computing.

About 1% of those on the blind register are also deaf; most of these people are elderly. A small number of people are deaf and blind without speech, mostly as a result of congenital defects. This small group of handicapped people require very specialised help and a number of aids have been devised to meet their needs. Most will qualify for attendance allowance at the lower rate.

Primary care and community services

Many of the services for disabled people already described in this section are delivered to people living in the community. Most people with disability will be registered with a general practitioner. Through this, they will have access to the services provided by the practice and the wider primary care team, including home nursing, dietetic and chiropody services, as well as general medical care. However, many people with disability may not be in regular contact with their general practitioner. Thus, whilst general practitioners provide a logical point of contact for disabled people, the numbers and requirements of disabled people in the practice population may not be clearly identified. Community social care services such as meals on wheels, home helps and care assistants which are most often provided for the elderly (described in chapter 8) can also be provided to younger disabled people.

Day care

Day care is an important component in the network of services for disabled people. It is mainly provided by either social services departments or by certain voluntary organisations, although specialist hospital facilities may develop a day care service alongside acute work.

Regular attendance at a day care centre helps disabled people to structure their time. It also facilitates important social contact and access to other specialist services. On a more practical level, meals are usually provided in the day care setting. Such measures also provide a safe and comfortable environment. Some day care, particularly that provided by voluntary organisations, has social integration as its main aim. It focuses on providing social activities for both able-bodied and disabled people. Such organisations tend to operate on an informal, drop-in basis.

Support for carers

Adequate support for those providing informal care to people with special needs is an increasingly important aim of statutory services. It is a key feature of the Community Care component of the NHS and Community Care Act 1990, described at various points in this book in relation to other care groups. The White Paper 'Caring for People' which resulted in this legislation made it particularly clear that carers should be fully involved in the assessment process, not only as partners with statutory agencies in providing care for disabled people, but also as individuals who themselves may have special needs.

The support which carers need has two dimensions. The first is aimed at providing the carer with a break. Services such as sitting services, respite care services, emergency cover and holiday care are all examples of what is required to enable the carer to be relieved of the task of caring for a short time. It is particularly important that respite services are available when carers want them, and that there is continuity of care among respite personnel. The second type of support for carers is aimed at helping the carer directly in the caring role. Examples would be education about lifting the disabled person and preventing pressure sores or in managing incontinence. Opportunities to form and participate in carers' support groups are also useful. Here, as is the case with all disability services, it is extremely important that health and social services agencies work together so that the full spectrum of carers' needs can be addressed.

Residential care

Different agencies are involved in providing residential accommodation: local authorities, voluntary organisations and the private sector. The type of residential accommodation needed by disabled people depends on individual requirements. Under the new Community Care legislation implemented in full from April 1993, social services departments as the lead agency are responsible for assessing need and determining the type of care required, including residential care.

LEGISLATION

National Assistance Act 1948

This Act was one of the main pillars of the welfare state established at the end of World War II. It was a wide ranging legislative measure dealing with various people in need, including disabled people. Amongst its measures it included powers for local authorities to provide for the welfare of "persons who are blind, deaf or dumb and other persons who are substantially and permanently handicapped by illness, injury or congenital deformity or such other disabilities as may be prescribed by the Minister".

Under the Act, the arrangement which local authorities may make include:

- advice on available services to those concerned;
- instruction in ways of overcoming the effects of disability;
- provision of workshops and hostels for handicapped workers;
- provision of work for handicapped persons;
- assistance in the disposal of the produce of such work;
- the provision of recreational facilities;
- compilation and maintenance of a register of handicapped persons.

Although most of the powers in the Act were discretionary, it was made a duty to provide welfare services for blind people, as had been the case in previous statutes. The Act also gave local authorities powers to contribute to the funds of voluntary organisations and use them as their agents to provide certain services.

The Education Act 1944

This Act was a second pillar of the post-war welfare state and placed a general duty on local education authorities to provide educational provision for all children of school age, including all those with special needs.

Chronically Sick and Disabled Persons Act 1970

This Act was a further major extension and improvement of services for disabled people. It was introduced as a Private Member's Bill and was intended to make it compulsory for local authorities to provide welfare services for disabled people. It set out the legal framework for wide ranging measures including welfare, housing, access to and facilities at premises open to the public, provision of public sanitary conveniences, public signs, access to and facilities at educational establishments, badges for display on motor vehicles and special educational treatment for the deaf, blind, autistic and dyslexic individuals.

Section I of the Act places a *duty* on every local authority (having functions under Section 29 of the National Assistance Act 1948) to inform themselves of the numbers and needs of disabled persons to whom Section 29 applies in their area. They are also required to publish information about the services they provide and *ensure* that disabled people are informed of other services relevant to their needs.

Under Section II of this Act such Authorities *must* make arrangements for any or all of the matters listed that are necessary to meet the needs of the disabled who are ordinarily resident in their area:

- practical assistance in his home;
- assistance in obtaining television, library or similar recreational facilities;
- lectures, games, outings or other recreational facilities outside his home or assistance in taking advantage of educational facilities;
- facilities for or assistance in travelling to and from his home for the purpose of participating in any services provided under these arrangements by the Authority;

- assistance in arranging for the carrying out of any works of adaptation in his home or for the provision of any additional facilities designed to secure greater safety, comfort or convenience;
- facilitating the taking of holidays;
- provision of meals for the disabled person, whether in the home or elsewhere;
- assistance in obtaining a telephone and any special equipment necessary to enable him to use the telephone.

Other provisions include the separation of the younger long-term disabled people from the elderly in hospital and local authority residential accommodation and the appointment of disabled people or those with experience of their needs to serve on advisory bodies and local authority committees. Permitting the use of pavements and footpaths by wheelchairs, whether motorised or not and the issue of badges for motor vehicles is another function of the local authorities in meeting the needs of disabled people.

The Education Act 1981, Education Reform Act 1988

These two pieces of education legislation specify the procedures to be followed by local education authorities when undertaking the assessment and statementing of children with special needs. The Reform Act encourages inclusion of children with special needs in mainstream teaching of the national curriculum.

The Disabled Persons (Services, Consultations and Representation) Act 1986

This Act is an attempt to strengthen the legal backing for the provision of support and services for disabled people. The individual is involved much more in decisions. A disabled person has a right to be assessed by the local authority and to receive a written statement of needs and of the services available to meet them. If the authority decides the person has no need, then they must give an explanation for this.

Other provisions of the Act relate to ensuring that official bodies work together, particularly in the context of disabled people, who are leaving education or being discharged from hospital.

Arrangements can be made for an authorised representative to act for the disabled person. Other Sections of the Act are concerned with the ability of carers and with the supply of helpful information by social services departments, concerning not only their own services but those available from other bodies.

NHS and Community Care Act 1990

With the full implementation of this Act in 1993, local authorities are required to meet social care needs of disabled people in new ways. They have lead responsibility for carrying out an appropriate assessment of an individual's need for social care (including residential and nursing home care). They must collaborate with appropriate health agencies in this task. They are also the lead agency in developing packages of services to meet the assessed need: in securing the delivery of services; in monitoring the effectiveness of services.

Before the implementation of this Act, disabled people could find that their social care needs were not assessed or adequately met because neither health nor social services agencies would accept responsibility for the work. The Act sought to remedy this situation by a clear allocation of responsibility to local authorities strengthened by the creation of a unified social care bridge for the purchase of individual packages of care.

The Children Act 1989

The Children Act 1989 clarifies and emphasises the unique situation of the child with disability. Local authorities have a requirement to open and maintain a register of local children with disabilities, and to provide services to minimise as far as possible the effects of disability. The Act imposes new duties on social services departments with regard to children 'in need' and their families, and specifies that the definition of in need includes all children with disabilities. A fundamental focus of the legislation and its associated policy guidance is that every effort should be made to work collaboratively in multi-agency structures so that an effective network of services is available for children in need.

Limitation of Statutory Powers

Section II of the 1970 Act, made it a duty to provide a wide range of services provided the local authority was satisfied that the individual's need existed. Thus, local authorities can create their own criteria for the existence of need. Over the years, local authorities have complained that they do not have adequate funds to provide all the services required, thus there is ample evidence which indicates that all the needs of disabled people are not being met. Although the Disabled Persons Act 1986 has gone some way towards strengthening the 1970 Act and to provide an adequate and uniform standard of service throughout the country, the situation is still far from satisfactory.

EMPLOYMENT AND TRAINING

Work, though a means of financing household necessities and leisure pursuits, also provides status and self-esteem for the individual and is the basis of many social contacts. Indeed, for some it represents the main focus of their lives. The work orientation of many modern societies is a source of additional pressure for disabled people. Even those who are very severely disabled may perceive work as a means of drawing closer to normal members of society.

Under the Wages Act 1986 a disabled person must not be employed on terms less favourable than someone who is not disabled. However, the main legal framework underpinning the employment of disabled people is laid down in the Disabled Persons Employment Acts 1944 and 1958.

The 1944 Act defines a disabled person as "one who, on account of injury or disease (including a physical or mental condition arising from imperfect development of any organ) or congenital deformity, is substantially handicapped in obtaining or keeping employment or undertaking work on his own account of a kind which apart from injury, disease or deformity would be suited to his age, experience and qualifications".

The Act provides for the setting up of a register of disabled persons. The Secretary of State for Employment may designate certain categories of work as being reserved for registered disabled people. It is an offence for an employer to engage an unregistered person for these kinds of work without permission. The Act also makes provision for training and rehabilitation courses.

The 1958 Act empowers local authorities to provide sheltered employment for disabled people. The Act also allows a disabled person who objects to his name appearing on a register to have it removed (no provision had been made for this in the earlier Act).

Most of the policies and responsibilities for employment, including those for disabled people, are controlled centrally. The government department concerned is the Department of Employment but the services are run by an agency known as the Employment Service. The Employment Service provides a range of services to help disabled people to get jobs. Another agency of the Department of Employment is responsible for training, the Training Agency.

A new, more coordinated employment service for disabled people was introduced in the early 1990s following the publication by the Department of Employment of a consultative document called 'Employment and Training for People with Disabilities'.

The service created comprises two main features. The first was the establishment of Placing, Assessment and Counselling Teams (PACTs) which are responsible for helping people with disabilities who face particular difficulties in the labour market to go into open, sheltered or self-employment or to retain their present employment. PACTs also promote the value of people with disabilities to employers and market the range of the Employment Service's facilities which are available to disabled people.

PACTs are staffed on a multidisciplinary basis and take over functions of the previous organisation (including, for example, the Disablement Resettlement Officer). The second feature of the present service is the Disability Resource Centre which seeks to improve the quality of specialist help for people with disabilities, and to provide training for those involved in this aspect of employment services.

Types of employment available to registered disabled people

Employment in open industry under the quota arrangements

The quota is currently 3% of all employees and the regulations apply to all firms employing more than 20 people. Although it is not an offence to be below the quota, an employer in this situation must not engage a non-disabled person to fill a quota place without a permit from the disablement resettlement officer.

Employment in designated jobs

Two occupations are reserved specifically for registered disabled people: car park attendants and passenger electric lift attendants. For these jobs an employer must obtain permission from the disablement resettlement officer to employ a non-disabled person.

Sheltered employment

For those disabled people who are so handicapped that they are unable to work in open employment, a number of opportunities are available.

Remploy is the best known in this field and is a limited company established by the government in 1946 to provide meaningful work for severely disabled people who are unable to obtain it in open industry. The company produces a wide range of products, including textiles, furniture and leather goods. It employs about 9,000 severely disabled people in 94 production units.

Some sheltered workshops are also provided by local authorities and voluntary organisations. Examples of the latter are the Royal British Legion and the Spastic Society. There are about 150 such workshops in Britain employing over 6,000 severely disabled people.

Special schemes to assist in employment of disabled people

The following are some of the schemes available:

Job introduction scheme

This is intended to encourage employers to give a trial period of employment (usually six weeks) to disabled people to assess their suitability for a job. During this time a contribution by the Employment Service is made towards their wages. This scheme is open to all disabled people and not limited to those on the register.

Sheltered placement scheme

This scheme has the advantage of providing sheltered employment in areas where sheltered workshops are not available but even more important it allows the disabled person to work alongside able-bodied workers. A sponsor (voluntary organisation, Remploy or a local authority) employs the disabled person and a host employer provides the work. The employer contributes to the wages on the basis of the disabled person's output.

Special aids to employment

Special tools or equipment, which an able-bodied person doing the same work would not need, are available on permanent loan (and free of charge) to assist a disabled person.

Adaptations to premises and equipment

Grants may be given to employers towards the cost of adapting premises and equipment to enable them to recruit disabled workers more easily.

Assistance with fares to work scheme

This scheme recognises the additional expense of getting to and from work for disabled people who cannot use public transport. People must be on the Disabled Persons' Register to qualify for this assistance.

Training

The main training facilities for disabled people are summarised below. Some are open to all employees. The Training Agency and other agencies are involved in this process.

Job training scheme

This scheme offers opportunities for unemployed adults to update their existing skills or learn new ones. It is open to people aged 18 and over who have been unemployed for at least six months.

Employment rehabilitation centres

The Training Agency has 27 of these centres located in various parts of the country in or near centres of population. Courses are arranged for individuals and so vary in length as well as content, although their usual duration is six to eight weeks. Specialist advice can be obtained from occupational psychologists, social workers, occupational therapists and physicians. The centres are equipped with modern factory and office facilities. Free meals are provided and travelling and subsistence allowances are available.

Residential training colleges

For those disabled people who need training under residential conditions, four colleges are provided by voluntary organisations, supported by the Training Agency. They are located at Durham, Exeter, Leatherhead and Mansfield and have over 1,000 places. Disabled people aged between 16 and 58, from any part of the country can attend courses and admission is arranged through the local disablement resettlement officer. They are not intended however, for blind people, for whom there are separate facilities.

Training for younger disabled people

Local education authorities provide a career service which is especially designed for young people who are attending full or part time educational institutions (except universities) or have just left them. It provides vocational guidance as well as help in obtaining employment. Many education authorities appoint special careers officers to work with handicapped secondary school children and to counsel them and their parents about employment. Confidential medical reports are obtained from local doctors and from the Employment Medical Advisory Service of the Health and Safety Executive. Careers officers also work closely with other agencies concerned with disabled young people, such as social workers and voluntary organisations. Education authorities have a duty to inform local social services departments when a disabled person is about to leave full time education.

BENEFITS AND ALLOWANCES

Many people with disability have a lower earning capacity than other members of society and are over-represented in the lower socio-economic groups. By the nature of their disability as well as on the basis of their level of income, disabled people are entitled to a wide range of benefits, special payments and income support. People who care for those with a disability also have certain entitlements. The whole system of financial support is quite complex and, therefore, an important component of services for people with disability and their carers is a mechanism to ensure that they are receiving their full entitlements. In practice, this means the provision of leaflets and other printed information in an easily readable form coupled with access to people who are skilled in the interpretation of the regulations and who can give specific advice and help. It is not surprising that specialist advisory staff are often in great demand where they are part of a Disabled Living Centre.

The benefits and income support field is a rapidly changing one and so the main features of the present framework are described in this section rather than all detailed aspects.

Statutory sick pay, sickness benefit and invalidity benefit

A number of benefits arise from the payment of national insurance contributions at work. Statutory sick pay is for people who are off sick for four or more days in a row up to a maximum of 28 weeks. Thereafter, the person is entitled to Invalidity Benefit which is paid automatically. Sickness benefit is for people who are employed but either cannot get statutory sick pay from their employer, are self-employed, or unemployed but entitlement is dependent upon the person having made the appropriate National Insurance contributions previously.

Severe disablement allowance

The Severe Disablement Allowance is a tax-free benefit for people aged 16 years and over who have not been able to work for at least eight weeks because of long term sickness or disability and who do not normally get sickness benefit because they have not paid sufficient National Insurance contributions. The allowance is not means-tested and does not depend on National Insurance contributions.

People who become incapable of work after their 20th birthday must be assessed as at least 80% disabled for a minimum of 28 consecutive weeks. There are certain criteria which mean that a person will be automatically regarded as 80% disabled. Otherwise, a medical assessment can be carried out using a scheme similar to that used for war and industrial injuries. Each disability is given a percentage and the percentages added together to give a total assessment. It does not follow that someone has to be housebound or requiring continuous attention to qualify for the Severe Disablement Allowance. For example, someone who is profoundly deaf or totally blind will be assessed as 100% disabled. Similarly, so will someone who has lost both arms or legs, however well they may manage with artificial limbs. Some kinds of disablement vary too much to be covered by hard and fast rules and there are no set percentages for some conditions.

Disability living allowance

The Disability Living Allowance is a tax-free benefit for people aged under 65 years and is not dependent on National Insurance contributions having been made.

It is designed for people who need help with personal care because of illness or disability and also for those who need help with mobility. The allowance is paid in two separate components (personal care, mobility) and each at different rates depending on the amount of help required.

Attendance allowance

A tax-free weekly Attendance Allowance can be paid to people who are disabled from 65 years of age and who need help with their personal care. Like the Disability Living Allowance it is not dependent on National Insurance contributions but a person must usually have needed help for six months before they became entitled to it.

Benefits for disability through injuries sustained at work, at war or in the armed forces

A variety of benefits is paid to workers who become disabled or injured at work. Industrial Injuries Disablement Benefit is paid at different rates (depending on the extent of disablement) to people who were in an accident at work. Compensation schemes also exist for payments due to injuries or industrial diseases as a result of negligence on the part of an employer. Disease benefits for pneumoconiosis, byssinosis and certain other diseases can be paid to people who sustained them before 1948. After this date, payments are usually made under the Industrial Injuries Disablement Benefit.

It has long been a principle that people who serve in the armed forces should be adequately compensated for injury or disablement sustained in the course of their duties. In the case of the War Disablement Pension the amount payable depends on the degree of impairment and this is assessed medically. The rate is also related to the rank of the recipient and thus, is earnings related. This pension continues after retirement age, is paid in addition to the old age pension and is unaffected by other sources of income. There are also allowances for dependants. The amount of pension paid is reduced only if there is an improvement in the disabling condition.

Disability working allowance

People who are 18 years or over and who have an illness or disability which limits their ability to earn, may be entitled to Disability Working Allowance. The allowance is tax-free and is not dependent on National Insurance contributions. The amount paid depends on the income of the disabled person and his or her partner. The amount paid is also affected by the size of any savings of the person and partner together and beyond a certain level of savings, the person becomes ineligible for the allowance.

Vaccine damage

People who have been severely disabled as a result of vaccination against diphtheria, tetanus, whooping cough, tuberculosis, poliomyelitis, mumps, measles, or rubella may be entitled to compensation as a lump sum payment.

Invalid care allowance

Someone who is of working age and providing a caring role for a person in receipt of Attendance Allowance may be eligible for an Invalid Care Allowance. This is not dependent on National Insurance contributions. To be eligible the person must be spending at least 35 hours per week in the caring role, be below a particular earnings threshold and be caring for a person who is receiving Disability Living Allowance at the middle or higher rates for the care component (or who fulfils certain other criteria of severe disability).

Parking concessions

The Orange Badge scheme enables people with certain categories of disability to apply for, and obtain, a display badge which entitles them to park in some restricted areas.

Disabled facilities grant

Under the Local Government and Housing Act, 1989, local housing authorities are able to give disabled facilities grants to disabled people to help them with the cost of adaptations in their home. The main principle is that disabled people should be able to enjoy comparable facilities in their homes to those enjoyed by able-bodied people. Mandatory grants are available for essential work and discretionary grants are available for work going beyond basic housing requirements. These grants are means-tested awards.

Other financial support

People with disability, depending on their circumstances, can be entitled to a wide range of other financial support through the social security and allied arrangements. These include Income Support, Family Credit, the Social Fund, Housing Benefit and help with NHS charges.

CONCLUSION

The value attached to disabled people and the extent to which they are regarded and treated as full members of the population is an important indicator of how caring a society is. Identifying the numbers of people in the population who are disabled, describing the nature of their disability and the needs which result from it has not been accorded a high priority in the past. Assessing need at both individual and population level is a key pre-requisite to the provision of appropriate services and requires attention being given to gathering and maintaining high quality information. Services for people with disability will be most effective when they are based on such needs assessment and when they are founded on team work – both at the organisational (health, local authority and voluntary agency) and at the individual (doctors, nurses, therapists, social workers) level.

6 Mothers and children

INTRODUCTION

Until about 70 years ago, childbirth was an event which threatened the life of both mother and baby. Deaths of women in labour were not uncommon and children's funerals were a prominent feature of everyday life.

Throughout the ages, children have been subjected to harsh and inhuman treatment and, until fairly recently, infanticide was regularly practised. Not everyone appreciates that the famous politician and Prime Minister of the last century, Benjamin Disraeli (1804 – 1881), was also a novelist. A quotation from *Sybil; Or The Two Nations* is an eloquent commentary on life at that time for some mothers and children in England.

> 'About a fortnight after his mother had introduced him into the world, she returned to her factory and put her infant out to nurse: that is to say, paid threepence a week to an old woman, who takes charge of these newborn babies for the day and gives them back at night to their mothers as they hurriedly return from the scene of their labour to the dungeon or the den, which is still by courtesy called 'home'. The expense is not great: laudanum and treacle, administered in the shape of some popular elixir, affords these innocents a brief taste of the sweets of existence and, keeping them quiet, prepares them for the silence of their impending grave. Infanticide is practised as extensively and as legally in England as it is on the banks of the Ganges: a circumstance which apparently has not yet engaged the attention of the Society for the Propagation of the Gospel in Foreign Parts.'

From the beginning of the present century up to modern times there has been a steep decline, both in maternal deaths and in mortality in the early years of life and later childhood. There is still considerable scope for improvement. In particular, many traditional inequalities between different sections of the population persist.

This chapter deals with the health of children and of mothers around the time of childbirth. The main ways of assessing health and need in these sections of the population are described. The scope for the promotion of health in the early years of life is discussed in terms of the prevention of fetal loss and of fetal abnormalities as well as the measures required to improve health amongst women of childbearing age. The range of services which are provided for mothers and children are described and where appropriate, set in their statutory framework.

BIRTH AND FERTILITY

Registration and notification of births, stillbirths and neonatal deaths

Registration of births, stillbirths and neonatal deaths is a legal requirement. The information is collected by the local Registrar of Births, Marriages and Deaths and transmitted to the Office of Population Censuses and Surveys. Statistics are derived from these data about live births and stillbirths, fertility, duration of marriage and other demographic information.

Every birth must be registered:

- With the local Registrar.
- By a parent or other informant.
- Within 42 days of birth.

Information collected as part of birth registration covers: date and place of birth, the baby's name and surname and its sex, the name, address and place of birth of parents, the occupation of the father and the mother's maiden name (or surname at marriage). Confidential information is also collected (but not entered in the register) which includes dates of birth of mother and father, date of parents' marriage (if the child is a legitimate birth), whether the mother was previously married, number of previous children (with present and previous husbands) distinguishing whether live or stillborn.

As with live births, the same legal obligation exists to ensure registration of all stillbirths and neonatal deaths. The legal definition of a stillbirth as amended by the Stillbirth (Definition) Act 1992 is:

'A child which has issued forth from its mother after the 24th week of pregnancy and which did not at any time after, having been completely expelled from its mother, breathe or show any other signs of life.'

A neonatal death is a baby born alive but who died within the first four weeks of birth. Recorded by the local Registrar are the same details about the father and mother as with live births. In addition a death certificate is obtained which is signed by a midwife who attended the birth or examined the body.

From the beginning of 1986, new stillbirth and neonatal death certificates were introduced in England and Wales which accorded with World Health Organisation guidelines. Amongst other issues, the new certificate sought to allow mention by the certifying doctor of both maternal and fetal causal factors (Table 6.1), although it is not now possible to select a single underlying cause of death.

In addition to birth registration, a parallel process of birth notification takes place. The midwife, doctor or other attendant at the birth is legally required to notify within 36 hours the health authority in which the birth occurred. The information usually reported in this notification includes: birthweight, length of gestation, parity and the presence of congenital malformation.

It is important to understand that registration and notification of births serve different purposes. Registration is essentially intended to collect information for statistical purposes. Notification is intended to alert Health Authorities to the birth

Table 6.1: *Cause of death categories in the certification of stillbirth and neonatal death*

- Main diseases or conditions in the fetus or infant
- Other diseases or conditions in the fetus or infant
- Main maternal diseases or conditions affecting the fetus or infant
- Other maternal diseases or conditions affecting the fetus or infant
- Other relevant causes

of the child so that the necessary services can be brought into action to support the mother and her new baby. Here there is a need for urgency in passing on the information about the birth of the child. There is also an exchange of information between the Health Authority and the Registrar of Births and Deaths. The Health Authority passes brief information of the notification of births to the Registrar as they are received in order to assist in obtaining full registration. The only medical information which is transferred is birthweight. It is incorporated with the co-operation of the Registrar and is not a legal requirement. When added to the other data collected at birth registration, it allows statistics of live and still births to be compiled to include this important dimension.

Indices of fertility

Crude birth rate

The number of live births, expressed as a rate per 1,000 total population per annum, is the annual crude birth rate. Although often quoted, it is a poor indicator of fertility because included in the denominator are males, children and post-menopausal women, (the limitations of 'crude' rates are discussed in chapter 1).

General fertility rate

A better denominator is used in the general fertility rate, which is calculated by expressing the number of live births per 1,000 women in the population of child-bearing age (by convention this is usually taken as those aged 15–44 years).

Age-specific fertility rates.

Because there are differences in levels of fertility amongst women of different ages within the child-bearing years, an even more precise measure of fertility is obtained by calculating the number of births to a specified age group per 1,000 women of that same age group. For example, the fertility rate for women aged 20–24 years is calculated by taking the number of live births occurring to mothers aged 20–24 years and expressing them per 1,000 women aged between 20 and 24 years in the population.

Total period fertility rate

The total period fertility rate is a convenient summary of all the age-specific rates. This rate is the sum of the age-specific fertility rates, in this case expressed as live births per woman of a single age, rather than per 1,000 women. It measures the average number of live-born children per woman which would occur if the current age-specific fertility rates applied over the entire 30 years of the reproductive span. It therefore takes account of differential fertility within the different reproductive age groups, whilst providing a convenient summary measure in a single figure. It enables comparisons to be made between countries and within the same country over time. The replacement of the British population requires a total period fertility rate of 2.1. This figure is 2.1 and not 2.0 as might first be thought because it is necessary to allow for deaths which occur before the reproductive years are reached. Hence the replacement rate varies from country to country.

Cohort measures of fertility

All indices of fertility so far described have referred to births at a specific period of time, most often a single year. However, births in any given year occur to a cross-section of women, married at different ages and with differing numbers of previous children. Temporary fluctuations in 'period' indices, may simply reflect the timing of child births within a reproductive lifespan, without any important change in the number of children women will have by the time they have come to the end of their reproductive years. A cohort of women is a population of women who were born in a particular year (generation or birth cohort) or married in a particular year (marriage cohort). Studies of fertility, following such cohorts of women, observe the occurrence and timing of births in their reproductive lifetime. The cohort fertility rate (which gives the completed family size for women born around the same time) provides a much more stable basis for commenting on trends and predicting future levels of fertility than do measures based on a specific period of time. The cohort fertility rate has the disadvantage that it cannot properly be calculated until the cohort concerned has completely passed out of the childbearing years.

Trends in fertility

A fall in fertility in Britain during the economic depression of the 1930s, stimulated considerable national concern about the long term growth of the population. An increase in the birth rate occurred after the Second World War, since when fertility has been dominated by two distinct trends. During the decade between the mid 1950s and the mid 1960s, the number of births, the crude birth rate, the general fertility rate and total period fertility rate, all rose to a peak in the mid 1960s. The succeeding decade showed a sharp fall in the same indices of fertility. In 1977, the crude birth rate, the general fertility rate and the total period fertility rate, all fell below their corresponding values in 1933, the previous lowest level of this century. Trends in these indices over the last several decades are shown in Table 6.2. By the beginning of the 1990s, fertility had increased well above its low point in 1977 but not to the high level of the 1960s. Changes in the fertility rates in the 1960s and 1970s have not been properly explained and were largely unpredicted.

The greatest number of births occur in the 25–29 year old age group but fertility rates amongst older women have increased and the gap between the traditionally higher rates of fertility in younger women and those in older women had narrowed by the beginning of the 1990s (Figure 6.1). As a consequence, the average age of women at childbirth has increased gradually. At 27.5 years in 1990 it was at its highest since the early 1960s. Completed family size has gradually declined for successive cohorts of women; a family of two children is now the average.

There has also been an increase in childlessness (presumably voluntary) over successive cohorts of women. Amongst the 1955 cohort, 20% were still childless at 35 years of age compared with 12% for the 1945 cohort. There may be some catching up in the later years for this cohort but not enough to reverse what seems to be the genuine option of childlessness for more couples (Figure 6.2).

Table 6.2:   *Changes in various indices of fertility for selected years, England and Wales*

| Fertility index* | Year or period | | | | | | | |
	1933	1940/42	1950/52	1960/62	1970/72	1978	1980/82	1990
Crude birth rate	14.4	15.6	15.6	17.6	15.6	12.1	12.9	13.9
General fertility rate	59.4	61.3	72.1	88.9	81.4	60.1	61.8	64.3
Total period fertility rate	1.72	1.81	2.16	2.77	2.31	1.73	1.81	1.84

Source: Office of Population, Censuses and Surveys.
*See text for definitions

Factors affecting fertility

In few societies do women produce the maximum number of children of which they are physiologically capable. The number of children they will actually produce is influenced by a wide range of factors inherent in particular societies, such as marriage and cohabitation patterns, sexual mores and practices, contraceptive usage, and levels of economic prosperity, all of which are closely interwoven and complex to interpret.

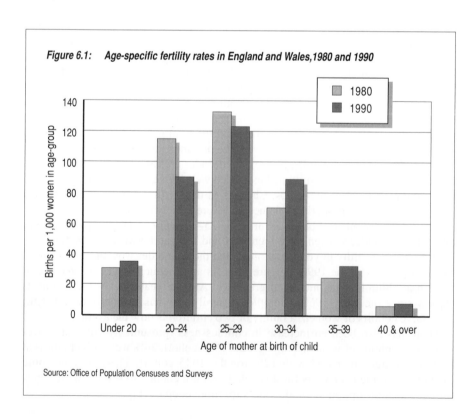

Figure 6.1:   *Age-specific fertility rates in England and Wales,1980 and 1990*

Source: Office of Population Censuses and Surveys

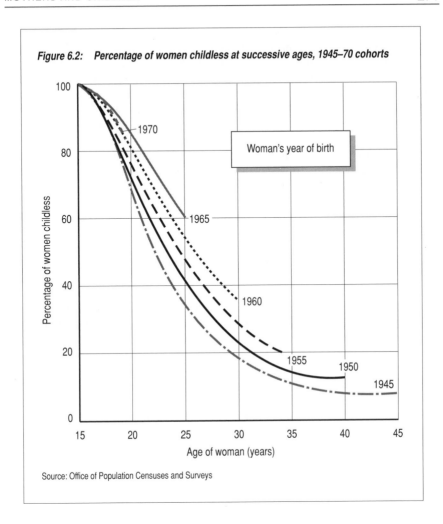

Figure 6.2:   Percentage of women childless at successive ages, 1945–70 cohorts

Source: Office of Population Censuses and Surveys

Factors which determine sexual behaviour in society are also wide-ranging and complex. They include the influence of society's norms and expectations, the family, the law, social or psychological factors in individuals, religion and lifestyle.

The term fecundity means the biological or physiological ability of a woman to become pregnant (i.e., her reproductive capacity). In the usual clinical setting a woman who remained childless, despite wanting and trying to have a child, would be described as 'infertile' or 'sterile'. The term 'fertility' used elsewhere in this chapter is a description of the number of babies who are actually produced by a population of women. Thus, it takes into account, not only their fecundity (basic physiological potential) but the impact of other factors, such as sexual activity and the use of contraception.

There are various formal definitions of 'infertility', most of which embody concepts of exposure to the risk of pregnancy over a certain period of time: for example, 'a failure to become pregnant over a period of a year whilst cohabiting and engaging in sexual intercourse without contraceptive use'.

There are a number of important influences on fertility. Factors both inherited and acquired, and of a short or long term nature, affect the physiological reproductive capacity of both males and females. Examples of acquired factors amongst women are infections, such as gonorrhoea, tuberculosis or other pelvic inflammatory conditions which may prevent conception by causing scarring and blockage of the fallopian tubes. All too often we stress the female causes of infertility, many of which are at least partly understood, but forget the male causes which are less well understood and less easy to treat. The advent of techniques such as in vitro fertilisation and Gamete Intrafallopian Transfer (GIFT) have widened the scope of infertility treatment.

Changes in marriage and cohabitation practices are another influence which will determine the number of babies born to a population of women of childbearing age. By the early 1990s, just over a quarter of all births in Britain occurred outside marriage, doubling the number of those in the late 1970s. However, the evidence would suggest that a substantial proportion of such births occur to couples who are cohabiting, with both parents caring for the child, even though not formally married. In over three-fifths of the cases of illegitimate births, both parents register the birth.

There are three main aspects of marriage which have important implications in terms of fertility. They are the proportion of women who marry, the average age of marriage and the degree of restriction of family size within marriage. Other demographic forces play a part in determining the proportion of people who will marry at any one time. The availability of partners for marriage is important. In the United Kingdom this has varied in this century because of excessive mortality of young males in wartime, as well as outward migration. Economic circumstances also affect the tendency of people to marry. The impact of marriage on fertility is now complicated by the fact that an increasing number of marriages are remarriages and that women may have children with their new partners. Divorce rates have risen particularly sharply in England and Wales compared with some other European countries, a feature to some extent, of differences in divorce legislation.

A number of explanations have been put forward to account for the changes in fertility which have occurred since World War II. Three common interpretations of the trends are as follows:

a. *Contraceptive availability*
    The widespread availability of modern contraceptive methods, particularly the introduction of oral contraception in Britain in the early 1960s. However, fertility fell in a similar way in the 1930s, when contraceptive technology was primitive. Trends in fertility, similar to those seen in Britain over the last 20 years, occurred in other industrial societies in Western Europe, North America and Australia and not all had well developed Family Planning Services. It seems unlikely that the availability of the oral contraceptive pill is the entire story. If a couple decide to limit the size of their family, they can do so with or without modern contraception. However, modern contraceptive methods have made the limiting of the family size much easier without curtailing sexual activity.

b. *Level of affluence*
    Levels of income and attitudes towards future prosperity are said to be influential. Hence, a parallel is drawn between the economic depression of the

1930s, which is considered to have been largely responsible for the reduction in fertility at that time and the downturn in fertility in the early 1970s when an economic recession also prevailed. However, the decline in fertility had started well before the financial crisis brought about by the increase in oil prices in 1973 so, once again, this cannot be the whole explanation.

c. *Working women*
More women of childbearing age now enter the labour force. It is believed that women restrict their family size in order to remain at work. However, the upward trend in the proportion of married women at work, was just as steep during the rise in fertility in the early 1960s as it was during the decline in the 1970s.

It is probable that all three factors, as well as others, influence fertility in a complex manner that is not fully understood, which illustrates the difficulty in predicting trends in fertility, even in the relatively short term.

HEALTH AND NEED AMONGST CHILDREN AND WOMEN IN PREGNANCY

An important aspect of the health of the population of children as well as women who are pregnant is the number of deaths which occur and their causes. Childhood mortality must be examined around the time of birth, in the early period of life as well as in the older children's age groups. Fortunately, death in childhood is now relatively uncommon in Britain so that a health needs assessment also entails reviewing the pattern of disease and disability in childhood. Increasingly, family factors such as lifestyle and behaviour, as well as social and environmental determinants of disease, are recognised as fundamental in assessing overall health status of the childhood population.

Maternal mortality

Improvements in the health of pregnant women, general medical advances (for example, the advent of antibiotics and blood transfusion), a reduction in the number of illegal abortions, together with improved standards of obstetric care, have all contributed to a major decline in maternal mortality during the present century. (Figure 6.3). At the turn of the century, in Britain, one in 200 women died in or around the time of childbirth, whilst by the beginning of the 1990s, the figure was around one in 13,000.

A maternal death is defined by the World Health Organisation as:

'the death of a woman while pregnant or within 42 days of termination of pregnancy, from any cause related to or aggravated by the pregnancy or its management, but not from accidental or incidental causes.'

Since 1952, a detailed confidential enquiry has been carried out into all maternal deaths in England and Wales. Separate enquiries have operated in the constituent countries of the United Kingdom but information was brought together as a single report for the first time in 1991. Maternal deaths are subdivided into 'direct', 'indirect' and 'fortuitous' (Figure 6.4). Direct maternal deaths are those resulting

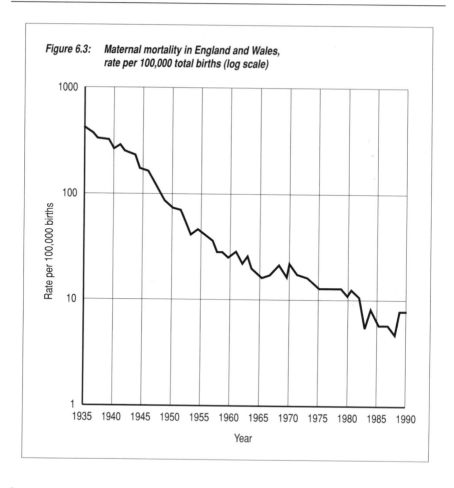

Figure 6.3:   Maternal mortality in England and Wales,
                rate per 100,000 total births (log scale)

from obstetric complications of pregnancy, labour and the puerperium. Indirect maternal deaths are those arising from an existing disease or from one which developed in pregnancy. Fortuitous maternal deaths are those resulting from causes not related to or influenced by pregnancy.

The enquiry into a maternal death is voluntary and initiated in England by the Director of Public Health (DPH) of the district in which the woman was usually resident (or equivalent officers in other United Kingdom countries). Using a standard enquiry form, information is collected from the various health staff concerned with the care of the woman. These may include general practitioners, midwives, health visitors, consultant obstetricians and anaesthetists.

The completed form, together with the Director of Public Health's comments is forwarded to an obstetric assessor who is a Consultant Obstetrician (and, where appropriate, to Anaesthetic or Pathology Assessors). The Assessors add their comments and opinions regarding the cause of death. The forms are then sent to the Chief Medical Officer. Central Assessors review all the recorded information and act as final arbiters in evaluating the factors which may have led to death. There are minor differences in the procedure between the different United Kingdom countries. Strict confidentiality is observed at all stages and reports based on the

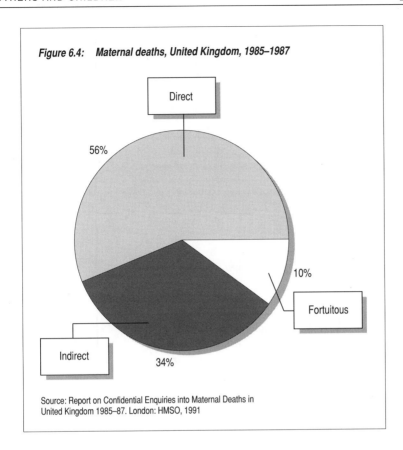

Figure 6.4:   Maternal deaths, United Kingdom, 1985–1987

Direct

56%

10%

Fortuitous

Indirect   34%

Source: Report on Confidential Enquiries into Maternal Deaths in
United Kingdom 1985–87. London: HMSO, 1991

analysis are published every three years. The reports draw general conclusions about causes of maternal deaths and changes over time and they make recommendations for action based upon the lessons learned.

Since the 1970s, the two leading causes of direct maternal death have been pulmonary embolism and hypertension in pregnancy. There has been a major decline in the proportion of anaesthetic deaths despite a rise in the number of mothers receiving anaesthetics (Table 6.3). This undoubtedly reflects improved standards of care provided by obstetric anaesthetists.

Despite the relatively low level of maternal deaths compared to the past, reports of the confidential enquiries into maternal mortality continue to make recommendations which, if implemented, would bring about further improvements. Reports have highlighted issues such as: the need for better communication between doctors, midwives and other professional staff involved in caring for pregnant women, greater involvement of consultants during pregnancy and labour and a failure to recognise and act upon potential problems when they develop.

Mortality in early life

Death rates in infancy are constructed differently from the mortality rates of later childhood and adult life. Births occurring during the same period as the deaths, not

Table 6.3: Causes of direct maternal deaths (percentage of total): England and Wales 1970–1987

Period	Pulmonary embolism	Hypertensive disorders of pregnancy	Anaesthesia	Amniotic fluid embolism	Abortion	Ectopic pregnancy	Haemorrhage	Sepsis excluding abortion	Ruptured uterus	Other direct causes	All deaths
1970–72	14.9	12.5	10.8	4.1	21.3	9.9	8.7	8.7	3.2	5.8	100(343)
1973–75	14.5	15.0	11.9	6.2	11.9	8.4	9.3	8.4	4.8	9.7	100(227)
1976–78	19.8	13.4	12.4	5.1	6.5	9.7	11.1	6.9	6.5	8.8	100(217)
1979–81	12.9	20.2	12.4	10.1	7.9	11.2	7.9	4.5	2.2	10.7	100(178)
1982–84	18.1	18.1	13.0	10.1	8.0	7.2	6.5	1.4	2.2	15.2	100(138)
1985–87	19.8	20.7	4.1	7.4	5.0	9.1	8.3	5.0	4.1	16.5	100(121)

Source: Report on Confidential Enquiries into Maternal Deaths in the United Kingdom 1985–87. London: HMSO, 1991.

the population of a particular age group, is the denominator. 'Infancy' is taken as the first year of life and thus, the *infant mortality* rate in a given period of time (usually a year) is the number of deaths of children under the age of one year (numerator) per 1,000 live births in the same period.

The infant mortality rate has long been regarded as an important measure of the health of a community. However, it is a rather crude indicator because deaths occurring during different periods of the first year of life usually reflect different groups of causal factors.

It has become customary to consider infancy in a number of different time periods:

(a) The perinatal period – from the 24th week of gestation to the end of the first week of life (after birth).
(b) The early neonatal period – the first week of life (after birth).
(c) The late neonatal period – from the end of the first week to the 28th day of life (after birth).
(d) The neonatal period – the first 28 days of life (after birth).
(e) The post-neonatal period – from the 28th day to the end of the first year of life (after birth).

The formal definitions of these rates are shown in Table 6.4.

Table 6.4:   *Definitions of annual mortality rates of infancy*

Stillbirth rate	Number of stillbirths per 1,000 *total* births per annum.
Perinatal mortality rate	Number of stillbirths together with deaths in the first week of life per 1,000 *total* births per annum.
Early neonatal mortality rate	Number of deaths in the first week of life per 1,000 *live* births per annum.
Late neonatal mortality rate	Number of deaths between the 7th and 28th day of life per 1,000 *live* births per annum.
Neonatal mortality rate	Number of deaths in the first 28 days of life per 1,000 *live* births per annum.
Post-neonatal mortality rate	Number of deaths after 28 days but before the end of the first year of life per 1,000 *live* births per annum.

The various mortality rates are constructed around these different periods of infancy (Figure 6.5). The numerator is all deaths occurring within the period of infancy in question (usually during a calendar year), the denominator is the number of registered live births during that same calendar year. The exceptions to this general rule are stillbirths (babies born dead after 24 weeks of gestation) and perinatal deaths (stillbirths plus babies dying in the first week after birth) where the denominator in each case is total births (i.e., both live and stillbirths). In other words, when stillbirths are included in the numerator then the denominator is total births, not live births alone. Records of infant deaths are routinely linked nationally to their birth certificates. This enables such deaths to be analysed using data collected at birth registration (which is more extensive).

Perinatal deaths

Amongst the reasons for using this index, which groups together stillbirths and deaths in the first week of life, is that the factors responsible for these two types of death are often similar, being those operating before or around the time of birth. Another practical reason is that it overcomes some of the difficulties (particularly in making international comparisons) of variation between different localities as to which conceptuses are regarded as stillborn and which as having been born alive but died shortly after birth. Information on perinatal deaths is determined from national death certification and birth registration data. In addition, each region in England, together with Wales and Northern Ireland is required to participate in a confidential enquiry of stillbirths and neonatal deaths. In this way, causes of death are established and potentially avoidable factors can be identified.

Trends in perinatal mortality

Just fifty years ago in Britain, one in every 20 babies was either born dead or died within the first week of life. By the beginning of the 1990s, these major risks of fetal life and of birth had receded to the extent that only one in 120 babies failed to survive the first week of life. The last decade in particular, has seen a major improvement in the survival of newborn babies in Britain. However, whilst the perinatal mortality rate has fallen steadily (Figure 6.6) Britain still lags behind some other countries. A statutory change to the definition of stillbirths (commencing from the 24th week of gestation not the 28th as previously), introduced in October 1992 has implications for the interpretation of trends over time.

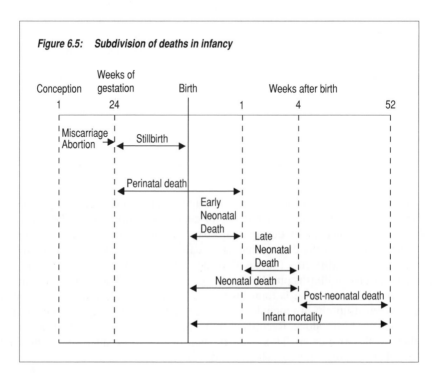

Figure 6.5:   Subdivision of deaths in infancy

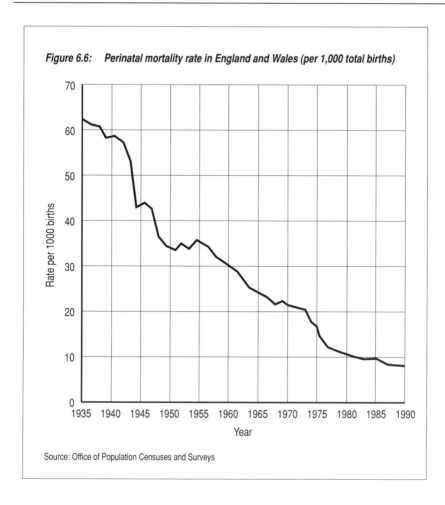

Figure 6.6: *Perinatal mortality rate in England and Wales (per 1,000 total births)*

Source: Office of Population Censuses and Surveys

Much of the reduction in perinatal mortality has been associated with an overall improvement in the health and nutrition of the population, also far fewer women are having a large number of pregnancies. In addition, over the last several decades, there have been major technological advances in the care of pregnant women and the newborn. Such treatments are now accepted as commonplace today but at the time of their introduction may have appeared to be as unnatural as some of the techniques used in the care of women in labour or very tiny babies today. Natural childbirth arguments have led to the acknowledgement that high technology care is not necessarily appropriate for all but recent improvements in perinatal mortality would have been hard to achieve without it.

The perinatal mortality rate varies between localities and fluctuates from year to year. Conclusions based upon comparisons between places and within places over time must be very cautiously drawn because the variations observed may be arising from very small numbers. Nevertheless, using data aggregated for several years (for local populations) or for larger areas, it can be seen that marked differences do occur (Figure 6.7).

Factors associated with perinatal loss

Low birthweight is the most important factor which is linked to perinatal death. Survival of babies with very low birthweight has improved over the last twenty years, although the most marked change did not occur until after 1980. This improvement is due in part to the wider availability of intensive care facilities for newborn babies together with advances in technology in this field of care.

It is important to understand the factors which contribute to, or are directly associated with, low birthweight or perinatal mortality and to identify those elements where there are clear associations and opportunities for improvement. If lethal congenital malformations are left to one side, the major factors associated with low birthweight are plural pregnancy, poor nutrition, low socio-economic

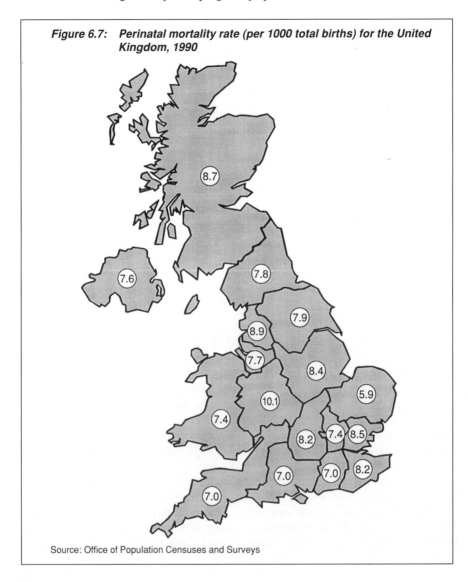

Figure 6.7:   Perinatal mortality rate (per 1000 total births) for the United Kingdom, 1990

Source: Office of Population Censuses and Surveys

status, teenage pregnancy and smoking and drinking in pregnancy. Many of the factors associated with low birthweight and perinatal mortality are inter-related. Their independent contribution is hard to assess.

The association between smoking and low birthweight was first reported in 1957 and there is now no doubt that smoking during pregnancy has an adverse effect on the unborn child. The more the mother smokes, the greater the risk to the baby. The average reduction in birthweight of a baby born to a smoker is of the order of 15–250 grams. Smoking is also associated with impairment of the child. The increased risk of perinatal mortality due to smoking has been estimated at 28%.

Drinking alcohol is also potentially damaging to the developing fetus. Heavy alcohol consumption, particularly in early pregnancy, can lead to a baby being born with fetal alcohol syndrome. This is characterised by retarded growth, abnormalities of the face and of the nervous system, as well as abnormal behaviour of the baby in the period after birth.

Women from poorer social backgrounds are one and a half times more likely to produce a low birthweight baby or suffer a perinatal death than those in the other social classes. Similarly, the youngest and the oldest women who are pregnant have much greater risks of poor outcomes of their pregnancies. For teenage pregnancies, the opportunities to effect change include better sex education, easier access to contraception and wider availability of counselling and support services as well as enhanced antenatal care for young expectant mothers.

Some parts of Britain have large ethnic minority populations. Some women within ethnic minority communities are at higher risk of perinatal loss than pregnant women as a whole. The factors contributing to such differences are not fully understood but include the presence of certain mother and baby illnesses, dietary practices and the availability, or otherwise, of services which are responsive to the special needs of women in ethnic minority groups, including interpreters, translations of written materials and familiarity of health care professionals with cultural and religious beliefs. Innovative approaches to this problem have already been taken in some parts of Britain such as special link workers to ensure that the needs of ethnic minority mothers are more comprehensively met. In areas where ethnic minority populations are present, the need for services to be appropriately targeted and designed to respond to these mothers and their families should be recognised and actively addressed.

Immediate causes of perinatal death

The immediate causes of perinatal death are identifiable and provide another means of assessing the scope for their prevention. This can be seen by examining the component parts of perinatal mortality in one health region (Figure 6.8), as an example. The data cover the whole of the 1980s for babies weighing 1 kg or more at birth, (the form of analysis recommended for comparative purposes by the World Health Organisation). The recorded major improvements to the perinatal mortality rates were due to reductions in the numbers of babies with malformations and in the number of babies dying during labour or as a result of factors encountered at the time of labour or delivery. This is one way of assessing the scale of improvement. Another is to look at the extent to which any one contributory factor seems to have reduced in the last ten years (irrespective of how common the problem is). If this is

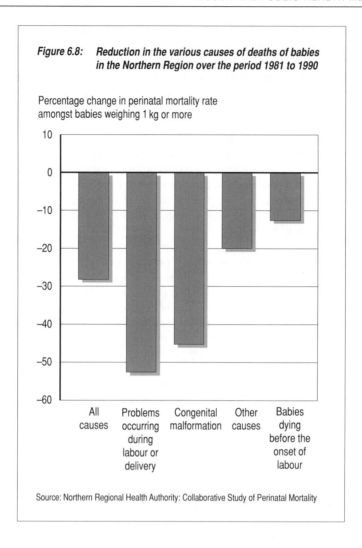

Figure 6.8: Reduction in the various causes of deaths of babies in the Northern Region over the period 1981 to 1990

Percentage change in perinatal mortality rate amongst babies weighing 1 kg or more

Source: Northern Regional Health Authority: Collaborative Study of Perinatal Mortality

done, then it is death as a result of problems encountered during labour or delivery that are seen to have declined most, deaths of babies with congenital malformations next and deaths occurring before the onset of labour least. In fact, by the end of the decade, only 31 of the 40,547 babies of 1 kg or more born alive in the health region concerned, who did not have either a lethal congenital malformation or experience distress during labour, died in the seven days following birth. This represented a major fall and was undoubtedly due to successful intensive care in the neonatal period.

Altogether there are four causes which account for just over 40% of all perinatal deaths. These are congenital malformations, high blood pressure in the mother, asphyxia or injury to the baby during labour or birth and respiratory disease or infection. Many such losses could be avoided if it were possible to eliminate all the deaths due to raised blood pressure in the mother; poor fetal growth; problems developing for the first time during labour; and, if antenatally recognisable but untreatable malformations had been identified through screening and the parents opted to terminate the pregnancy (Figure 6.9). Techniques for supporting the breathing of small babies immediately after birth have improved so much that the risk of delivering a baby ten weeks early is now often less than the risk of allowing some pregnancies to continue. Good antenatal care at this time makes it possible to monitor the baby's health as well as the mother's.

Other causes of pregnancy loss present a greater challenge. Deaths before the onset of labour in the absence of any serious malformation now account for half of all perinatal loss amongst babies weighing 1 kg or more at birth. High blood pressure in the mother accounts for some such deaths. Raised blood pressure can develop rapidly and without warning between the 28th and 32nd week of pregnancy, especially in a mother's first pregnancy. This can easily go unrecognised (especially if there is any ambiguity as to how care is being shared between the hospital and general practice services). Signs of poor fetal growth at this time, even in the absence of any problem with the mother's blood pressure, can point to a situation where the risks of early delivery are less than the risk of leaving the pregnancy to run its normal course.

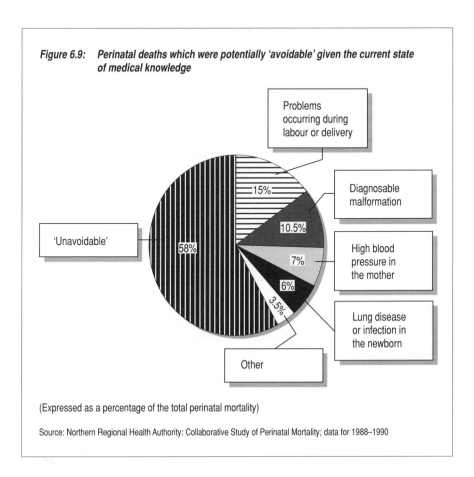

Figure 6.9:   Perinatal deaths which were potentially 'avoidable' given the current state of medical knowledge

Problems occurring during labour or delivery

Diagnosable malformation

15%

10.5%

'Unavoidable'

58%

High blood pressure in the mother

7%

6%

3.5%

Lung disease or infection in the newborn

Other

(Expressed as a percentage of the total perinatal mortality)

Source: Northern Regional Health Authority: Collaborative Study of Perinatal Mortality; data for 1988–1990

Neonatal, postneonatal and infant deaths

At the end of the last century, about 150 children in every 1,000 live births died during the first year of life. The decline in this rate since then has been both consistent and dramatic. By 1936 it had fallen to 58.7; by the beginning of the 1960s it had halved again and by the beginning of the 1990s it was around eight deaths per 1,000 live births. The decline is unlikely to have been due to a single event. Better nutritional standards, better education and improved environmental conditions of the large working class population of late Victorian England, together with the emergence of the middle class, have all contributed. Improvements in medical care also played a part. For example, The Midwives Act, 1902 phased out the unqualified handywoman and improved the management of labour.

Deaths occurring in the first year of life are a fair reflection of the health of a population generally. For descriptive epidemiological purposes, infant deaths are usually divided into neonatal and postneonatal deaths (definitions given above). The factors affecting neonatal deaths have many similarities with those which influence perinatal mortality.

Postnatal deaths are more strongly related to social and economic factors as reflected by place of residence, father's occupation and social class. Even since the mid-1970s, there have been further sharp declines in neonatal and postneonatal mortality and in infant mortality as a whole (Table 6.5). The data are presented in tabular, rather than graphical form to show the extent of fluctuation in these rates. Whilst neonatal mortality fell for each successive year of the observation period, the postneonatal mortality rate has declined over the whole period but less steadily. Indeed, in 1986, there was much concern that infant mortality had apparently risen due to an increase in postneonatal deaths.

Table 6.5:   *Trends in various components of infant mortality, England and Wales*

Mortality rate*	Year										
	1980	1981	1982	1983	1984	1985	1986	1987	1988	1989	1990
Stillbirth	7.3	6.6	6.3	5.7	5.7	5.5	5.3	5.0	4.9	4.7	4.6
Neonatal	7.6	6.6	6.2	5.8	5.5	5.3	5.2	5.0	4.9	4.7	4.5
Post-neonatal	4.3	4.3	4.4	4.2	3.8	3.9	4.2	4.0	4.0	3.6	3.2
Infant	11.9	10.9	10.6	10.0	9.3	9.2	9.4	9.0	8.9	8.3	7.7

Source: Office of Population, Censuses and Surveys.
* See text for definitions

Undertaking analyses using routinely available national data shows that infant mortality varies according to birthweight, multiple pregnancy, marital status and social class as defined by occupation. The assessment of marital status has been made more complex by the fact that more children are born outside marriage but statistics can distinguish registrations of birth which are made by both parents (even if unmarried) or by the mother alone.

As a result of rules for certification of stillbirth and neonatal death (introduced in 1986) causes of neonatal deaths are analysed by the main maternal and fetal conditions but not by a single underlying cause. The conditions cited most often for neonatal deaths are congenital malformations, prematurity and respiratory distress syndrome.

For post-neonatal deaths, where certification rules are different, a single underlying cause can be analysed. The leading causes of death in this period are: 'sudden infant death syndrome', diseases of the respiratory system, other infections and congenital malformations (Figure 6.10).

Since the early 1970s, death certified with terms such as 'cot death', 'sudden unexpected death in infancy' or 'sudden infant death syndrome' (SIDS) have been separately identified and analysed for epidemiological purposes. The category is defined as 'sudden death of an infant or young child, which is unexpected by history, and in which a thorough postmortem examination fails to demonstrate an adequate cause of death'.

The whole issue of sudden unexpected deaths in apparently healthy babies is one which has caused a great deal of public concern. At the same time as interest in this syndrome has risen, its frequency as a certified cause of death has also increased, whilst respiratory causes have declined. This suggests a change in certification practice. The postneonatal mortality rate as a whole is strongly influenced by changes in the occurrence of the sudden infant death syndrome, since the latter now accounts for 45% of all post-neonatal deaths.

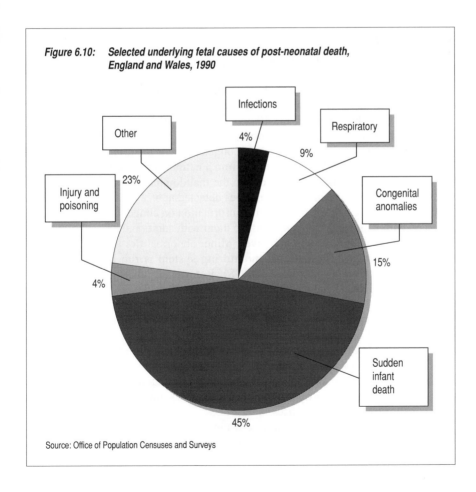

Figure 6.10: *Selected underlying fetal causes of post-neonatal death, England and Wales, 1990*

Infections 4%

Respiratory 9%

Other 23%

Injury and poisoning 4%

Congenital anomalies 15%

Sudden infant death 45%

Source: Office of Population Censuses and Surveys

The United Kingdom incidence of the sudden infant death syndrome was 1.5 per 1,000 live births in 1990. Over 70% of such deaths occurred in babies between one and four months. Boys were more commonly affected than girls and it was more often seen in the winter months. Babies at greatest risk were those born to younger mothers who already have two or more children and the risks were increased if the mother smoked. The prone sleeping position is associated with an increased risk of sudden infant death as is a very hot environment and the presence of cigarette smoke. Advice to mothers on the sleeping position (babies should be placed on their backs unless there is a medical contradiction) and environment for babies is now issued routinely by the Department of Health.

Dramatic improvements in the infant mortality rate has occurred in most of the countries in the European Community. Whilst England and Wales fares quite favourably in comparative terms, the scope for further improvement is evident from the lower rates of some other countries (Figure 6.11). Developing countries and Eastern European countries have much less favourable rates whilst Japan at the end of the 1980s had 4.8 per 1000 live births for boys and girls, the lowest infant mortality rate in the world.

Fetal abnormalities

An important cause of fetal death as well as impairment, disability and handicap is the disorders which develop during intra-uterine life. The decline in other causes of death over the last several decades has meant that congenital abnormalities have accounted for an increasing proportion of infant deaths, estimated as a quarter of all such deaths at the beginning of the 1990s. Such abnormalities also cause some of the deaths which occur in later childhood.

Some information on the frequency of congenital malformations and other fetal abnormalities in the population is derived from a national monitoring system which was introduced in the mid-1960s following the thalidomide tragedy. The system is voluntary and takes account of abnormalities detected at or within 10 days of birth. It relies upon health authorities extracting information on congenital malformations contained within birth notifications made to them with additional information being supplied by doctors, nurses and midwives. Minor abnormalities are excluded from the reporting system. The national monitoring system is run by the Office of Population, Censuses and Surveys (OPCS). Returns are analysed monthly and subjected to statistical analysis and any significant increases are reported to the health authority concerned. The system is primarily a method of surveillance to compare trends over time. It is of less value exploring variations in incidence between different localities, testing aetiological hypotheses and detecting overall prevalence. Problems with under-reporting, with accuracy of notification, and the fact that late detections cannot be included are serious drawbacks. Despite these limitations, congenital malformation statistics from the national monitoring scheme yield much valuable information. Table 6.6 shows rates of congenital malformations for some selected causes.

Surveys at regional or local level, where a higher degree of ascertainment can be achieved, can provide better data for exploring differences in prevalence and risk factors.

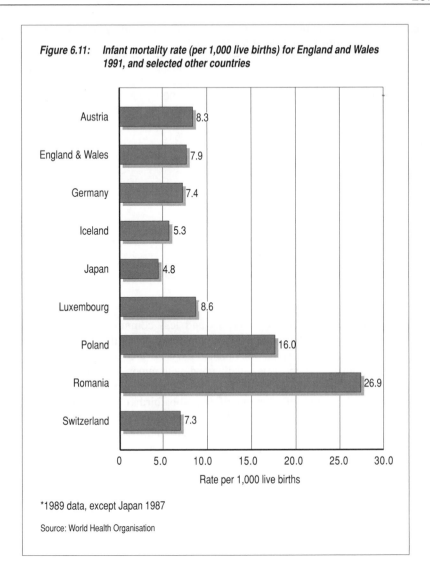

Figure 6.11:   Infant mortality rate (per 1,000 live births) for England and Wales
1991, and selected other countries

*1989 data, except Japan 1987

Source: World Health Organisation

An important cause of fetal abnormalities is a group of conditions called neural
tube defects which occur in differing forms, including that of spina bifida. Neural
Tube Defects (NTD) arise from a failure of normal development of the central
nervous system during the first few weeks of embryonic life, specifically the failure
of proper closure of the neural tube. A spectrum of disorders may result depending
on the site and severity of the defect:

Anencephaly – failure of development of the forebrain, its coverings and the
skull. This defect is incompatible with life; most affected infants are stillborn,
whilst the remainder usually die within hours of birth.

Spina bifida occulta – failure of fusion of the vertebral arches with no protrusion
of tissue and seldom any neurological impairment.

Table 6.6:   Rate of babies born (per 10,000 total births) with selected congenital malformations, England and Wales

Condition	Number	Rate
Talipes+	1,090	15.4
Hypospadias and epispadias	869	12.3
Cardiovascular malformations*	612	8.6
Cleft lip (with or without cleft palate)	542	7.6
Down's syndrome	415	5.9
Central nervous system malformations	360	5.1
Cleft palate	217	3.1

Source: Office of Population, Censuses and Surveys.
+Talipes is a condition of variable degree with marked fluctuation in reported prevalence.
*These conditions are underestimated as many conditions only come to light some time after birth.

Spina bifida cystica in two forms:

(a) *Meningocoele* – This less serious and less common form consists of a protrusion of meninges, but not the spinal cord, through a defect in the vertebral column. The sac consists of spinal membranes and is covered by skin ('closed' NTD). After surgical closure, prognosis is usually good, with minor residual impairment.

(b) *Myelomeningocoele* – This type is more serious and more common (accounting for 80 – 90% of all spina bifida cystica births). In this 'open' NTD the protruding sac contains spinal cord which is partly uncovered. This defect often results in severe handicap of the nervous, urinary and locomotor systems, even if surgical treatment is undertaken, (although this depends on the spinal level at which the defect occurs). Hydrocephalus and mental handicap may also be accompanying features.

NTD is a worldwide phenomenon. Its aetiology is not fully elucidated. It has declined sharply in Britain (Figure 6.12) and a number of other countries. There is a strong social class gradient for the prevalence of NTDs: they occur more frequently in social class IV and V than in I and II. In part, the fall has been due to a reduction in the natural incidence of the condition for reasons which are so far unexplained but which may be due to dietary and environmental factors. Support for this theory came from an important seven year Medical Research Council study which showed that the risk of conception of a second child with such a defect is decreased by 72% if the mother takes folic acid supplements prior to conception of the next child. The Department of Health subsequently issued guidance that all women planning a pregnancy should consume additional folic acid prior to conception and in the first 12 weeks of pregnancy in the form of folate-rich foods supplemented by a daily dietary supplement of folic acid of 0.4 milligrams. The guidance stipulates that women who have already had a NTD-affected fetus should take folic acid supplements of 5 milligrams daily to aim to prevent a recurrence.

Another factor which has contributed to the decline in NTD affected babies is the advent of techniques for detecting open neural tube defects during pregnancy.

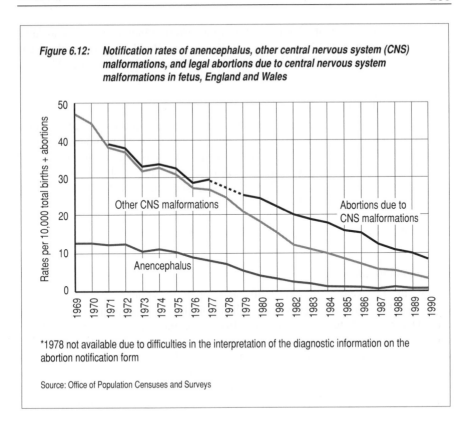

Figure 6.12: *Notification rates of anencephalus, other central nervous system (CNS)*
malformations, and legal abortions due to central nervous system
malformations in fetus, England and Wales

*1978 not available due to difficulties in the interpretation of the diagnostic information on the
abortion notification form

Source: Office of Population Censuses and Surveys

This approach enables parents to be offered the option of terminating the pregnancy
and so avoid giving birth to a severely handicapped baby or one who may die in the
perinatal period. About one third of the reduction in the number of babies born
with open neural tube defects in the last ten years is estimated to be due to
screening and termination.

Possibly the most important genetic abnormality is Downs Syndrome. It is
important because of the stigma, the disability and the social implications attached
to the condition but in itself is not a major cause of death in the first year of life.
Other chromosomal abnormalities, severe bilateral renal malformations and some
of the more severe forms of congenital heart disease have a greater impact on infant
mortality. The risk of a baby with Downs Syndrome increases markedly to mothers
over 35 years of age but because the majority of babies are born to mothers under
35 years old, the absolute number of babies born with Down's syndrome to
younger mothers is much greater. Down's syndrome is discussed more fully in
chapter 7.

Illness and disease in childhood

Childhood is a time of substantial minor illness which may result in a great deal of
contact with the family's general practitioner, most commonly for respiratory
illness and gastrointestinal problems.

A small proportion of children have more serious illnesses, such as asthma, diabetes, epilepsy, coeliac disease and cystic fibrosis. Problems such as these can have serious effects on the family as a whole as well as on the affected child.

Lifestyle and behaviour

Childhood is the time when people establish lifestyles and internalise values which will have a bearing on their health for the rest of their lives. The guidance children are given by parents and other adults with respect to smoking and use of alcohol can influence whether they smoke or drink to excess later in life. Similarly, their approach to diet and nutrition is likely to be shaped by early experiences.

This is not to say that children can simply be educated into a healthier lifestyle. Childhood is also a time of risk-taking, particularly in the teenage years. These are issues which are discussed more fully in chapter 3.

Mortality in childhood

Beyond the first year of life, mortality rates for the remainder of childhood (until the age of 15 years) are expressed in relation to the numbers in the population at risk. Deaths in childhood, like mortality in infancy, have undergone major decreases since the turn of the century. The main reason for this improvement has been a substantial reduction in the importance of infectious diseases as a cause of death in this age group. In the 1930s, one in every two childhood deaths were attributed to one of five diseases: pneumonia, tuberculosis, diphtheria, measles and whooping cough. By the beginning of the 1990s, these diseases accounted for about one in 150 deaths. The change has been brought about by a combination of socio-environmental changes (such as improvements in standards of nutrition, housing and sanitation), preventive measures (immunisation) and therapeutic medical advances. The decreased importance of infectious diseases means that the mortality rates, within the different phases of childhood (conventionally 1–4, 5–9 and 10–15 years of age) are lower than at any other period of life.

Whilst this overall improvement in childhood mortality has occurred other conditions have assumed greater importance (Figure 6.13). Injuries and poisoning are now responsible for one-third of childhood deaths (half of these are road accidents) between the ages of one and 14 years. Cancers account for a substantial minority of the remainder (particularly in older children) with leukaemia prominent amongst them.

In childhood mortality, inequality amongst different social groups persists. There is a marked upward gradient in mortality for both boys and girls from Social Class I to Social Class V. For boys, the ratio of mortality in Social Class V as compared to Social Class I is about two to one and somewhat less for girls. The gradient is less marked as children become older. The steepest gradients are for accidents and respiratory disease.

FAMILY PLANNING SERVICES

The widespread availability of safe, effective methods of contraception is an essential component of the range of health services which must be provided.

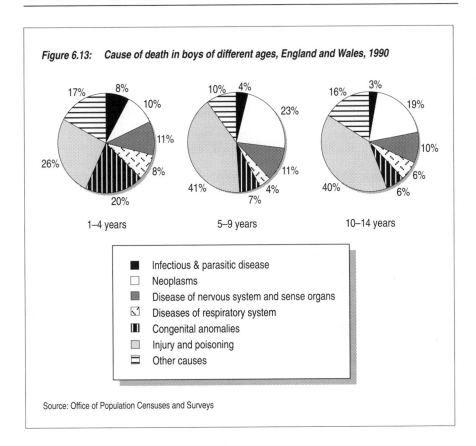

Figure 6.13:   *Cause of death in boys of different ages, England and Wales, 1990*

1–4 years   5–9 years   10–14 years

Legend:
- ■ Infectious & parasitic disease
- ☐ Neoplasms
- ▨ Disease of nervous system and sense organs
- ▨ Diseases of respiratory system
- ▥ Congenital anomalies
- ▨ Injury and poisoning
- ▤ Other causes

Source: Office of Population Censuses and Surveys

Contraceptive Methods

Since the 1960s contraceptive methods have been dominated by the, so called 'high technology' measures – the oral contraceptive pill and to a lesser extent, the intrauterine device (IUD).

Data indicating the usage of these different methods are available from routine statistics collected on people receiving family planning services. This is a selected group not representative of the whole population. An impression of contraceptive practices of the general population is obtained from special surveys.

The pattern of contraceptive use by women is shown in Figure 6.14. The contraceptive pill is used by the younger age groups and sterilisation is the most popular method with older women. Since 1986, however, the use of condoms has increased substantially. This trend is largely accounted for by the advent of the Acquired Immune Deficiency Syndrome (AIDS).

The effectiveness of various methods of contraception is illustrated in Table 6.7. The estimates are based on the percentage of women who became pregnant using the method for one year. A major feature is the variation between failure rates of careful and consistent users and those who are less attentive. For example, use of the cap varies from 2% failure rate to 2 to 15% with less careful and consistent use.

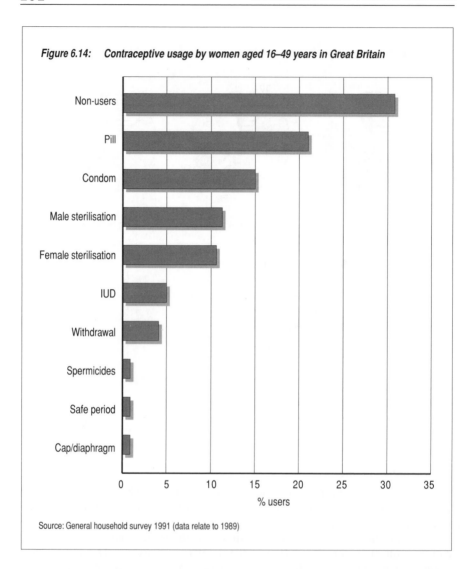

Figure 6.14:   Contraceptive usage by women aged 16–49 years in Great Britain

Source: General household survey 1991 (data relate to 1989)

Safety of methods

Most published data about mortality from the use of contraceptives, concentrate on the risk from the method itself. Some investigators, however, deal with the wider aspect and calculate cumulative mortality. Thus, not only is there inherent risk of death from the method included but also risk from pregnancy as a result of method failure. Additionally, in the case of the oral contraceptive, the beneficial effects of reducing the risk of ovarian and endometrial cancer are taken into account.

Precise risks of methods related mortality are difficult to determine and are limited to oral contraceptives, intrauterine devices and sterilisation. Risk related to the oral contraceptives has been most studied in this and other countries. There is good evidence for increased risk from myocardial infarction, stroke and deep vein

Table 6.7: Efficacy rates of various contraceptive methods

Method	Pregnancy rate per annum	
	Careful and consistent use	*Less careful and consistent use*
Progestogen-only pill	1 in 100 women	1–4 in 100 women
Male condom	2 in 100 women	15 in 100 women
Female condom	n/a	n/a
Intrauterine device (IUD)	1–3 in 100 women	n/a
Injectable methods	1 in 100 women	n/a
Cap	2 in 100 women	2–15 in 100 women
Sponge	9 in 100 women	25 in 100 women
Natural methods	2 in 100 women	2–20 in 100 women
Male sterilisation	1 in 1000 operations	n/a
Female sterilisation	1 in 200 to 1 in 1000 operations	n/a

n/a = not applicable or data not available
Source: Family Planning Association.

thrombosis, with greater risk for older women, especially cigarette smokers. In addition, a strong adverse influence has been shown for hepatocellular adenoma. There is also less convincing evidence for carcinoma of the cervix. This information has been available for a number of years and corrective measures have been applied so that for example, the 'lower' dosage pills are available and doctors are much less likely to prescribe the pill for older women.

Overall, method related mortality varies from different studies. For example, deaths resulting from the use of intrauterine devices arise from sepsis as a complication of accidental pregnancy and from pelvic inflammatory disease not associated with pregnancy. The risk from this complication is very low and has been estimated to be less than one death per 100,000, fertile married women of reproductive age.

Sterilisation involves a one time risk associated with surgery, unlike the sort of continuous exposure of the other two methods. It has been estimated to be four deaths per 100,000 operations, for women undergoing tubal sterilisation and 0.1 per 100,000 procedures for vasectomy.

Provision of services

Family planning services in Britain are provided in three main ways: by general practitioners, in community family planning clinics and in departments of obstetrics and gynaecology of local hospitals. Despite the move, during the 1990s, towards more family planning services being delivered by general practitioners, it has been national policy to maintain a choice of service and hence the community family planning clinics have been preserved (albeit in smaller numbers than in the past). Women may prefer to visit such a clinic rather than their general practitioner for a number of reasons. They may prefer anonymity, it may be easier to see a woman doctor, there may be a fuller range of contraceptive techniques and they will often regard the staff of the family planning clinic as 'specialists' who have more detailed knowledge. Moreover, community clinics are increasingly widening their role to incorporate other aspects of sexual health such as advice on sexually transmitted disease, premenstrual tension and the menopause.

A number of principles underlie the provision of good family planning services (Table 6.8). These include ensuring that certain quality criteria are fulfilled, providing good access and enabling groups with traditionally low uptake (but who may be in particular need) to receive services. Services have a variety of aims. Of particular importance are the problems of sexual health amongst teenagers where the risks of unwanted pregnancy and sexually transmitted diseases are particularly high. In addition, effective family planning services must seek to reduce the occurrence of pelvic inflammatory disease which can be a cause of infertility.

Table 6.8: Factors to be considered when organising family planning services

- Ensure the number, times and locations of clinics meet the needs of users.
- Provide choice of male and female professional staff.
- Make available a wide choice of contraceptive methods.
- Ensure the service is staffed by those with skill and knowledge of contraceptive methods and sexual health.
- Provide opportunities to discuss related subjects (for example premenstrual tension, HIV).
- Offer an appointments system with flexibility to allow walk-in attendances (especially for emergencies).
- Provide facilities for children.

Aside from teenagers, most family planning services will be advising and helping two broad groups of women: the young, relatively geographically mobile women and older women who have had previous pregnancies. The needs of these two groups are different both in terms of the kind of advice and help they will need and in terms of accessibility to clinics and opening hours. Family planning services will also offer an emergency contraceptive service to deal with 'morning after' and other problems.

Infertility

Failure to conceive may produce as much distress as an unwanted pregnancy. Formerly, adoption was the sole resort of couples who were childless. The widespread availability and use of effective contraceptive methods, and changes in the law relating to termination of pregnancy, have had the effect of reducing the number of babies offered for adoption. This has, to some extent, been countered by the development of methods of assisted reproduction in couples of low fertility, and by the acceptance of the use of donor sperm for men who are infertile.

With treatment, approximately 40% of infertile couples can achieve a successful pregnancy. The investigation of sub-fertility and infertility should involve both partners. Approximately 30% of problems relate to the male partner, 30% to the female and in the remainder there is no apparent cause.

In general terms, infertility and subfertility are usually due to failure to produce sperm or to ovulate, or to a mechanical blockage in the vas deferens or the fallopian tubes. Treatment of female subfertility and infertility may include tubal surgery or drug induced ovulation. The latter may result in multiple pregnancy.

More recent developments have included in vitro fertilisation (test tube babies), where ovulation is artificially induced, the eggs are harvested, fertilised under artificial conditions and placed in the uterus. A further development of this technique is gamete intrafallopian transfer (GIFT) where ovulation is also artificially induced, the eggs are harvested and are then mixed with semen and returned directly to the fallopian tube. Because more than one ovum may be used in order to give an increased chance of pregnancy, both of these methods may also give rise to multiple pregnancy.

Artificial insemination by donor (AID) is also available where the problem is male infertility. The whole question of artificial fertilisation has been addressed by the passing of the Human Fertilisation and Embryology Act 1990, which has detailed requirements for regulation.

Childless couples may go to very considerable lengths to acquire a child. Recent years have seen the appearance of surrogacy where a fertile woman is willing to bear a child for one who is infertile. There are a number of ethical questions surrounding this issue which have still to be addressed, particularly where the surrogate mother is paid.

Abortion

Abortion is defined as "the emptying of a pregnant uterus up to the 24th week of pregnancy" although in certain circumstances the Human Fertilisation and Embryology Act 1990 places no limit on legal abortion. A spontaneous abortion (often referred to as a 'miscarriage') is one which occurs as a result of an accident or disease, estimated as 9–15% of recognised pregnancies. A criminal abortion is one procured deliberately and unlawfully. A termination of pregnancy is the legal ending of a pregnancy.

The Abortion Act 1967 became law in April 1968. It enabled the legal termination of pregnancy (by a registered medical practitioner) to take place in a National Health Service hospital, registered nursing home or other approved premises. In the intervening period, some amendments have been made, including those introduced by the Human Fertilisation and Embryology Act, 1990. The current requirements are that two registered medical practitioners should certify that certain defined indications for abortion have been met (Table 6.9), that the abortion should be performed by a registered medical practitioner, and that the procedure should be undertaken in a National Health Service hospital or other approved premises. In England, all cases of abortion must be notified to the Chief Medical Officer of the Department of Health and in Wales, to the Chief Medical Officer at the Welsh Office, within seven days of termination.

From the advent of the Act to the beginning of the 1990s, over three million terminations of pregnancy were carried out in England and Wales (Figure 6.15). The proportion of terminations undertaken on non-residents of England and Wales reached a peak of 34% in the mid-1970s. The proportion has fluctuated however, being partly influenced by the liberalisation of abortion laws in countries from which a high proportion of non-resident abortions were drawn. The impact of these factors is well illustrated by the position of women from the Republic of Ireland (which prohibits abortion). Between the beginning of the 1970s and the start of the 1990s, there was a sixteen-fold increase in the number of women from that country having abortions in England and Wales.

Table 6.9: *Statutory grounds for abortion under the Abortion Act 1967 and amended by the Human Fertilisation and Embryology Act 1990*

A	The continuance of the pregnancy would involve risk to the life of the pregnant woman greater than if the pregnancy were terminated.
B	The termination is necessary to prevent grave permanent injury to the physical or mental health of the pregnant woman.
C	The pregnancy has NOT exceeded its 24th week and that the continuance of the pregnancy would involve risk, greater than if the pregnancy were terminated, of injury to the physical or mental health of the pregnant woman.
D	The pregnancy has NOT exceeded its 24th week and that the continuance of the pregnancy would involve risk, greater than if the pregnancy were terminated, of injury to the physical or mental health of any existing child(ren) of the family of the pregnant woman.
E	There is a substantial risk that if the child were born it would suffer from such physical or mental abnormalities as to be seriously handicapped.

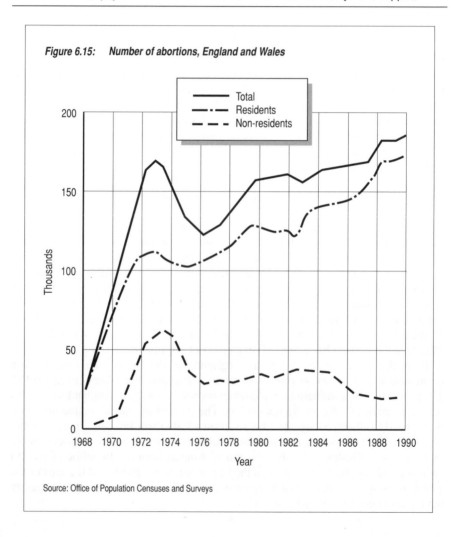

Figure 6.15: *Number of abortions, England and Wales*

Source: Office of Population Censuses and Surveys

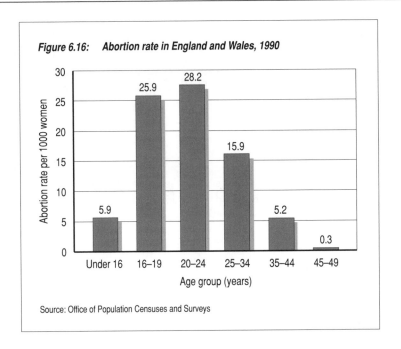

Figure 6.16:   Abortion rate in England and Wales, 1990

Source: Office of Population Censuses and Surveys

The highest rates of abortion are amongst the 16 to 19 year old and the 20 to 24 year old age groups (Figure 6.16). There is marked variation in the extent to which different health authorities provide services for termination of pregnancy, as evidenced by the number of women having abortions outside their region of residence and in non-National Health Service facilities (Table 6.10). In part this reflects the fact that obstetricians and gynaecologists are free to follow their consciences in respect of whether or not they are prepared to perform terminations.

The proportion of conceptions overall which end in termination of pregnancy is around 20%. However, the figure is much higher for young and older women: 53% (for the under 16s) and 45% (for the over 45s) respectively. The figure for the latter group reflects indirectly, screening for Down's syndrome which is offered to older women who become pregnant.

Critics of the abortion law have considered that liberal interpretation of the grounds for abortion has led to termination of pregnancy on demand. In addition, it has been suggested that abortion encourages promiscuity as it can be regarded as a method of contraception. It is often asserted that lack of availability of a well publicised Family Planning Service is reflected in an increase in the termination of pregnancy rate. However, the relationship is not straight-forward because many pregnancies become unwanted after conception. There is ample evidence from surveys of women who have had abortions that they do not regard it as a substitute for contraception but rather as a last resort in the case of failure or mistake. A wide variety of factors can potentially affect the rate of abortion at any one time, some of which are shown in Table 6.11.

Table 6.10:　**Places where women obtain legal abortions in relation to their health region of usual residence, 1990**

English Health region	Place where abortion obtained and type of premises (Percentage)				Rate per 1000 women aged 14–49 years
	Own region NHS	Own region non-NHS	Outside region NHS	Outside region non-NHS	
Northern	83%	1%	1%	15%	9.5
Yorkshire	37%	41%	1%	21%	11.1
Trent	56%	16%	3%	25%	10.6
East Anglian	77%	4%	0%	18%	10.0
North West Thames	29%	16%	3%	52%	20.0
North East Thames	47%	32%	1%	19%	22.3
South East Thames	32%	49%	2%	18%	18.4
South West Thames	27%	18%	3%	53%	15.8
Wessex	36%	51%	1%	13%	11.1
Oxford	40%	1%	1%	58%	11.9
South Western	67%	4%	1%	27%	9.9
West Midlands	14%	80%	1%	5%	14.1
Mersey	38%	39%	2%	22%	12.5
North Western	38%	42%	1%	19%	12.4
Wales	58%	1%	2%	39%	10.5
England and Wales	42%	58%	0%	0%	13.6

Source: Office of Population Censuses and Surveys.

Table 6.11:   Some factors which can influence the rate of abortion in a population

- Prevailing legislation
- Social attitudes
- Contraceptive efficacy and usage
- Scope for diagnosis of fetal abnormalities
- Fertility patterns
- Age structure of female population

MATERNITY SERVICES

Care provided to pregnant mothers and their babies is increasingly being seen in terms of promotion and maintenance of good health and not as a problem-based patient care service. The health of the mother and her child depends upon her lifestyle before she becomes pregnant, during the period of gestation and afterwards. The role of health services is to ensure that appropriate advice, help and support are given at all stages. This will involve the application of the most up-to-date medical technologies to detect and treat abnormalities but will also entail giving advice and guidance on the measures which can be taken by the mother and the family themselves.

Antenatal care

The whole process of antenatal care is geared to a healthy outcome of pregnancy both for mother and baby. In practice, this means preventing fetal death, disease or abnormality by the early identification of problems in the mother and fetus, their treatment and control. Increasingly, the traditional antenatal period (which follows conception) is being embraced within the wider concept of prenatal care. Women in the childbearing years are now encouraged to think about the prospect and implications of pregnancy before it happens. Well women and pre-conception clinics provide a focus for discussion about lifestyle, contraception, and the timing of conception. It is now recognised that a diet rich in folates prior to conception is important in the prevention of neural tube defects.

When pregnancy does occur, it is important that the woman is enrolled into a programme of antenatal care as early as possible. The most common model of antenatal care is a shared approach between the midwife, general practitioner as well as the wider primary care team and the local hospital department of obstetrics and gynaecology.

Antenatal care encompasses a wide range of activities including: advice on lifestyle (for example, smoking, alcohol intake, sexual activity, diet); assessment of fetal size, development and well-being; screening for maternal illness (for example, hypertensive disease, diabetes, infection); the recognition and treatment of abnormalities in pregnancy (for example, bleeding), the detection of fetal abnormality; and psychological preparation for delivery (including antenatal classes). The content of antenatal care has evolved over time as a development of medical and midwifery practice rather than on the basis of evaluating the efficacy of specific interventions on the outcome of pregnancy.

The prevention and recognition of fetal abnormalities

A number of general and specific measures can be taken during the antenatal period to reduce the occurrence of fetal abnormalities. Good diet, non-smoking and moderate alcohol intake before and during pregnancy will reduce risks. For high risk mothers, the use of skilled genetic counselling can often prevent a pregnancy affected by congenital malformation. Similarly, the use of folic acid supplementation (discussed above) may reduce the risk of a neural tube defect pregnancy. Once a pregnancy is established, advances in medical technology have enabled a higher proportion of fetal abnormalities to be detected early enough for the parents to be offered the choice of termination of the pregnancy. This has come about because of improved ultrasound methods and (for some abnormalities) blood and amniotic fluid tests, chorion villus biopsy, placentesis, and fetal blood sampling.

Rhesus haemolytic disease in the newborn

This disorder arises from a genetic difference between a mother and her baby. Each member of the population belongs to one of four main blood groups: A, B, AB and O but also falls into two other broad groups, rhesus-positive and rhesus-negative. In Britain, 85% of the population is rhesus-positive carrying the rhesus antigen (commonly the 'D' antigen) on their red blood cells. A rhesus-negative woman can conceive a rhesus-positive baby if she is fertilized by the sperm of a rhesus-positive man.

If at some time during, or at the end of the ensuing pregnancy, fetal (i.e., rhesus-positive) red blood cells pass into the maternal circulation, then the (rhesus-negative) mother may respond by producing antibodies against the rhesus protein which has entered her blood stream. This can happen even if pregnancy ends in miscarriage or abortion. The risk is that antibodies can then cross the placenta and haemolyse the red cells of the fetus, producing anaemia, jaundice, cerebral impairment and even death in any subsequent pregnancy.

In the 1950s, haemolytic disease of the newborn accounted for over 1,000 stillbirths and neonatal deaths each year. The development of postpartum exchange transfusion, intra-uterine transfusion, and early induction of labour, reduced the number of deaths to 708 by 1969, but the introduction of Anti-D Immunoglobulin prophylaxis in the early 1970s was a further major advance. If it is shown that a rhesus-negative woman has borne a rhesus-positive child, she is injected with rhesus antibody (Anti-D gamma globulin) within 72 hours of delivery. This destroys any rhesus positive fetal red cells before they can stimulate continuing maternal antibody formation. Any rhesus-negative woman who has an abortion or other procedure (for example, amniocentesis) during pregnancy should also receive antibody in the same way. The virtual elimination of rhesus haemolytic disease could be achieved by a well organised and well administered programme. Unfortunately, women are still sensitised each year in Britain, many due to transplacental bleeding in pregnancy. The treatment of this may call for the use of immunoglobulin during as well as at the end of pregnancy (and this is currently being evaluated).

Detection of neural tube defect

The possibility of early detection of open neural tube defect (NTD) came in the early 1970s when it was noted that a substance called alpha-feto protein (AFP) was present in increased amounts in the amniotic fluid of women carrying babies with anencephaly or spina bifida. A later discovery, that raised AFP levels could be detected in the serum (blood) of mothers carrying NTD fetuses, meant there was a potential for a screening test. The earlier finding, of the association between raised levels of AFP in the amniotic fluid and a fetus with an open NTD had a much more limited application. Amniocentesis is an invasive procedure which would prove impractical to carry out routinely on all pregnancies.

Initial serum testing must be undertaken between 16 and 18 weeks of pregnancy and should be combined with counselling when it is necessary to spell out to the patient the possible implications of a raised level of AFP. The accurate dating of a pregnancy is essential to the diagnostic process. Since the level of AFP alters as a normal pregnancy progresses, it could be thought of as abnormal if the stage of gestation was incorrectly estimated or in the presence of twins. Ultrasound examination enables a more accurate estimation of gestational age to be made and to exclude twins. A positive serum AFP result, indicating abnormality, is dealt with by repeating the serum screening test, checking on gestational age and searching for the presence of other abnormalities or of twin pregnancies (which can produce raised levels of AFP). If the test is still positive and alternative explanations have been eliminated, an amniocentesis will be performed, a procedure carrying a risk of induced abortion estimated at 1%. With the advent of more sophisticated methods of ultrasound scanning in the antenatal period, this method of screening is superseding AFP assay as the primary method of detection of NTD. If a fetus is found to have a NTD, the parents will be offered the choice of terminating the pregnancy during appropriate counselling and most will elect to do so.

The detection of Down's Syndrome

Diagnosis of Down's Syndrome can be made in the antenatal period by amniocentesis, chorion villus sampling, placentesis and fetal blood sampling. Such invasive procedures carry a risk of miscarriage and cannot appropriately be offered to all pregnant women. The offer is usually limited to older mothers or those who had a previously affected child or one partner with known chromosomal abnormalities. However, because most cases are born to women aged below 35 years, the screening of older women makes a limited impact on the overall number of Down's Syndrome babies born. Current studies hold out the promise of testing the mother's serum for biochemical markers of a Down's Syndrome fetus which will provide the basis for an effective antenatal detection programme.

Intrapartum care

One of the most important issues in maternity care, and one of the most contentious is the choice of place of delivery. Over the last thirty years, there has been a growing trend towards deliveries taking place in specialist obstetric units within general hospitals.

Over more recent years, around the country, there has been progressive closure of smaller local maternity units, often on the basis that they could not fulfil professionally set standards for care during labour. This trend has taken place with professional support and has accorded with Department of Health policy. Although, on the face of it, larger, specialised well-staffed and equipped general hospital units would seem safer, there is little hard evidence of poorer outcome of pregnancy amongst women delivered in smaller units. Moreover, many women, when asked about place of delivery express the view that they want to be cared for in an environment which is not dominated by the high technology aspects.

Place of delivery

There will always be some mothers for whom underlying medical problems or complications of pregnancy mean that any idea of delivery away from immediate obstetric or paediatric assistance entails such a risk that it would be out of the question. There will similarly be many mothers whose delivery will be so straightforward as to entail virtually no risk at all. Those who argue, often passionately, for or against home or hospital delivery can always cite the exception to these rules; the patient with toxaemia who delivers safely at home; the patient whose third uncomplicated pregnancy results in a handicapped baby following a totally unforeseen problem in labour at home.

In between these two are a group of mothers who face a higher risk of complication in labour because of, for example, their age or that it is their first baby and it is these women, who, were they to be given a free choice, would truly have to weigh up the risks and the advantages of either having their baby at home or in hospital.

Those in favour of home delivery would argue that labour should take place in the more intimate atmosphere of their own home with those members of their family or friends that they might wish around them. They would also argue that the technology of a modern labour ward dehumanises what is an intense, emotional and essentially normal experience.

There are others who would argue that the risk of something going wrong at very short notice is such that they are willing to trade the familiar and comforting environment for safety. Evidence can be produced on both sides to support the arguments advanced for both points of view. There is even a suggestion that intervention in hospital deliveries may produce more complications than would occur in home deliveries. The definitive study has yet to be conducted.

These matters were brought to a head in 1992 with the Report of the House of Commons Select Committee on Health which dealt with Maternity Services. The Select Committee made a number of conclusions and recommendations on place of delivery and related issues and was critical of the organisation and philosophy of maternity care in Britain at the time. In particular, the Select Committee did not think the policy of encouraging all women to give birth in hospital was justified on the grounds of safety. It considered that the centralised hospital-based system of maternity services reduced choice for women and that the option of birth in a small maternity unit was not readily available for many women. It recommended that midwives, rather than doctors, should provide a higher proportion of care.

The role of specialist obstetric units

It seems unlikely that there will be any major shift away from the specialised obstetric unit as the main focus of care. However, there is greater flexibility and choice in provision than in the past. When women do choose to have their baby in a specialist unit, it is essential that they receive the highest standards of care available. This includes, for example, access to the equipment necessary to detect fetal distress and the availability of epidural anaesthesia. In turn, this means ensuring that units are well equipped and staffed with highly trained personnel.

A number of general practitioners, who receive training in obstetrics, offer maternity care to patients on their lists. The concept of shared care involves the assessment of women by a consultant obstetrician during pregnancy but the majority of care, and in many cases, the delivery is undertaken by the general practitioner, either in a consultant-run obstetric unit or in a local general practitioner-run community or cottage hospital. There are many local and small maternity units around Britain, particularly in rural areas, which offer a service which is often perceived as more friendly and less clinical than the maternity unit attached to a district general hospital. For many mothers it can provide a compromise between the more natural setting of a home delivery and the safety of a hospital environment.

A safety-net in the form of an obstetric flying squad, is provided for those mothers delivering at home or in the smaller more remote rural maternity units. Traditionally this has consisted of an obstetric team comprising, usually a midwife, an obstetrician and an anaesthetist who could be available almost immediately to go out by ambulance to an obstetric emergency. However, obstetric flying squads are decreasing in number, partly because of less frequent calls due to fewer home deliveries, partly because in many cases it is a paediatrician who is required, (rather than an obstetrician) and partly because of an increase in the use of paramedics in the ambulance service.

Maternity care tends to face a dilemma in that there is a public expectation that the outcome of every pregnancy will be a normal baby, but at the same time there is a desire to ensure that the emotional experience of giving birth is not marred by the intrusion of an overly technological environment. Some maternity units are now arriving at a compromise of having delivery suites which are furnished much more in the style of the average home than the normal hospital environment.

The size of a maternity unit may also affect the mother's choice in terms of, for example, anaesthesia during labour. The Royal College of Anaesthetists recommends that epidural anaesthesia should only be offered if there is a resident anaesthetist in the hospital. This must, of necessity, limit the choice of mothers who choose to have their babies in those small hospitals which do not have a resident anaesthetist.

The majority of newborn babies require no additional management in a special care nursery. However, for those who do, pre-term survival may depend on tube feeding and, in particular, ventilation to counter the effects of lung immaturity and lack of natural surfactant, which tends to lead to respiratory distress syndrome (RDS). Improved technology has led to smaller and more pre-term babies being successfully ventilated. This, in turn, has resulted in the need for additional high dependency or intensive care cots for neonates because the earlier these babies can be successfully ventilated the less they are then likely to need respiratory support. This situation has been exacerbated to some extent by the increase in multiple births produced by assisted reproduction.

In addition, recent developments in extra corporeal membrane oxygenation (ECMO) have meant that it may be possible to keep babies from even earlier gestation alive until they are mature enough to survive independently. This particular technique, like others such as the renal dialysis of pre-term babies is an example of medical technology which requires careful and full evaluation.

There are four categories of babies requiring quite high dependency or special care:

High dependency care

(a) Infants requiring artificial respiratory support.
(b) Infants requiring 40% oxygen or more; or whose entire fluid intake is provided intravenously; or whose current weight is less than 1.0 kg.

Special care

(c) Infants receiving less than 40% supplemental oxygen; or receiving some intravenous fluid; or receiving tube feeding; or whose weight is between 1.0 kg and 1.75 kg.
(d) Bottle or breast fed infants, weighing more than 1.75 kg, admitted for observation only.

The majority of district general hospitals which have an obstetrics service are equipped to deal with babies in categories (c) and (d) in special care baby units. In addition, they are almost all capable of dealing with babies in categories (a) and (b) in the short-term. However, for very tiny and very pre-term babies there is no doubt that the outcome is better if they are treated in units where long term ventilation is a standard procedure. The development of such regional or sub-regional units has also led to the establishment of neonatal flying squads which consist of an experienced junior paediatrician or consultant, accompanied by an experienced neonatal nurse who go out with a fully equipped incubator to peripheral hospitals and stabilise and then supervise the transfer of the baby requiring high dependency care back to the sub-regional centres.

Whilst in the short-term, facilities need to be available to ventilate babies with respiratory distress in all hospitals offering an obstetric service, current evidence suggests that given the medical and nursing expertise required to deal with babies who need long-term ventilation, high dependency neonatal care should, for the foreseeable future, be provided in a smaller number of centres in each health region.

The increased workload produced by low birth weight survivors means that many hospitals providing this type of care have experienced great pressure on their facilities. An example of this trend in one health region is shown in Figure 6.17.

SERVICES FOR CHILDREN

Services, exclusively dedicated to the welfare of children, developed slowly and sporadically in Britain during the eighteenth century. A dispensary for children of the poor was established in London in 1769 and, as part of its service, children were visited at home. A hundred years later this feature was developed when a home visiting service by 'respectable working women', to help and advise on child welfare matters, was established in Manchester and Salford. At the beginning of this century, a comprehensive Health Visiting Service was established in Huddersfield to combat the high infant mortality rate. A local Act made notification of birth to the Medical Officer of Health compulsory so that a home visit could be

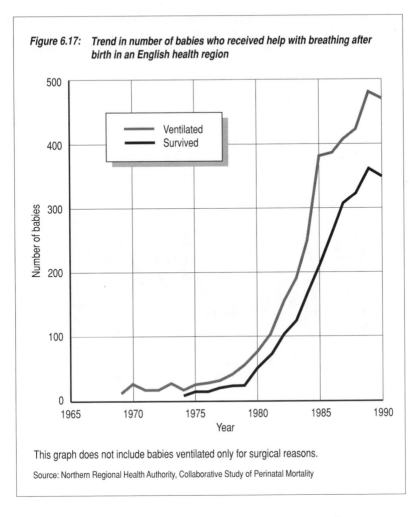

Figure 6.17: Trend in number of babies who received help with breathing after birth in an English health region

This graph does not include babies ventilated only for surgical reasons.

Source: Northern Regional Health Authority, Collaborative Study of Perinatal Mortality

made shortly after the birth. This pioneering service was followed by national legislation which was, at first, permissive but later, through the Notification of Birth Act 1915, made compulsory. A few years later, local authorities were empowered to make arrangements for safeguarding the health of mothers and children, including the provision of free antenatal and postnatal clinics. Child Welfare Clinics provided by local authorities became more numerous and a national scheme for training health visitors was inaugurated. Universal compulsory education introduced in 1870 and 1880, revealed the extent of poor hygiene, malnutrition and handicapping conditions prevalent amongst school children. Further legislation was soon passed to give powers to local authorities to make provision for blind, deaf, mentally handicapped and epileptic children. The first full-time School Medical Officer was appointed in London in 1890 and other places followed suit. However, it was the disquiet about the nation's health, following the discovery of the poor physical condition of recruits for the Boer War, which finally persuaded the government to introduce a school health service.

Medical inspection of school children was made compulsory in 1907 and as there was no National Health Service, provision was also made for the treatment of school children. This arrangement continued until the National Health Service was established in 1948.

In the eighteenth and nineteenth centuries, young children were often admitted to women's hospital wards, usually accompanied by their mothers who helped to care for them in hospital. In 1852, the Hospital for Sick Children in Great Ormond Street, London, was opened and shortly afterwards, many other children's hospitals were built. A register for Sick Children's Nurses was established in 1919 and the emerging new specialty of Paediatrics assumed increasing importance during the late 1920s and early 1930s.

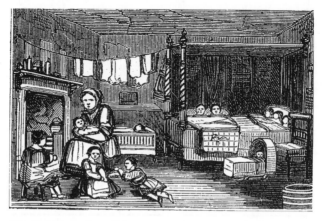

Woodcut: a mother and ten children in a damp and dilapidated room; anon., c. 1864. Source: George Godwin, Another blow for life, London: 1864

Beyond birth, services for children cover a range of functions. They encompass surveillance (the process of monitoring a child's developmental progress and identifying abnormalities); preventive interventions (for example, immunisation against the communicable diseases of childhood); the promotion of healthy behaviours; the recognition, diagnosis and treatment of disease, illness and other disorders; the management and care of children with chronic disease, disability and handicap; the recognition of abuse and neglect and the protection and care of the child; the care of other children who cannot be with their families.

Child health surveillance

For the past thirty years or more, the regular surveillance of children's growth and development has been an integral part of the child health service. The scope of such surveillance has varied over the years, particularly when the value of some kinds of screening of apparently healthy children to detect abnormalities has been challenged. A full discussion of the principles of population screening can be found in chapter 3. In the late 1980s, the place of child health surveillance was fundamentally reviewed and redefined as:

'The oversight of physical, social and emotional health and development of all children; measurement and recording of physical growth; monitoring of developmental progress; offering and arranging intervention when necessary; prevention of disease by immunisation and other means and health education.'[1]

The review analysed the procedures used in child health surveillance and classified them in the light of current knowledge as, of definite value and should be continued, of uncertain value and should be further evaluated and of little value and should be discontinued. On the basis of this, the recommended functions of child health surveillance are described below.

Physical examination

A programme of physical examination of all children should be carried out at birth, at discharge from hospital (or within 10 days of birth), at six to eight weeks, at six to nine months and pre-school. The content of these physical examinations varies at different ages. The examination after birth should incorporate a full physical examination, weight and head circumference measurement, a check for congenital dislocation of the hip, for undescended testes and an examination of the eyes. The ten day examination should also incorporate a second check for congenital dislocation of the hip. The six to eight week review should again include a full physical examination, further measurement of weight and head circumference. Gait should be specifically assessed between 18 and 24 months. Examination for congenital heart disease should be incorporated in the birth, the neonatal and the six week examinations and also at a re-examination at some point before the child is five years of age.

Screening tests

Neonatal screening for phenylketonuria and hypothyroidism are of value and should be carried out. Evidence in favour of other screening programmes, for example, to detect iron deficiency anaemia, hypertension, and scoliosis are not of clearly established benefit.

Vision and hearing

Examination of the eyes to detect abnormalities such as squint should be carried out at the neonatal and the six week examinations. Tests for visual acuity in the young child are of limited value and this is best assessed at school entry. For sensory neural hearing loss, a distraction test at eight months of age and sweep test at school entry should be carried out. It is important that parental concern about a child's hearing or vision is always taken seriously.

Growth and development

The weight of all babies should be measured and recorded at birth and at the six to eight week review. Although regular weighing of babies thereafter is commonplace, there is little evidence that it is of value unless the baby or child has problems. Nevertheless, it can act as a focus for the doctor or health visitor to discuss parenting issues with a mother. Height should be measured at around the age of three years, again at school entry and more regularly if there is concern. In recording weight and height, it is essential that properly calibrated instruments are used and that measurements are recorded on standard developmental charts to allow deviation from the normal range to be clearly recognised and acted upon.

Communication and information

Effective child health surveillance requires high quality communication and information systems at a number of levels. Firstly, there is a need to ensure good databases to identify children at birth, to ensure that they are called up for their regular assessments, for immunisation and vaccination and to enable the findings of examinations as well as immunisation status to be recorded. Secondly, there is a need for exchange of information between all health care professionals involved in child health: for example, the general practitioner, the health visitor, the paediatrician and the community health doctor. Increasingly, parent held child health records are being developed as a way of overcoming some of the traditional logistic difficulties of maintaining continuity and accuracy of records.

Staff providing child health surveillance

Responsibility for ensuring that effective child health surveillance is carried out within a local population rests with district health authorities and family health services authorities (see chapter 4 for a full description of their roles). The service is delivered by general practitioners, consultant community paediatricians, community health doctors, health visitors, school medical officers and school nurses. The organisation of the service varies around the country but services mainly differ in the extent to which the service is based with general practice or whether there is greater emphasis on community health services (outwith general practice). In either case, general practitioners, other members of the primary health care team and community health service staff work closely together.

Health promotion in childhood

The subject of health promotion and the importance of developing healthy lifestyles and behaviours early in life is described fully in chapter 3. It is important to recognise the opportunities available for health promotion, through health education, as a result of the regular contacts with children and their parents which occur throughout childhood. This applies whether the child is presenting with a problem to the general practitioner or to the hospital service or for routine child health surveillance. Opportunities for health education on issues such as immunisation and vaccination, accident prevention, safety, nutrition, passive and active smoking, drug and alcohol misuse should be taken by health professionals whenever possible.

The School Health Service

The creation of a National School Health Service represented an important landmark in the progress towards better health for children. It arose largely because of recommendations published in 1904 by the Interdepartmental Committee on Physical Deterioration, following the discovery of high levels of unfitness amongst recruits for the Boer War. The Education Act, 1907, placed a duty on local authorities to arrange systematic medical inspections of school children.

The original objectives of the School Health Service were twofold. They were to supervise the growth and development of school children and to identify those with physical or mental abnormalities or other specific disorders which might affect their learning capacity. As well as routine medical examination of school children, the service provides additional screening procedures, ensures immunity levels against communicable diseases are maintained and promotes health education programmes. Staff provide a consultation service for all children, their parents and teachers and also act in a supervisory and advisory role for children with special needs. Whilst the School Health Service's main focus is the promotion of health, treatment can also be provided from health care professionals in dentistry, speech therapy, physiotherapy and chiropody.

For many years, routine medical examinations of children were carried out on three occasions: at school entry, before entering secondary school (about 10 years of age) and before leaving school (about 14 years of age). It became apparent that medical examination of the entire school population at this frequency was not justified and that attention should be concentrated on those children most likely to benefit from medical screening and referral. Hence, some schemes for selective medical examination have been introduced but, at present, opinion differs about which criteria should be used for selection.

The orientation of the school health service varies from place to place. Some suggest that it is anachronistic to have a school health system running in parallel to services provided by general practitioners and paediatricians. It is likely in the future that greater emphasis will be placed on the school nurse with medical intervention being used more selectively.

The 1981 Education Act has important implications for school health services. The Act required local education authorities to identify services for a disabled child to meet his or her 'special educational needs'. These should be provided in a mainstream school so long as this is compatible with parental wishes and the efficient use of resources. In order to establish the child's special educational needs an assessment must be undertaken with reports submitted from parents, teacher, educational psychologist and school medical officer and if appropriate from others such as nurse or therapist. The child's requirements are then formally recorded in a 'statement'. Parents must be fully involved in all stages of the assessment and there are formal appeal mechanisms should they disagree with the assessment or provision made.

The protection of abused and neglected children

Although injury to children by their parents is not a new phenomenon, it only became widely recognised in the early 1970s. In 1962, the term 'battered child syndrome' was first used by an American paediatrician, Dr. Kempe and was taken up by the media.

In Britain, widespread attention was first focused on child physical abuse in 1974, following an inquiry into the death of seven year old Maria Colwell. This inquiry uncovered serious deficiencies in professional practice and in the response of services. Its main historical importance is that it acted as a stimulus to the establishment of a procedure for dealing with the problem.

There has since been at least one major public inquiry per year into a child death in the home. These inquiries have discovered a consistent pattern of failure of professional practice, lack of communication and poor co-ordination of services.

Recognition of the widespread nature of child sexual abuse was much slower in coming. Although it was recognised amongst professionals who were dealing with the issue, the public were largely unaware of it, at least as a major problem. All this changed in the late 1980s when the sexual abuse of children became a prominent issue for the public, the media and for politicians. Esther Rantzen, the broadcaster, launched 'Childline', a free telephone counselling service for child victims of sexual abuse.

In Cleveland in 1986, the admittance to hospital of large numbers of children suspected of being sexually abused led to an inquiry. The subsequent report stated that there was not only lack of communication but also a lack of understanding by the agencies involved, of each others' functions in relation to child sexual abuse, as well as fundamental differences in approach amongst professionals of the same discipline.

The crisis in Cleveland raised new issues. Firstly, it brought into the open the fact that child sexual abuse might be a much greater problem than had previously been realised. Secondly, it drew attention to the need for a balance between the rights of parents and the power of professionals to take action to protect children. Although the Cleveland Inquiry report was far-reaching and was a force for the introduction of much new guidance (and parts of the Children Act 1989) on the detection and management of child sexual abuse, the lessons were not fully learned. Further controversy surrounded incidents in Orkney and Lancashire in the early 1990s.

The key to successful child protection services is effective working between all the agencies involved, particularly the local authority Social Services department, the local health services, the police, and the courts. In some parts of the country the local branch of the National Society for the Prevention of Cruelty to Children (NSPCC) plays a prominent role in child protection services.

These agencies have a duty not just to safeguard and promote the interests and welfare of children but also to work with families.

Size of the problem

The spectrum of child abuse is now recognised as extensive. It covers physical injury to the child, sexual activities involving a child, emotional ill-treatment, and severe neglect. There are no reliable data to describe the size of the problem of child abuse in the population. By its nature it is a problem that may not be recognised or which may be concealed.

Children recorded on child protection registers provide an estimate of the problem, although undoubtedly it is an underestimate. In 1991, there were 45,200 children and young people on child protection registers in England, a rate of 4.2 children per thousand aged under 18 years. There was a marked variation in age for cases already on the register and cases newly registered. The peak occurrence of newly registered children was in those under one year, whilst the peak for those already on the register was in the age range one to four years (Figure 6.18).

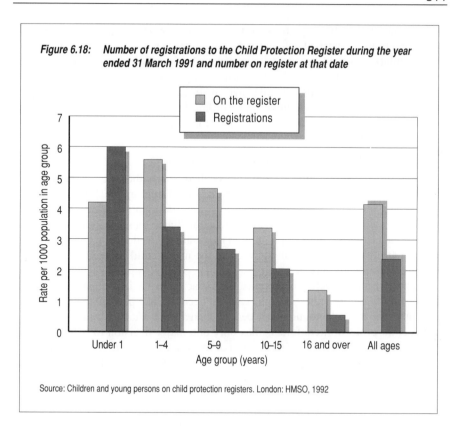

Figure 6.18:   Number of registrations to the Child Protection Register during the year
ended 31 March 1991 and number on register at that date

Source: Children and young persons on child protection registers. London: HMSO, 1992

Recognition and referral of cases

A potential case of child physical abuse may present to a general practitioner or to a
hospital Accident and Emergency department. Alternatively, cases of both physical
and sexual abuse may be detected by a professional worker (for example, health
visitor, social worker, school teacher) or a suspected case may be brought to the
attention of the social services department or the police through a wide variety of
concerned sources (for example, a relative, friend or neighbour). It is important
that any suspicion of child abuse reported to one of the agencies is taken extremely
seriously. Also professionals working in each of the agencies should be skilled in
recognition of the signs of abuse and neglect.

Investigation and assessment

An early decision needs to be taken as to whether the child is in need of urgent
protection. If so, an application can be made to the court for an Emergency
Protection Order (see later in the chapter for discussion of legislation relating to
child protection). Such action will not usually be warranted and the first step will be
a strategy discussion between representatives of the various agencies to plan the
investigation of the suspected abuse. There is always the possibility that legal
action may be taken by either the social services department (to protect the child) or
by the police (to prosecute an alleged perpetrator of abuse) or by both agencies.

Staff undertaking this type of work from whatever agency must be appropriately skilled and trained. Detailed national and local guidance covers how the various types of investigation should be carried out, especially in relation to interviewing and examining the child. It is essential that this is done with great sensitivity otherwise the investigation process could further damage an already vulnerable child.

High standards are also required in recording findings and evidence which may be required subsequently for the child protection conference and by the court.

The child protection conference and registration of cases

The child protection conference (sometimes called simply the case conference) is a vital part of the child protection procedures. It is the forum in which representatives of all agencies concerned come together to review information related to the child and to plan the action required. The conference will also seek advice on assessment from relevant experts (for example, a child psychiatrist, an educational psychologist).

There are two main types of conference: the initial child protection conference and the child protection review.

An initial child protection conference takes place after the investigation and initial assessment. Its timing varies. In some cases, it needs to take place extremely quickly but in any case it would not normally be later than a week after the initial referral.

The child protection conference has only one major decision to make which is whether to register the child. The process of registration leads to the designation of a key worker who is a social worker from the social services department or the NSPCC. He or she is responsible for the development of a plan for the protection of the child, co-ordinating all other agencies as well as co-ordinating further assessment and if necessary preparation of the application to court for a Care Order. It is important to realise that it is not the purpose of the child protection conference to establish whether abuse has taken place.

Children, parents and other family members should usually be involved in some part of the conference though this can be problematic and not all care professionals agree with such an approach.

The Chair of the child protection conference is by a senior representative of the lead agency (either social services department or NSPCC). The skills and knowledge of the chairperson are very important. Poor chairing can make the difference between a child being adequately protected and being left vulnerable to further abuse. Representatives from each agency and each care professional should be invited to attend the child protection conference.

The review conference serves a different purpose. It assesses the current status of the child, reviews the current child protection plan, the level of risk and decides whether registration should continue.

A key feature of the approach to the problem of child abuse at a local level is the establishment and maintenance of child protection registers to record all cases of abuse and those in which a child is at risk of abuse. It is a requirement that such a register is maintained in each social services area.

There are three broad objectives of such a register:

- To provide a record of all children in the area who are currently the subject of an interagency protection plan and to ensure that the plans are formally reviewed at least every six months.

- To provide a central point of speedy enquiry for professional staff who are worried about a child and want to know whether the child is the subject of an interagency protection plan.
- To provide statistical information about current trends in the area.

A child's name can only be entered onto the register after a child protection conference if there is significant risk of harm leading to the need for a child protection plan or a likelihood of such harm.

The categories of abuse for registration are:

- Neglect.
- Physical injury.
- Sexual abuse.
- Emotional abuse.

The removal of a child from the register is considered at every review child protection conference but all those present at the conference must agree that the abuse (or risk of it) is no longer present for de-registration to occur. Other aspects of register maintenance include ensuring confidentiality, communication of changes of registered details, updating with additional reports and notification of details to another area if the family moves house.

Area Child Protection Committees

The Area Child Protection Committee is the body in which all the agencies come together to formulate, review and monitor child protection policies. The main functions of the Area Child Protection Committee are set out in Table 6.12.

Table 6.12: Main functions of Area Child Protection Committees

- To establish, maintain and review local inter-agency guidelines on procedures to be followed in individual cases.
- To monitor the implementation of legal procedures.
- To identify significant issues arising from the handling of cases and reports from inquiries.
- To scrutinise arrangements to provide treatment, expert advice and inter-agency liaison and make recommendations to the responsible agencies.
- To scrutinise progress on work to prevent child abuse and make recommendations to the responsible agencies.
- To scrutinise work related to inter-agency training and make recommendations to the responsible agencies.
- To conduct reviews required in cases where there are adverse incidents.
- To publish an annual report about local child protection matters.

Source: Working Together Under the Children Act 1989. London: HMSO, 1991.

Prevention of child abuse

As in so many fields involving human behaviour, successful preventive measures are very difficult to establish.

If better methods could be devised to identify families where violence is likely to occur, then the necessary corrective measures could be taken. It has been suggested that this could begin in hospital obstetric departments by making a concentrated effort to identify mothers who are at risk of maltreating their child. More frequent visiting to give support to isolated families may reduce the risk. As more attention is focused on the problem of child abuse, various schemes are being established, such as 'self help' groups and the 'crying baby' 24 hour service, where health visitors respond to crises.

A longer term measure is to develop the teaching of parenthood in schools, with emphasis on child development and the emotional needs of babies and children.

Where sexual abuse is concerned, there is general agreement that it should be openly discussed with young children and their families, both before it occurs, in sensitive prevention programmes and afterwards, in the form of therapy. It is also necessary to educate preschool and day care managers and teachers about the recognition of symptoms and the kinds of threat that children might receive to prevent them from revealing the abuse.

Children in care

At any one time, some 60,000 children in England will be in the care of local authorities. Care in this context encompasses a wide variety of settings ranging from fostering through various types of residential care to secure institutions

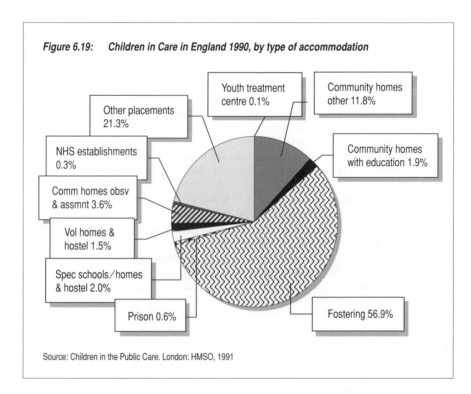

Figure 6.19: Children in Care in England 1990, by type of accommodation

Youth treatment centre 0.1%

Community homes other 11.8%

Other placements 21.3%

NHS establishments 0.3%

Comm homes obsv & assmnt 3.6%

Vol homes & hostel 1.5%

Spec schools/homes & hostel 2.0%

Prison 0.6%

Community homes with education 1.9%

Fostering 56.9%

Source: Children in the Public Care. London: HMSO, 1991

Table 6.13:   *Main purpose of residential care for children*

A home for children who:
- Have decided that they do not wish to be fostered
- Have had bad experiences of foster care
- Have been so abused within the family that another family placement is inappropriate
- Are from the same family and cannot otherwise be kept together

Source: Children in the Public Care: London: HMSO, 1991.

(Figure 6.19). Children need care of these kinds for a variety of reasons. For example, they may have been abused or neglected, their parents may not be able to cope with their upbringing, they may have severe behavioural or emotional disturbance, or their family may have broken down and fragmented.

A child being considered for care by the local authority should have a full assessment so that the choice of placement can be made in a way which reflects his or her individual needs. The preferred placement for many children today is fostering with various types of residential care underpinning the fostering system. Residential care is usually the best option in certain situations (Table 6.13). In the early 1990s concern over the treatment of children in residential care and the competency of staff running children's homes led to a number of rigorous reviews of staff recruitment and training policies as well as the organisation of residential care itself. A number of general principles of good practice should govern the operation of residential care (Table 6.14).

Day care of children

Arrangements for day care of children under school age are both formal and informal and broadly encompass: nurseries and nursery schools, playgroups and childminding. The purpose of these schemes is either to allow mothers to go out to work or to give some respite from the heavy burden of looking after young children.

Table 6.14:   *General principles governing the provision of residential care for children*

- The purpose of the establishment and the objectives for individual young people should be clear
- The home should provide an ambience in which residents feel valued, encouraged to want to stay and not to have to consider moving on too soon; and in which staff are willing and able to accept dependent relationships with children and young people
- The residents should have some influence over the regime; controls should be related to their needs as well as to the maintenance of the institution; trivial confrontation should be avoided
- The physical surroundings should be pleasant and comfortable and everyone should be interested in maintaining them in that condition

Source: Children in the Public Care. London: HMSO, 1991.

Day nurseries are provided by Social Services departments of local authorities, for children of preschool age. They usually have between 30 and 60 places and are open from Monday to Friday from about 7 a.m. to 6 p.m. Charges are made in accordance with the parents' income. Most of the staff have a nursery nurse qualification and health visitors have a responsibility to ensure that adequate measures are being taken to prevent the spread of infection. Many nurseries have teachers available to advise and help with the children's educational needs.

Most Social Services departments assign priorities in deciding how to allocate places in day nurseries. Such categories might include children of one parent families, children at risk of non-accidental injury, children of families where the mother or family are under particular stress, children whose home circumstances are poor and handicapped children.

Private nurseries are provided by individuals or organisations for profit. They are run on the same general lines as day nurseries. The purpose and clientele varies with the locality. Local authority Social Services departments are responsible for the registration and supervision of private nurseries, under the provision of the Nursery and Childminders Regulations Act 1948, as amended by the Health Service and Public Health Act 1968.

A small proportion of full-time day care nurseries are provided by employers such as industrial firms, hospitals, universities and colleges and these are established at or near the work site. The organisations concerned subsidise the schemes and charges vary. They are popular because mothers are nearby and able to see their children during the day. They tend to be cheaper than local authority day nurseries and the hours match the working hours. The disadvantages of such schemes, however, are that travel to work with young children can be difficult and it makes changing jobs less straightforward. Local Social Services departments are responsible for registration and supervision.

The nursery school has a different orientation to the day nursery. It is the responsibility of the Education department, rather than the Social Services department, although close links exist between the two. Its aim is to provide part-time education for children between three and five years of age.

A childminder is a person who looks after children under the age of eight in his or her own home for two hours or more per day, for which they receive a fee or reward. Local authority Social Services departments are responsible for maintaining a register of childminders and their premises. Before registration, they must be satisfied that the person is fit to act in this capacity and that the premises are suitable. An upper limit on the number of children to be cared for is also fixed and conditions set out concerning safety. Some local authorities employ childminders on a salaried basis.

Playgroups offer informal sessional care to children under the age of five. Children usually attend for a two and a half hour session and a fee is charged towards the cost.

LEGISLATION RELATING TO CHILDREN

In the Autumn of 1991, The Children Act 1989, came into effect. It was a far reaching reform of child care law. Its aim was to simplify the many complex aspects of old child care legislation and to produce a more practical and consistent law. In so doing, the law relating to the care, protection and upbringing of children was, for the first time, integrated with the responsibilities of public authorities, in

Table 6.15: Key principles of the Children Act 1989

- Makes children's welfare a priority
- Recognises that children are best brought up within their families wherever possible
- Aims to prevent unwarranted interference in family life
- Requires local authorities to provide services for children and families in need
- Promotes partnership between children, parents and local authorities
- Improves the way Courts deal with children and families
- Gives rights of appeal against Court decisions
- Protects the rights of parents with children being looked after by local authorities
- Aims to ensure children looked after by local authorities are provided with a good standard of care

Source: The Children Act and Local Authorities: A guide for Parents: London: Department of Health, 1991

particular, local authorities. The Act itself rests on the belief that children are generally best looked after within the family and intervention by the State, in the form of the court or local authority, should not occur unless it is necessary to safeguard the welfare of the child. The Children Act 1989 also establishes the child's rights and interests at the centre of the care process (Table 6.15).

The key concepts of the Act are outlined below.

Local authority responsibilities

The main role of the local authorities outlined by the Children Act 1989, is to provide a range of services and when necessary, accommodation for children in need. As a category 'children in need' is wide, covering children who need services to secure a reasonable standard of health and development and includes children with disabilities. Each local authority must attempt to identify the children in need in their areas, publish information about specific services available and try to ensure this information reaches those who might benefit from it. Such services include advice and counselling, home help, assistance with travelling to use a service, the provision of family centres and appropriate daycare facilities and, in exceptional circumstances, cash (this may be by way of a loan , repayable in whole or in part). Local authorities are also required to establish simple, easily accessible complaints procedures.

Children and the courts

In court cases involving children, the Children Act 1989 sets out principles which must be followed by the courts in dealing with their cases. The court is always mindful of the child's interests and will weigh up a number of factors (Table 6.16).

Court orders and procedures

A distinction must be made between court cases involving children which concern private law (for example, marital and custody disputes) and those which concern

Table 6.16: Main features taken into account by courts in dealing with cases involving children

- The child's own wishes
- The child's physical, emotional and educational needs
- The child's age, sex, background and other relevant considerations
- Any harm which the child has suffered or might suffer in the future
- How able the child's parents (or other relevant persons) are to meet his or her needs
- How the child might be affected by any change in circumstances
- The powers available to the Court

Source: The Children Act and the Courts: A guide for parents. London: Department of Health, 1991.

public law (for example, where the local authority wishes to take action to protect the child). Broadly, the procedures adopted in both types of law are similar and the court action will usually involve an order (a set of legally binding conditions) on what action must be taken. The Children Act 1989 requires that where a child is party to a private law and public law suit, both actions should be heard together. Cases involving children and families are heard in a relatively informal atmosphere by courts which have special expertise in family law.

In cases involving the local authority, the court will appoint a person to represent the child's interests and to make sure that his or her voice is heard. Such a person, the *guardian ad litem*, is independent of the local authority.

Orders issued in private law cases cover such matters as the child's place of residence (where divorcing partners cannot reach agreement) or deal with access arrangements.

In public law cases, the local authority may apply to the court for an order to protect the child or promote his or her welfare in various respects. The main types of such orders are described below.

A **Care Order** places the child into the care of a local authority where the court believes that a child is likely to suffer (or is suffering) significant harm through lack of parental care and control. While a Care Order is in force, the authority has parental responsibility for the child, but it must share this with the parents. Parents are involved in local authority decision-making and must be allowed reasonable contact with the child. Although the local authority has the power to limit the parental responsibility retained by the parents, it may only do so if it is satisfied that this is necessary to safeguard or promote the welfare of the child.

A **Supervision Order** places a child under the supervision of a local authority if the court believes that the child is likely to suffer (or is suffering) harm due to lack of parental care and control. The time limit for a Supervision Order is one year. This is renewable on application to the court but may not exceed a total period of three years. The supervisor is usually a social worker and he or she has a duty to advise, assist and befriend the supervised child. Obligations are imposed on the person responsible for the child to ensure that the child follows the supervisor's directions. The parents still have parental responsibility for the child.

An **Education Supervision Order** can be implemented where a child is not attending school. This order is supervised by the local education authority.

A **Child Assessment Order** can be applied for by a social worker where he or she is concerned about a child and needs further information which the parents refuse (for example, medical or psychological) before deciding on the appropriate type of application to the court.

If a local authority is informed, or has reasonable cause to suspect that a child is in **immediate danger** and must be urgently protected, an application can be made for an emergency protection order or a secure accommodation order.

Any person can apply to the court for an **Emergency Protection Order**. The duration of an Emergency Protection Order is not more than eight days, though the court may extend it once for a further seven days, if necessary. Children, parents or other carers may apply for an order to be discharged after 72 hours.

A **Secure Accommodation Order** can be applied for by the local authority where the child's behaviour is so serious that it is the only method of preventing harm either to the child or to others. The child can be legally represented at the hearing and usually a *guardian ad litem* will be appointed.

CONCLUSIONS

The health of a population's children is an important indicator of its overall health status. Over this century, the industrialised world has witnessed a major reduction in the number of babies lost around the time of childbirth. Despite the fact that a high proportion of pregnancies now have a successful outcome for mothers and babies, a minority of babies still die or survive in a damaged or impaired state. A small number of mothers also die because of pregnancy or childbirth. An important role for public health is to identify the scope for further reductions in this pool of potentially avoidable death, morbidity and disability. Health services working alone or with other agencies have a responsibility to improve the health and well-being of children. This can be through the promotion of health; the application of preventive interventions (such as immunisation); the maintenance of good surveillance; the provision of high quality diagnostic, treatment and rehabilitation services; or making available alternative forms of care, protection and support for children in need.

More than at any other time of life, health and disease in childhood encompasses emotional, psychological, environmental and social influences as well as specific risk factors. Responding to the health challenges of the future will involve a vigorous and imaginative public health approach to the needs of mothers, infants, children and adolescents. For it is amongst these groups that the foundations of a Nation's health are laid.

7 Mental health

INTRODUCTION

Mental health is not just the absence of mental disorder. It is a state in which a person is able to fulfil an active functioning role in society, interacting with others and overcoming difficulties without suffering major distress, abnormal or disturbed behaviour.

Mental disorder is a generic term which includes the very different conditions of mental illness and mental handicap (also called learning disability). It encompasses a heterogeneous collection of conditions which together represent one of the major health and social problems of today.

Whilst attitudes in society are changing, both mental illness and mental handicap continue to carry a stigma for those who suffer from them, and, to a lesser extent, those who care for people who suffer from them. Many health professionals still find the pursuit of a career in this field of care unattractive compared with alternatives involving the care of acutely ill patients in high technology surroundings. Yet, this group of the population has special needs which can pose formidable challenges for those seeking to provide the most appropriate care. The field of work can offer scope for innovation just as great as in the other therapeutic fields of medicine and surgery.

This chapter deals with the extent and range of mental disorder found in the population, the needs of people who suffer from them, and the spectrum of services available to meet those needs.

THE NEEDS OF THE MENTALLY ILL

The spectrum of psychological disorders which can incapacitate people and interfere with their ability to function normally is very large. Whilst distinctions are often made between major and minor mental illnesses, disorders of the mind can be very distressing and disruptive to individuals and their families, even when they do not amount to a full blown psychiatric illness. For example, a thirty year old woman with three small children who develops uncontrollable panic attacks when she enters a shop can be so incapacitated by this problem that she is unable to go outdoors unaccompanied. Moreover, she may be so distressed that she needs to ask her husband to stay away from work to be with her, thus putting his employment position in jeopardy. Similarly, the teenage girl who develops an eating disorder at the time of school leaving examinations can perform so badly that she may lose important career opportunities, yet her condition may not amount to anorexia nervosa.

Many so called 'minor' mental illnesses are treated in general practice or do not necessarily come to the attention of medical services, so that routine data are not available to enable them to be quantified within the population.

A smaller number of people suffer from very serious psychiatric disorders which can have a major social impact. Schizophrenia is an example of this kind of condition. It is usually a long-term illness for which people require medication, support and several episodes of hospital care during the course of many years. Whilst most people who have developed the disease over the last twenty years have been able to maintain a home outside hospital, there is a group of people with chronic schizophrenia who were diagnosed at a time when modern drugs were not available. Many such people are long-term residents within large psychiatric hospitals which have, in effect, become their homes. Their inability to lead an independent life is in part a feature of the long-term nature of their illness but in part also caused by a dependence on the routines and habits of institutional life. With the advent of programmes of care which seek to phase out the large long-stay psychiatric hospitals, this group of chronically mentally ill people must be considered as having special needs.

Also amongst the more severe mental illness problems within the population is the group of people whose disorder of the mind makes them commit crimes such as assault, rape, murder, theft and arson. Although the numbers of mentally ill people in this category is small, they pose problems which are complex to solve and have needs with require highly specialised forms of care.

Describing the size and nature of the problem of mental illness in the population, and the range of needs experienced by people with mental illness, is very difficult. Not least are the problems of diagnosis and disease classification. Whilst variation between psychiatrists in the use of disease labels is not of major importance when addressing the needs of individual patients, it causes difficulty when it is necessary to aggregate diagnostic information to produce estimates of the size of particular pools of psychiatric morbidity at population level. There is also a lack of routinely available population-based information. Traditionally, information on psychiatric morbidity has been based on contacts with services, usually hospital services.

Establishing the frequency of psychiatric morbidity in the general population has been a major area of epidemiological research since the 1960s and the subject of important studies even before that. Early studies concentrated on people already in contact with mental health services but it was quickly realised that this represented only a small proportion of total psychiatric morbidity (Figure 7.1). Findings of early community-based surveys suffered from the difficulties of operationalising psychiatric diagnoses so that survey instruments could be applied to large populations, by non-medical (but trained) interviewers and then yield valid assessments of morbidity in the population.

One of the most influential early studies of mental illness in a population was carried out in New York in the mid-1950s. The Mid-Town Manhattan Study was based on a single home interview of a randomly selected sample of 1.7% of households to idenjfy adults aged 20 to 59 years, together with information from searching records of hospitals and other agencies (to identify people who could have been missed in the household survey). The survey questions covered 120 manifestations of mental illness, mainly drawn from symptom-based psychiatric screening tools of the day. Psychiatrists then classified the responses gathered by the field interviewers. The results were presented in terms of a continuum of mental health (Table 7.1) not as a series of diagnostic categories. As a result, the prevalence of mental 'illness' appears quite high. For this reason, the study is often

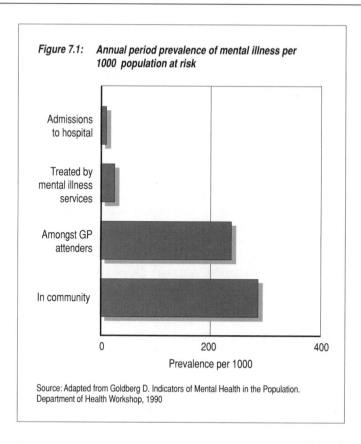

Figure 7.1: *Annual period prevalence of mental illness per 1000 population at risk*

Source: Adapted from Goldberg D. Indicators of Mental Health in the Population. Department of Health Workshop, 1990

criticised by those who seek to establish the prevalence of mental illness in terms of precise diagnostic groups. Yet, it would have been impractical at the time to carry out a full psychiatric assessment on each member of the sample. Moreover, the variation in diagnostic approach between psychiatrists would have limited the generalisability of the findings.

Table 7.1: *Classification of people's mental health status in an early community study; mid-town Manhattan*

Mental health	Percentage of sample
Well	18.5
Mild symptom formation	36.3
Moderate symptoms	21.8
Marked symptoms	13.2
Severe symptoms	7.5
Incapacitated	2.7
	100
	N(100%) = (1660)

Source: Srole L et al. Mental Health in the Metropolis. New York: McGraw-Hill, 1962.

In more recent years, views have differed as to the approach which should be used to establish the prevalence of mental illness in the population. Broadly, when the aim is to explore causation, disease categories are more useful. When the aim is to examine need for services, functionally-based measures are usually preferable.

The development of standardised diagnostic and assessment scales has greatly improved the value and comparability of population-based studies of mental illness. For example, Table 7.2 shows the results of studies in different populations of the world using such a standardised scale (the Present State Examination, PSE) to determine the prevalence of depression. Apart from the survey in Uganda, the prevalence figures are of a similar order of magnitude and differences may reflect genuine variations in the frequency of the problem. Table 7.3 gives a broad indication of the prevalence of the main mental disorder in the adult population, based on various survey data.

Table 7.2: Prevalence of depression in various studies (using a standardised assessment scale)

Location	Prevalence (%)
Uganda	18.9
Canberra	4.8
Athens	7.4
Nijmegen	5.5
Santander	6.2
Camberwell	7.0
Finland	4.6

Source: Adapted from Bebbington PE. Social Psychiatry and Psychiatric Epidemiology 1990; 25: 33–40 (in which references to the original surveys can be found)

Table 7.3: Estimated frequency of mental disorders in the adult population over 16 years of age

Mental disorder	Point prevalence (%)	Lifetime risk (%)
Schizophrenia	0.2 – 0.5%	0.7 – 0.9%
Affective psychosis	0.1 – 0.5%	1%
Depressive disorder	3 – 6%	>20%
Anxiety states	2 – 7%	N/A
Dementia (over 65)	5%	N/A
Dementia (over 80)	20%	N/A

N/A = not available or not applicable

Source: The Health of the Nation. London: HMSO, 1992.

Hospital statistics

As with other groups of hospital patients, Hospital Episode Statistics is the method by which statistics on psychiatric inpatients are collected from National Health

Service psychiatric hospitals and psychiatric units in England and Wales. Detailed information is collected about each admission and discharge and a notional census of all psychiatric inpatients is carried out once a year (see chapter 1 for a fuller description).

In addition to these routinely collected statistics, many surveys have investigated psychiatric illnesses using populations of psychiatric inpatients and outpatients. The danger in such studies arises when the assumption is made that admission rates to hospital for particular conditions are synonymous with their incidence in the population.

The fact that fewer people in one area are admitted to hospital than in another may not necessarily be an indication of a lower occurrence of mental illness. It may be reflecting the availability of facilities, the policy for admission, the social stigma attached to mental illness in general or to a particular institution for its treatment, or the tolerance of the community towards abnormal behaviour. Other factors determining whether or not people with a particular psychiatric illness come to the attention of hospital-based services may be the extent to which they or their relatives perceive an abnormality and consider it necessary to make contact with services. This, in turn, may depend upon whether the abnormality interferes with social functioning either in the person's job or in the discharge of other social responsibilities.

Psychiatric morbidity in general practice

No statistics are routinely collected on contacts of patients with general practitioners. However, a number of studies have looked at various aspects of psychiatric morbidity in general practice. Studies of the general practice population give an indication of the distribution of less severe psychiatric conditions and highlight the importance of the psychological components of illness to the work of the general practitioner. In addition, this population gives a fuller indication of the natural history of mental illness. There are, however, special difficulties which limit the conclusions which may be drawn from the results. Rates of psychiatric illness reported by general practitioners vary widely. The report of a single general practitioner is of little value when extrapolated to the whole population. The patients in the practice may not be typical, and the diagnostic criteria and classification adopted by the general practitioner may not be satisfactory. A survey of minor psychiatric morbidity and general practice consultation was carried out in West London in the mid-1970s (which reported in 1986). Random samples of adults were asked to complete a standardised assessment schedule, the General Health Questionnaire (GHQ), designed to identify and measure non-psychotic psychiatric illness. On the basis of previous methodological work with this questionnaire, respondents were classified by their assessment scores into 'probable cases' and 'probable normals'. Table 7.4 illustrates some of the findings and shows the relationship between minor psychiatric morbidity and employment status.

Psychiatric case registers

A case register records and collects information concerning contacts made by individuals residing in a defined geographical area which has a specified set of

Table 7.4: *Percentage of minor psychiatric morbidity amongst people of different employment status in a population survey in West London*

Employment Status	Men % cases	Women % cases
Employed	18.5	22.4
Not employed	51.1	27.8
Retired	66.7	66.7
Ill health	20.1	27.6
All	20.9	25.3

Source: Williams P, Tarnopolsky A, Hand D, Shepherd M. Psychological Medicine 1986; Monograph Supplement 9, 1–37.

psychiatric facilities. Having identified an individual making contact with services, a register monitors any future contacts so that the patient's record is cumulative.

Amongst the best known psychiatric registers developed in the United Kingdom are those in Camberwell, Salford and Aberdeen. They may be used to trace the natural history of disease, to identify groups at high risk and to determine the pattern of use of services as well as the extent to which needs are being met. The maintenance of registers is labour intensive if accuracy is to be achieved. Thus, there are few such registers in Britain as a whole. A fuller description of the concept of disease registers is to be found in chapter 1.

Risk factors for schizophrenia

Schizophrenia is one of the psychiatric illnesses which has been most extensively studied using epidemiological approaches. Studies of risk factors have yielded a fascinating range of influences on the frequency of the disease (Table 7.5). Familial risk is now well established and a great deal of subsequent work has been to elucidate whether this is due to genetic or environmental causes. Sociodemographic risk factors for schizophrenia have been classified into mutable (for example, marital status) and immutable (for example, ethnic origin). It must be remembered however that mutable risk factors may occur because of the disease and not vice versa. A good example of this kind of problem is the relationship between schizophrenia and social class.

One of the earliest and best known examples of the use of hospital admissions to study mental illness was the investigation of the relationship between schizophrenia and social class carried out in the 1930s in Chicago[1]. First-admission rates to hospital for schizophrenia were used to pinpoint differences in its frequency between parts of Chicago. The question of selection bias (discussed above) is not further raised here, except to say that first-admission rates for schizophrenia at that time are probably a fair approximation of incidence, since most people were hospitalised at some stage during the first illness. It was observed that the mental hospital admission rates for schizophrenia were highest in the central slum districts, with much lower rates in the outer residential areas of the city. One interpretation of these observations was that since the poor areas contained many people of lower socio-economic status, it was therefore the environment, lifestyle and living

Table 7.5:   Potential risk factors for schizophrenia

Risk factor	Approximate relative risk
Familial factors	
Schizophrenic parent	12
Two schizophrenic parents	37
Schizophrenic sibling:	
Monozygotic twin	55
Dizygotic twin – same sex	18
Other sibling	8
Schizophrenic second-degree relative	3
Mutable sociodemographic factors	
Low socioeconomic status	3
Single status	4
Immutable sociodemographic factors	
Ethnic group status	2
Modern industrialised nation	2
Other risk factors	
Rheumatic disease	0.2
Winter birth	1.1
Stressful life events	2.7

Source: Eaton WW. Epidemiology of Schizophrenia. Epidemiologic Reviews 1985; 7: 105–125.

conditions of people in the lowest stratum of society that predisposed them to the disease. This hypothesis seemed to be substantiated by a later study which looked at first-admission rates to all psychiatric services, including outpatients in a defined geographical area, New Haven, Connecticut[2]. The results appeared to show that people in lower social classes had a higher incidence of schizophrenia. This phenomenon became known as 'the breeder hypothesis'; adverse social circumstances being seen as generating mental illness. Some doubt was shed on this reasoning by the observation that poor areas and social isolation do not necessarily go together, at least in European cities, and that schizophrenic patients quite often moved into isolated areas before admission to hospital.

Table 7.6:   Social class distribution of schizophrenic patients and their fathers
            (males, first admissions aged 25–34 years, England and Wales, 1956)

Social Class	Patients at admission		Fathers at patient's birth	
	Observed	Expected	Observed	Expected
I	12	12	14	8
II	21	44	42	42
III	178	203	192	192
IV	52	55	66	68
V	90	39	55	59
Total	353	353	369	369
Not Stated	18		2	

Source: Goldberg EM, Morrison SL. Schizophrenia and Social Class. British Journal of Psychiatry, 1963; 109: 785–802.

British researchers then provided important new evidence. Their findings are presented in Table 7.6. They compared the social-class distribution of young male patients diagnosed with schizophrenia on first admission to mental hospitals with that of their fathers at the time of the patient's birth. It was found that although the patients had a marked excess of jobs in the lower social class categories, they had been born into families with a similar social-class distribution to that of the general population. The implication was that there had been a 'drift' downwards in the social classes of schizophrenic patients as a result of their illness. This contradicts the 'breeder hypothesis' which suggested that socio-economic deprivation is of major aetiological importance. It is now more generally believed that the preponderance of lower social class patients with schizophrenia is due to the disabling effect of the illness (the drift hypothesis) rather than through poor environmental circumstances (the breeder hypothesis), although the debate is one which has continued within the field of psychiatric epidemiology and some consider the question unresolved.

Suicide and parasuicide

Suicide

The classic work of the famous French sociologist, Durkheim (1858–1917) on suicides, during a period of over 30 years is a landmark in his own discipline and in social psychiatry.

Durkheim, by studying statistics from various European countries as well as by analysis of case records, concluded that suicide was a relatively stable characteristic with a fixed rate for a given society which reflected its culture. He considered that factors in society, such as the degree of social cohesion, exercised a powerful effect on the individual which might predispose him to suicide. Durkheim's studies were spread over many years and one of his conclusions was that suicide rates were higher amongst Protestants and the well-to-do and lower amongst Catholics and poor people. He also found suicide more frequent in males than females with an increased rate in elderly people.

Unnatural deaths are required to be reported to the Coroner who, on the assembled evidence, and if necessary with the aid of a court and a jury decides whether the verdict is suicide. The Coroner arrives at one of three verdicts for a possible suicide: suicide, open (i.e. undetermined as to whether suicide or accidental) or accidental. Misclassification is a particular problem with elderly people, as intent to die may be difficult to establish. Given that this is the principal source of data on suicide, it is inevitable that there is an underestimation of the true size of the problem.

Although published statistics rely solely on officially confirmed suicides, the potential sources of error should not affect the large, observed variations of suicide rates over time.

In the immediate post-war period, suicides in England and Wales increased to a peak in the mid-1960s and then fell until the mid-1970s. Thereafter suicides increased (Figure 7.2). These overall trends conceal a striking contrast between the age and sex groups. Suicides amongst younger males have increased whilst those amongst older males have fallen (Figure 7.3). For females, rates for all age groups except the under 25s have fallen (Figure 7.3).

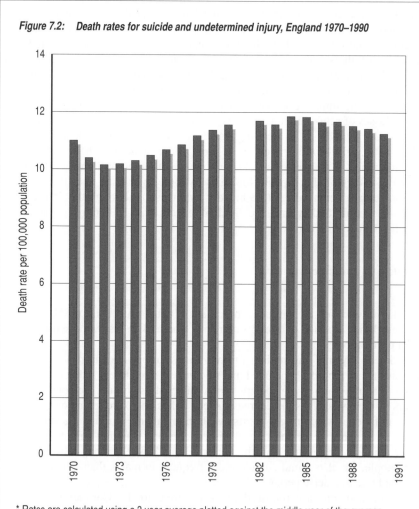

Figure 7.2:   Death rates for suicide and undetermined injury, England 1970–1990

* Rates are calculated using a 3 year average plotted against the middle year of the average

Source: The Health of the Nation. London: HMSO, 1992

Suggestions have been made that this increase is linked with unemployment in the 1980s, especially as a rising rate was linked with working age men (similar high suicide rates were observed in the 1930s). Increase in divorce is also cited as a factor. However, care must be taken in interpreting such trends over time.

Different countries have different criteria for attributing deaths to suicides, thus these data should be taken as providing a general comparison only. Nevertheless, there is considerable variation in suicide rates within Europe (Figure 7.4).

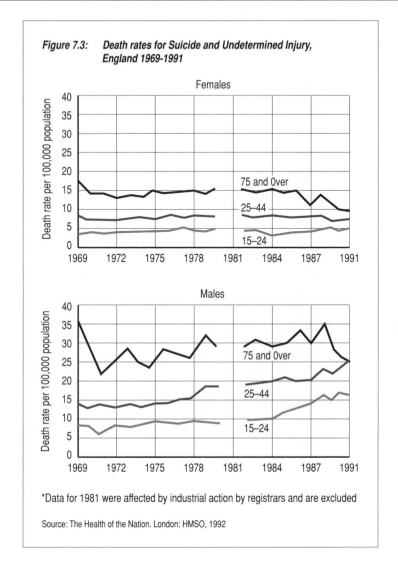

Figure 7.3:   Death rates for Suicide and Undetermined Injury, England 1969-1991

*Data for 1981 were affected by industrial action by registrars and are excluded

Source: The Health of the Nation. London: HMSO, 1992

Parasuicide

Parasuicide is a non-fatal incident in which a person causes self-injury or self-poisoning. The term 'attempted suicide' used to be applied to acts in which people tried to kill themselves but were not successful. It was then realised that some people, who were labelled attempted suicides, did not have death in mind as an end result but it was a 'cry for help' (this may not be an impulsive cry for help but the end result of a rather lengthy period of distress). However, the question of intent is extremely difficult to determine.

The frequency of parasuicide in the population is difficult to define accurately. Estimates are based on cases of poisoning or self injury admitted to hospital. However, from hospital data it is difficult to distinguish between accidents and admissions which result from a deliberate attempt at self harm. Furthermore, it has

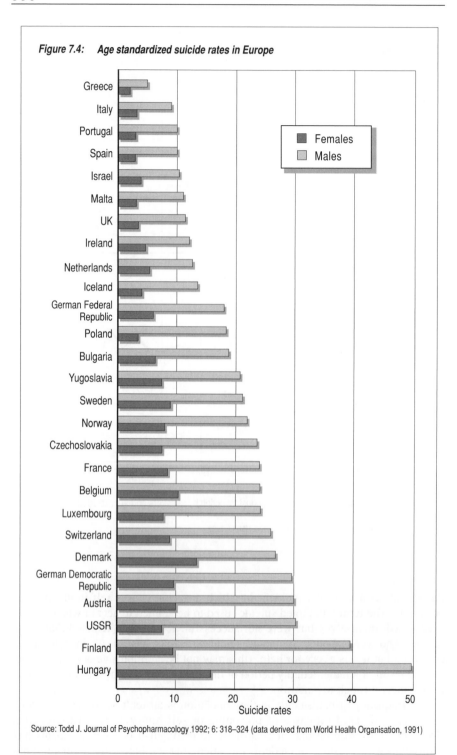

Figure 7.4: *Age standardized suicide rates in Europe*

Source: Todd J. Journal of Psychopharmacology 1992; 6: 318–324 (data derived from World Health Organisation, 1991)

been suggested that estimates based on hospital inpatient statistics may miss between one-fifth and one-third of cases. Those who sought help from their general practitioner or a hospital accident and emergency department will not be included nor will those who did not make contact with any medical authority. Thus, figures based on hospital cases for poisoning must be an underestimate of the true number of parasuicides in a population.

However, from any hospital statistics it is estimated that there are about 100,000 cases of adverse effects of medicinal agents (mainly overdose) each year in Britain and that parasuicide accounts for 10% of all acute admissions.

For the reasons just described, it is difficult to establish accurate, long-term trends. In addition hospital data were especially unreliable before 1961 when it was a criminal offence to attempt to commit suicide. Hence, information was concealed. Given these limitations, the rate of hospital admissions due to the adverse effect of medicinal agents increased until 1977 but since then there has been a downward trend. The incidence of parasuicide has also declined in many European countries.

Prevention

Whilst the scope for reducing mortality from suicide is self-evident, the measures to achieve such a reduction are far from clear. It is possible to identify high risk groups (for example, those with existing mental illness, those who have experienced major life events) but it is difficult to select those within high risk populations who will commit suicide. Improved detection and diagnosis of mental illness and enhancing the counselling skills of health professionals will undoubtedly contribute.

Other important primary strategies for prevention include the control of drugs of abuse, poisons, prescription of drugs which are dangerous in overdose and weapons.

Voluntary organisations also have a part to play in prevention. The Samaritans are the best known of the organisations which help people in distress. They provide a 24 hour telephone service, manned by trained volunteers, which is available to potentially suicidal people. The success of such agencies in reducing the number of suicides has not been clearly established.

TRENDS IN THE CARE OF MENTALLY ILL PEOPLE

Early practices

In the Dark and Middle Ages the treatment of mental illness was governed by ignorance and superstition. If the mentally ill had delusions of a religious nature, they were often revered; if their utterances were blasphemous they were held to be possessed by demons and treated, in the first instance, by exorcism by a priest. If this was unsuccessful, then they would be subjected to physical restraint, pain and degradation. This quasi-religious view of mental illness gave way later to the notion that insane people were practitioners of the Black Arts. In Britain alone, thousands of women and children were subjected to the ducking stool or burned at the stake as witches. The last woman to meet her death in this way did so in Scotland in 1722.

Britain in the eighteenth and nineteenth centuries

In the early years of the eighteenth century, a number of singularly unpleasant fates could befall the person who was mentally ill, depending on the circumstances in which he found himself. There was then no organised service to provide care for the mentally ill.

The pauper lunatic

If the manifestations of his illness led him into the trap of poverty, the pauper lunatic became subject to the conditions of the Poor Law. Under the old Poor Law, which dated from Elizabethan times, the responsibility for paupers rested with individual parishes, each of which had an overseer who raised money by taxation to provide for them. The standard of poorhouses varied greatly from one part of the country to another but in many of the larger cities the workhouse began to emerge as the principal type of provision. A report by the Poor Law Commissioners which gave rise to the Poor Law Amendment Act 1834, saw the workhouse as the fulcrum of the State's policy on the poor. There was almost an obsession on the part of the Authorities to prevent exploitation by malingerers. The workhouse with its frugal, and in many cases, inhuman surroundings, was seen as the way to deter the lazy and work-shy and to extract the maximum productivity from the able-bodied pauper. The policy on the pauper lunatic was expressly to exclude him from the workhouse. Nevertheless, the majority found their way into it, although they were not recognised or treated as a separate category. The law dealt with the vagrant very strictly and thus, the mentally ill who left their own homes to wander abroad as beggars would often find themselves in prison. Similarly, criminal insanity was not recognised. Hence, if a person's mental condition led him to commit a crime, he would be judged by penal law and usually find himself in one of the already crowded prisons.

Because of the deep shame attached to mental illness many families of poor and well-to-do alike sought to conceal its presence amongst their relatives. This led to the practice of keeping 'single lunatics' in remote places. It was not uncommon for a family member to be secured in a cellar like an animal for years at a time.

The private madhouse

For the wealthy, though escaping the indignity of the workhouse or the prison cell, insanity brought confinement in one of the private madhouses which proliferated in England at the time. These were run for profit and the fate of their inmates was scarcely better and, in many cases, worse than that of the pauper lunatic in the workhouse; shackling and deliberate ill treatment were often the order of the day.

Bedlam

Originally founded in 1247, as a priory by the Order of St Mary of Bethlehem, Bethlehem Royal Hospital in London was the largest, and for some time, the only public hospital in England devoted to the care of the insane. It existed largely on public subscriptions. The treatment meted out to inmates was as harsh as that in the private madhouses. The mentally ill were chained in confined surroundings and often subjected to bizarre and whimsical therapies, such as bleeding, purging or the induction of vomiting. Towards the end of the eighteenth century the general

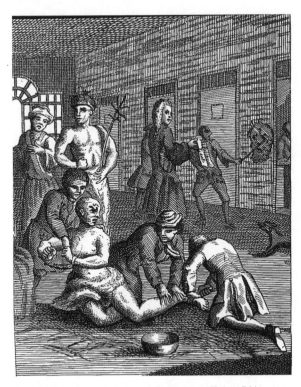

A ward in Bethlem about 1745. Source: Tuke, DH. Chapters in the history of the insane. London: Kegan Paul, 1882.

public could be admitted to the hospital and for the fee of one penny amuse themselves by watching the antics of the inmates. The name of the hospital, corrupted in common parlance to 'Bedlam', gave the English language a new word which was synonymous with mindless disorder and chaos. Discharged patients were given badges to allow them legitimately to exist as beggars without falling foul of the harsh vagrancy laws of the time. These 'Toms O'Bedlam' soon found their ranks swelled by imposters who had forged their badges.

The humanitarian movement

At the beginning of the nineteenth century, concern began to grow amongst a few enlightened reformers and to a lesser extent by public opinion about the appalling way in which the mentally ill were treated. In part, this came about through the existence of islands of compassion in the approach to mental illness. Outstanding in this respect was William Tuke, a Quaker, who founded the Retreat at York where the mentally ill were not manacled and restrained but were treated humanely. The success of this venture made a deep impression on attitudes to mental illness and its treatment.

Equally important were the revelations made by various select Parliamentary Committees of the circumstances of those housed in public asylums and private madhouses. One of the most well known examples is the visit made by Edward Wakefield, MP and his colleagues to Bethlehem Hospital. During their visit they discovered one of the inmates, William Norris, who was half naked and chained to the wall in such a way that he could stand up or lie down but not sit. This wretched man had been kept in this way for nine years and by the time he became a cause celebre was in the terminal phase of tuberculosis. Similar discoveries of conditions in private madhouses led to legislation bringing them under licence, although it must be admitted that conditions changed little at first. Another important advance was the County Asylums Act, 1808, which recommended that Local Authorities should build asylums to provide treatment for the mentally ill. The programme was not compulsory and consequently, implementation was very slow in most parts of the country but it was designed to cater mainly for the pauper lunatic, who would otherwise have found himself in the workhouse.

Under the Madhouse Act 1828 (with subsequent amendments), the Metropolitan Commissioners in Lunacy, consisting of medical practitioners, barristers and lay people appointed by the Lord Chancellor, became the guardians of insane patients and made reports.

The culmination of the reform movement was the passing by Parliament of the Lunatics Act 1845. In it, the power of the Lunacy Commissioners was greatly extended so that they were responsible for inspection, licensing and reporting on all places in which the mentally ill were housed or cared for. They were able to investigate and report the circumstances of the mentally ill in prisons and workhouses (which had previously been outside their jurisdiction), as well as in public hospitals, asylums, private madhouses and other licensed premises. Further measures introduced in the Act were the tightening up of procedures for certification of the mentally ill and the compulsory keeping of records by institutions treating them.

Into the twentieth century: the open door policy

During the early years of the twentieth century, the mental hospital, closed and often situated in a remote locality, served a predominantly custodial role with little attempt to treat mental illness or to forge links with the community. One of the first rays of light on this depressing scene was the widespread establishment of psychiatric outpatient clinics, which together with the move towards voluntary admission, were byproducts of the enlightened Mental Treatment Act 1930.

In 1948, mental hospitals, along with other types of hospital, became part of the National Health Service and were no longer the responsibility of the Local Authorities. The local authorities were given statutory responsibilities for providing community care, which comprised care and aftercare, as well as prevention.

Most of the hospital facilities for the mentally ill, inherited by the National Health Service, were in buildings erected during the last century and even earlier. These large mental hospitals had been designed to provide an isolated, self-sufficient community, often enclosed by high walls with the objectives of protecting society from the patient and of protecting the patient from the outside world. Few new mental hospitals have been built since the start of World War II so that serious overcrowding of existing hospitals reached crisis point by the mid 1950s. For instance, a typical large hospital designed to accommodate 1,800 patients might contain 2,700, be serving a catchment population of about one million covering four or five different local authorities and be staffed by three consultant psychiatrists. Thus, serious thought was being given to the idea of building new hospitals. The discovery of the psychotropic drugs, which helped to accelerate a trend in the reduction of psychiatric hospital inpatients (Open Door Policy), arrested this development. A similar picture was seen in the United States of America and other countries. This more optimistic outlook in treatment led to changing attitudes to mental illness amongst professionals and the public. Locked doors were opened and many more patients left hospital to live in the community, where local authorities began to provide an increasing quantity of supportive services.

In a way, the Mental Health Act 1959 served as the legislature's imprimatur on a wagon that was already rolling. In a relatively short space of time, the mantle of isolationism fell away from mental hospitals and a real working partnership sprang up between hospital and community services. It was as if a latter day Joshua had blown his trumpet and the high walls around the mental hospitals had fallen down.

The population of mental hospital inpatients reached a peak in England and Wales in 1954, at just over 152,000. By 1975, this figure had been reduced to 98,000 and by the beginning of the 1990s, there were 59,000 mental illness beds.

From before the beginning of this century until the end of the Second World War, there was a slow increase in the number of admissions to mental illness hospitals and units in England. From the late 1940s until the early 1970s, there was an increase in annual admissions from around 25,000 to 160,000. During the course of the 1970s, admission rates remained stable, varying only slightly in an upwards or downwards direction but from then onwards, episodes of inpatient care have increased and lengths of stay have decreased. In other words, modern psychiatric inpatient facilities are now used much more intensively than they used to be.

SERVICES FOR THE MENTALLY ILL

Current national policy on care of those with serious mental illness in Britain can be traced back to the White Paper, 'Better Services for the Mentally Ill' which was issued in the mid-1970s. It proposed a reduced role for the large mental hospitals, many of which were the former asylums of Victorian times. In turn, there was to be greater development of locally based services so that inpatient facilities for the mentally ill would be provided in the district general hospital alongside those for people with other illnesses. Greater emphasis on community care was seen as the best way to enable some patients who would formerly have been treated in hospital to be supported in their homes or in settings closer to their families and friends.

By the beginning of the 1990s, implementation of this policy had led to a much wider range of more flexible locally based services. Much hospital treatment of people with mental illness is now provided on an outpatient, rather than an inpatient basis, and many patients are now provided with care in their own homes or in residentially based settings within local communities.

On the other hand, progress on policy implementation viewed in the round, still has a considerable way to go. Whilst the ratio of beds in larger psychiatric hospitals to those for the treatment of mental illness in district general hospitals fell from 8 to 1 in the mid-1970s to about 2 to 1 at the beginning of the 1990s, there was still substantial reliance on the old psychiatric hospitals as a major provider of service. Over 80 such hospitals were still open in the country as a whole. The economic consequences of such closures are formidable with substantial capital expenditure as well as additional revenue required to develop replacement services in general hospitals and in the community.

In some parts of Britain, a failure to re-provide a sufficient range of community services in tandem with psychiatric hospital closure programmes has led to ex-hospital patients wandering the streets in a state of neglect. By the early 1990s, services for the mentally ill were still in the transitional phase. After twenty years of a programme based upon closure of large, old psychiatric hospitals, the alternative of acute hospital care in a general hospital setting, with associated day and outpatient facilities, together with smaller more local residential care and with packages of community care tailored to individual needs was still a goal to be striven for rather than a reality everywhere in the country.

A substantial part of the workload of general practitioners is made up of patients presenting with psychiatric symptoms. It has been estimated that mental health problems constitute 40% of all symptoms reported to general practitioners. The majority of these would fall into the category of minor psychiatric morbidity and be managed in the practice without recourse to specialist psychiatric opinion. The smaller number of patients with severe, intractable or psychotic symptoms are usually referred to a consultant psychiatrist. In addition to dealing with new episodes of mental illness, the general practitioner will have on his or her list psychiatric patients who have been treated by the specialist psychiatric services and require follow-up and aftercare. With the move towards larger group practices and the attachment of other professionals (such as home nurse, health visitor and social worker) the concept of a primary health care team has emerged. This multi-disciplinary team is an essential element in the provision of community care for many of the chronic disorders, like mental illness, and in providing a bridge with specialist teams in the psychiatric hospital unit. The team is uniquely placed to detect mental illness in its early stages and to provide or co-ordinate support for the established cases in the community.

Ideally, services for people with the more serious forms of mental illness are sited in district general hospitals and based upon a multidisciplinary professional team approach. Whilst the composition of such a team will vary from place to place, it will often be led by a consultant psychiatrist and will include psychiatric nurses, psychologists, occupational and other therapists as well as social workers. Hospital-based mental illness services will vary in the extent to which they have community outreach facilities but many will extend their activities to include the assessment and continuing care of patients in the community. Community psychiatric nurses are a key component of these kinds of services. In some parts of the country innovative forms of care have been developed such as crisis resource centres which are sited in the community and work on a 24 hour a day self-referral basis.

Length of stay for patients with mental illness has fallen substantially over recent years. However, because people with such illnesses often require long-term support, it is important that they are not lost track of and that aftercare arrangements are in place which enable them to be followed up within the community.

Continuing care facilities will always be needed for those people whose illnesses are too severe in impact, and chronic in nature, to allow them to live on their own. Rather than being provided in traditional hospital wards, these services should be available in more intimate and community-based care settings such as hostels, group homes and supported lodgings. Services provided in this way not only reduce the dislocation of the individual from society but also, when provided in a comprehensive network, allow easier progression to more independent forms of accommodation as the person's condition permits.

The spectrum of care for people with mental illness living in the community is quite wide. It ranges from independent living accommodation (for example, single flats in shared accommodation) to shared group accommodation (with or without support), to living as part of a family (including fostering), to hostels and staffed housing schemes.

There are some differences in the nature of services which need to be provided for the different groups of people with mental illness. The accurate psychiatric assessment of the condition and its effective clinical management can in many cases allow people to regain control over their own lives. Full, skilled assessment is critical for the small proportion of people with mental illness whose disease is so severe that the law requires them to be deprived of their liberty during the acute phase of their illness. Mental health legislation is based on the presumption of making the least restriction on liberty needed to safeguard the patient and the public.

The onset of mental illness is often accompanied by the inability of the individual concerned to participate fully in society. In severe mental illness, the resulting dislocation can be near total with the loss of friends and employment and, in some cases, estrangement from family. Care will usually be directed towards integrating the individual into society using services such as sheltered employment, day care, accommodation in the community and creating opportunities for social contact. Ideally, a key worker will ensure that the mentally ill person is receiving and benefiting from the various elements of the care package. The importance of a range of other components in a comprehensive network of services for people with mental health problems cannot be over-stated. Such services will include community psychiatric nursing, social work services, day resource centres and supported employment projects to help mentally ill people regain the ability to earn a living. In time, the development of such a comprehensive range of services will reduce the need for acute admissions as people's conditions will be monitored and stabilised in the community.

Users' views, advocacy and carers' needs

All services for people with mental illness must share the aim of allowing them maximum autonomy. It is increasingly recognised that people with psychiatric conditions should have influence over the care that they receive. Mechanisms like patients' councils have been established to facilitate this process. Advocacy and other schemes to involve users can help people with mental illness express their views on services.

Mental illness, particularly when it first develops in an acute form, can be extraordinarily stressful and difficult for families and friends of the affected person. As with other groups with special needs, the role of informal providers of care is of fundamental importance in the planning and delivery of services. Needs assessments of mentally ill people must also include an appraisal of their carers' needs. Statutory services should seek to involve carers in planning their response to the individuals' problems and also provide support to the carer.

LEGISLATION AND THE MENTALLY ILL

At the beginning of the present century, the basis of legislation for the mentally ill was the Lunacy Act 1890. In this Act, no distinction was made between mental illness and mental deficiency. The main failing of the 1890 Act was, however, that it was deeply entrenched in a legal framework. Asylums could only admit patients who had been certified and this was often performed only as a last resort. As a consequence, sufferers from mental illness were admitted only when the condition was severe and this served to enhance the stigma attached to mental illness in the mind of the public.

Gradually, after the First World War, a greater proportion of patients were admitted to mental hospitals without compulsory procedures being involved. This situation received legislative recognition in the Mental Treatment Act 1930, which had been preceded by a Royal Commission on Lunacy and Mental Disorder. Subsequently, the proportion of voluntary admissions to mental hospitals continued to increase. Compulsory admissions remained essentially a judicial procedure, with the final decision being taken by a magistrate. This situation continued until the Mental Health Act 1959 cleared the way for a more liberal approach. This Act was based on the report of a Royal Commission and embodied the basic principles of its recommendations, which were that the mentally disordered should be treated in the same way as those suffering from physical illness and that compulsory admission and detention should be used as infrequently as possible. The procedures became a mainly medical rather than a judicial affair.

Subsequent legislation has removed much of the general provisions for the care and treatment of the mentally ill and handicapped. This has been incorporated in other Acts. The Mental Health Act 1983 consolidated the Mental Health Act 1959, as amended by the Mental Health (Amendment) Act 1982. It is principally concerned with the grounds for detaining patients in hospital or placing them under guardianship and aims to improve patients' rights and to protect staff, in a variety of ways. A code of practice under Section 118 of the Mental Health Act 1983 is prepared from time to time for the guidance of professional staff in the implementation of the Act.

Terminology

The 1983 Act was mainly concerned with the admission procedure but also made certain amendments to the terminology introduced by the 1959 Act.

The generic term mental disorder embraces:

a) Mental illness.
b) Arrested or incomplete development of mind ('mental impairment' and 'severe mental impairment').
c) Psychopathic disorder. A persistent disorder or disability of mind (whether or not including significant impairment of intelligence), which results in abnormally aggressive or seriously irresponsible conduct on the part of the patient.
d) Any other disorder or disability of mind.

The Act defines 'mental impairment' and 'severe mental impairment' and psychological disorder but does not define mental illness. Promiscuity or immoral behaviour, sexual deviancy or dependence on alcohol or drugs are not, by themselves, regarded as mental disorders.

Procedures for admission under the Mental Health Act 1983

Informal admission (Section 131)

As the term implies, informal admission is the admission of patients to mental hospitals and similar institutions without any legal compulsion. It is by far the most common manner by which patients enter hospital. Of 197,000 patients entering mental illness hospitals and units in England during 1986, 92% were informal admissions.

Compulsory admissions

In 1986, there were 15,932 admissions to hospitals in England under specific Sections of the Mental Health Act. The procedures which exist for compulsory admission of patients may be summarised as follows:

Admission for assessment in cases of emergency (Section 4). This emergency procedure allows a patient, of any age, to be detained for up to 72 hours where he or his relative refuse informal admission and it is deemed necessary, either for the patient's welfare or to protect others. An application is made by an approved social worker or the nearest relative of the patient. In addition, a medical certificate is required, usually from a doctor who has previous knowledge of the patient. About 52% of all compulsory admissions fall under this Section of the Mental Health Act. At the end of the period of detention the patient may be discharged, continue on an informal basis or be further detained under Section 2 of the Mental Health Act.

Admission for assessment (Section 2). This allows the patient to be detained for up to 28 days, for assessment or for assessment followed by medical treatment. Application is made by an approved social worker or the patient's nearest relative and must be supported by two medical recommendations. One of the doctors must be approved by the relevant health authority as a person with specialist experience in the diagnosis and treatment of mental disorder. Approximately 30% of all compulsory admissions fall into this category.

Admission for treatment (Section 3). A similar application procedure to that required for admission under Section 2 is used here, although the recommendation is for a six months' period of compulsory treatment. Under certain circumstances the patient may be discharged before the end of six months or a further detention order may be procured. Only 3% of all compulsory admissions are under this Section of the Act.

Hospital and guardianship orders (Section 37). This is an order made by a Judge in a Crown Court for compulsory treatment in hospital of a patient convicted of a criminal offence. In the case of psychiatric disorder or mental impairment, this applies only where treatment is likely to alleviate or prevent deterioration of the condition. It must be supported by two medical recommendations, as under Section 2. About 5% of all compulsory admissions take place in this way.

Other provisions for compulsory admission. Other provisions for compulsory admission and detention are dealt with in the Mental Health Act 1983. These include emergency admissions involving the police, and concern prisoners, people under guardianship orders and patients already resident in mental hospitals. Together, these types of provision account for 9% of the total compulsory admissions.

In all, only 5% of patients in hospitals for the mentally ill and the mentally handicapped are detained compulsorily and less than 2% are under a court order.

Less than 10% of people remanded in custody by the police are found to be suffering from mental disorder, as defined by the Mental Health Act 1983. It would, however, be misleading to think this is a true reflection of the proportion of psychologically disturbed people coming before the courts. Many surveys suggest that up to a third of prisoners have some form of mental disorder.

Discharge of patients compulsorily detained

A number of people are authorised to discharge patients who are compulsorily detained but it is most commonly undertaken by the responsible medical officer. The nearest relative also has certain rights. Special restrictions on discharge may be imposed by Courts.

Mental Health Review Tribunal

The basic function of the Mental Health Review Tribunal is to consider applications for discharge of those patients compulsorily detained in hospital or under guardianship orders, and to ensure that no patient is detained compulsorily without good reasons. The appointment of the Mental Health Review Tribunal is the responsibility of the Lord Chancellor and three categories of members (legal, medical and lay) are recognised. A panel of members exists in each regional health authority, from which tribunals are formed to consider cases as necessary. Each tribunal comprises at least three members, one from each category, with the legal representative acting as chairman.

An application for discharge may be made by the patient himself, his next of kin, the Secretary of State or the Home Secretary, depending on the Section of the Mental Health Act under which the patient is detained. A patient detained under Section 2, may apply to the tribunal within 14 days after admission; a patient detained under Section 3, may apply once within the first six months, once within the second six months and once every subsequent year. A patient detained under Section 37, may apply once in the second six month period and once every following year. The Tribunal interviews the patient and his relatives and may seek evidence from medical and other health professionals who are involved in the care of the patient. The verdict of the Tribunal is communicated in writing to the patient.

Property of mentally ill patients

The Court of Protection is responsible for the protection and management of the affairs and property of patients who are incapable, because of mental disorder, of managing and administering their own affairs, irrespective of where the patient may be living.

Scotland

The Mental Health (Scotland) Act 1960 was amended by the Mental Health (Scotland) (Amendment) Act 1983, along broadly similar lines to the Mental Health Act 1983.

Mental Health Act Commission

This is a special health authority, set up by the 1983 Act. About 80 part-time members – Commissioners – are appointed by the Secretary of State for Health from the professions of medicine, nursing, social work and psychology, as well as lay members. The Commission has a wide brief. It can investigate complaints and keep under review, all aspects of the care and welfare of detained patients. Second independent opinions can be given by medical members of the Commission or by doctors appointed by the Commission. Furthermore, it can submit proposals for the content of a Code of Practice to the Secretary of State for Health.

THE NEEDS OF PEOPLE WITH MENTAL HANDICAP

Accurate and respectful descriptions of this sub-group of the population have proved difficult to establish. Early legislation used and defined terms, such as mental defective, idiot, imbecile and feeble minded. The Mental Health Act 1959 introduced the term 'subnormal' and the definition encompassed subnormality of intelligence as well as the concept of social incapacity. The term was traditionally confined to those individuals who were handicapped in childhood. It excluded those who acquired their mental handicap in later life, for example, people with permanent and severe impairment of the central nervous system caused by road accidents.

Taxonomies

Because mental illness and mental handicap are both included in the generic term 'mental disorder' there is often confusion between them. They are distinct conditions, although it is important to recognise that they may sometimes co-exist. For example, a mentally handicapped adolescent may exhibit psychotic symptoms and an older person with mental handicap may develop senile dementia. There was much debate about whether to include people with mental handicap in the 1983 Mental Health Act at all. Thus, it was something of a compromise that the concept of "abnormally aggressive and seriously irresponsible conduct" deliberately limited their inclusion to the minority of people with mental handicap who need some sort of legally supervised care because of their behaviour.

The Education Act 1981 introduced the term 'learning difficulties' but this does not recognise the social aspect of mental handicap. At the beginning of the 1990s, the Department of Health in England formally adopted, for use within the health and social services, the term 'people with learning disabilities' instead of 'mental handicap'. Both terms are still widely used. In the United States, the term 'mental retardation' is used despite its negative connotations.

Internationally, both scientific study and health service practice have yielded a bewildering diversity in terminology, conceptual frameworks and classification of this group of conditions. Different approaches are based on, for example, causes, disorder or injury to the brain, low intelligence on formal testing, social maladaptation and personality dependency. It is important to establish what taxonomy is being used. Without this, it is impossible to establish which people are being counted in epidemiological studies or in needs assessment of populations.

The framework used in the 1980s by the World Health Organisation to define disability is described fully in chapter 5 in relation to physical disability. The basic concepts – impairment, disability, handicap – are also applicable to mental handicap. Three approaches have been used for classification in this context (Table 7.7). The intellectual impairment approach, widely used in the past, is based upon the idea of

Table 7.7:   Taxonomy of mental handicap

Intellectual impairment	
Criteria	Intellectual: intelligence or development tests.
Main categories	Severe: IQ <50 (or 'severe and moderate'). Mild: IQ 50–69.
Learning disability	
Criteria	Usually educational: e.g. reading or numeracy tests but should reflect learning dysfunction, not merely achievements.
Main categories	Various, according to legal, administrative and professional contracts.
Mental handicap /retardation	
Criteria	Social: e.g. dependency or maladaptation scales.
Main categories	Severe: co-extensive with severe intellectual impairment, if IQ <50 is used as a necessary criterion. Mild: many factors in selection, varying in different communities.

Source: Adapted from: Fryers T. Epidemiology and taxonomy in mental retardation. Paediatric and Perinatal Epidemiology 1992; 6: 181–192.

low intelligence. Intelligence is measured by intelligence tests and usually expressed as the intelligence quotient (IQ). The IQ measure is distributed within the population in a way which has some similarities with other characteristics of people (such as height). This approach to classification has remained popular precisely because it is so readily measurable and can be expressed in terms of severity (based upon IQ scores). Thus, 'severe intellectual impairment' is the term used to describe people with an IQ less than 50 whilst the term 'mild intellectual impairment' is used for people with an IQ between 50 and 69.

The second approach to classification is to view the problem in terms of the resulting disability, principally in learning. Thus, the concept of 'learning disability' has emerged. Although valid ways of measuring learning disability are not well developed, it is important to recognise that it is not simply a case of assessing IQ (as for intellectual impairment). Not all sources of disabled learning in children and adults are associated with impaired intellect, although they are clearly closely related.

The term handicap in the World Health Organisation classification denotes social disadvantage for the mentally handicapped person just as it does for someone who is physically handicapped.

For the remainder of this chapter the term mental handicap is used. It is preferred to 'learning disability' (currently the accepted terminology in the British health and social services) because of its wider use in epidemiological studies and in other countries.

Frequency in the population

As will be evident from the discussion of the taxonomy and aetiology of mental handicap, assessing the size of the problem in a population and making comparisons between different places or over time, is particularly difficult because of the complexity of issues surrounding definition and classification.

Despite the limitations of measuring IQ and of relating intellectual impairment to handicap, the most comprehensive epidemiological data relate to the frequency of people in populations with an IQ less than 50 (severe intellectual impairment, but often also referred to in studies as severe mental handicap or severe mental retardation). Reasonably reliable estimates are also available for the more clear cut syndromes which are associated with mental handicap (for example, Down's syndrome).

The two most often used measures to express the frequency of mental handicap in the population are the birth prevalence (number of affected infants per 1000 births) and age-specific prevalence (number of affected people in particular age groups expressed per 1000 people of that same age living in the population concerned).

Most data on the frequency of mental handicap in the population are derived from epidemiological surveys. Routinely available health service data are not generally useful sources although the establishment of population-based mental handicap registers is becoming more common (see chapter 1 for a fuller description of case registers). Notifications of congenital abnormalities (see chapter 6) can provide estimates of the population frequency of some conditions which cause mental handicap.

When considering the frequency of severe intellectual impairment it is important to examine rates of occurrence in birth cohorts (children born in the same year) as well as within different age groups of the population. The prevalence of severe intellectual impairment varies between similar birth cohorts in different populations, both nationally and internationally. Similarly, birth prevalence shows changes over time. For example, it was relatively low in many developed countries of the world for birth cohorts of the early 1950s (1.8–4.0 per 1000) and higher for birth cohorts in the early 1960s (3.5–5.5 per 1000). Factors likely to affect birth prevalence at different times include: survival of impaired infants due to better neonatal intensive care, detection of fetal abnormalities through screening and termination of affected pregnancies, changes in maternal age. Differences in birth prevalence then work through to be reflected in age-specific prevalence ratios as the cohort concerned grows older. Changes in survival of affected children is the other main factor which affects such age-specific prevalence figures.

Table 7.8: **Key epidemiological features of severe intellectual impairment in developed countries**

- Geographical variation within similar birth cohorts.
- Variation over time in successive birth cohorts in the same population.
- Many countries experienced low prevalence in early 1950s births; high prevalence in early 1960s births.
- Variations in age specific prevalence due to cohort variations in incidence and mortality.
- Improved survival at all ages.
- More males than females.
- Social class gradient for incidence and mortality.

Source: Fryers T. Mental retardation in developing countries. Tantam D, Duncan A (Eds). Psychiatry for the Developing World. London: Gaskell Press, 1993.

Table 7.9:   *Estimated age-specific prevalence of severe intellectual*
             impairment in a United Kingdom health district, 1990

Age group (years)	Prevalence per 1000
0 – 4	2.5
5 – 9	3.0
10 – 14	4.0
15 – 19	4.5
20 – 24	5.0
25 – 29	4.5
30 – 34	4.0
35 – 39	3.5
40 – 44	3.0
45 – 54	2.5
55 – 64	2.0
65 – 74	1.0
75 and over	very few

Source: Fryers T. Applied epidemiology of mental handicap. In: Russel O, Johnston S
(Eds). Psychiatry of mental handicap. London: Gaskell Press, 1993.

It used to be thought that severe intellectual impairment was evenly distributed between the social classes. This no longer seems to be true with more recent evidence showing higher prevalence in lower social class groupings.

These main epidemiological features of severe intellectual impairment are shown in Table 7.8 whilst an estimate of its age-specific prevalence in a typical British population is shown in Table 7.9.

Aetiology of mental handicap

Causes of mental handicap are mostly multifactorial processes. When considering the impairment of individuals, it is important to recognise that the precise mechanisms of causation of many forms of mental handicap are not yet fully established, even though the principal causal agent can often be identified. For example, it is recognised that alcohol intake during pregnancy causes the fetal alcohol syndrome (which can include mental handicap). However, the amount of alcohol which will induce such damage is not well established nor is it clear which maternal or fetal characteristics predispose to the syndrome. When considering causes of mental handicap at population level they must be viewed more broadly. The influences on the population frequency of mental handicap in different places or over time can be diverse. For example, the frequency of mental handicap resulting from the fetal alcohol syndrome will vary according to the availability of alcohol in the society concerned, attitudes to pregnancy and childbearing, as well as the price of alcohol.

There is a wide range of factors and conditions associated with increased frequency of mental handicap. These include: causes of neurological impairment, factors concerned with general genetic endowment, deprivation and educational under-functioning. Causes of neurological impairment (i.e. organic causes of mental handicap) can be classified as pure primary disorders, primary disorders with secondary neurological damage and pure secondary disorders.

Pure primary disorders

A number of disorders which result in mental handicap are present at the time of conception and result from an abnormal chromosome formation. The nuclei of normal human cells contain 23 pairs of chromosomes: one of each pair is derived from either parent. There are two types of chromosome, one pair which determines sex (sex chromosomes) and the other 22 pairs which are called autosomes. Males have 44 autosomes, one X and one Y sex chromosomes; females have 44 autosomes and two X sex chromosomes. Chromosome abnormalities may involve either the sex chromosomes or the autosomes and may be due to abnormalities in chromosome number (more or less than the usual complement) or in their structure. Specific chromosomal abnormalities are associated with particular diseases.

Down's Syndrome. The physical characteristics of Down's syndrome (although each is not present in all cases) include narrow slanting eyes with prominent epicanthic folds; short stature; small ears; short broad neck; furrowing of the tongue and a tendency for the mouth to hang open; a single transverse palmar crease; prominent and characteristic skin ridges on the palms of the hand, fingers and soles of the feet. Congenital abnormalities of the heart and intestinal tract occur more frequently in these children than in other infants.

Within the spectrum of Down's syndrome there is a range of cognitive ability but the IQ usually lies somewhere between 20 and 55 with a small proportion of affected people having an IQ greater than 50. People with Down's syndrome are usually described as humorous, cheerful and affectionate. Whilst it would be wrong to accept this as a stereotype, many people involved in the care of children with Down's syndrome would agree with this description of their personalities.

People with Down's syndrome always possess extra chromosomal material in the cells of their bodies. The presence of an extra discrete autosomal (i.e. non-sex) chromosome is called 'trisomy'. In 94% of cases of Down's syndrome, all or part of an extra chromosome resembling the normal number 21 pair of chromosomes is present in the cell; this most common variant of Down's syndrome is called 'trisomy 21'. It arises because of a failure of separation of chromosomes (non-disjunction) during cell division in the formation of the ovum. The fetus developing from this ovum, when it is fertilized, has 47 chromosomes rather than the usual 46. In a less common form of Down's syndrome (3–5% of cases) the extra chromosomal material becomes joined to another chromosome: the so-called 'translocation type'. These are familial with a high risk of recurrence in families, so there are opportunities for prevention through genetic counselling. In a third rare form (1–3% of cases), non-disjunction occurs after fertilization so that only some of the cells of the body are abnormal (mosaicism) and people show some signs of Down's syndrome but not all. They may be of normal intelligence.

The incidence of Down's syndrome is of the order of 1 in 800 live births. The precise aetiology of Down's syndrome is unknown but the most striking feature is the strongly increased risk of trisomy 21 with increased maternal age. Recent trends towards earlier childbearing have led to a fall in the crude incidence of Down's syndrome live births. However, despite this falling incidence, the prevalence of the condition has risen over the same period of time. This is because life expectancy for people with Down's syndrome has greatly improved. Studies in various countries have confirmed this but also demonstrate that life expectancy in Down's syndrome is still much poorer than for the general population.

Fragile X syndrome. This is a sex chromosome disorder which can result in severe intellectual impairment although only in a minority of males and almost never in females. About 80% of boys will have an IQ less than 70, a smaller proportion of girls have impairment, mostly in the mild category. Females may carry and pass on the abnormality but be unaffected themselves.

Primary disorder with secondary neurological damage

A second group of disorders do not affect the constitution of the individual per se but a genetic abnormality leads to abnormal or arrested development.

Phenylketonuria. This is a rare recessively inherited condition (birth prevalence 0.05–0.2 per 1000 births) in which the absence of a specific enzyme leads to a failure in the ability of the body to convert the amino acid phenylalanine to tyrosine. Normal diet thus becomes a direct hazard to the child. Phenylalanine accumulates in the blood and tissues and has a toxic effect on the brain, leading to convulsions and, if untreated, severe damage. The deficiency of tyrosine leads to paucity of melanin formation and thus, lack of pigmentation giving rise to the other characteristics of the syndrome: blonde hair, blue eyes, pale skin and a tendency to infantile eczema. The treatment is to eliminate phenylalanine from the diet until the central nervous system is mature.

Since it is an essential amino acid, this cannot be done completely but if a special diet is instituted as early as possible, there is a chance of limiting the degree of damage resulting from the condition. This has led to the practice of screening all new-born babies by taking a few drops of blood and testing for excess phenylalanine (the Guthrie test).

Sporadic congenital hypothyroidism. Congenital hypothyroidism occurs sporadically within the population (birth prevalence 0.1–2.0 per 1000). It is important to realise that this results from a mutation and not from iodine deficiency (see below). Thyroid failure ensues and if the condition is not recognised early and treated with thyroid replacement therapy, severe intellectual impairment can result.

Pure secondary disorders

A third group of disorders arise because of an environmental factor interacting with a normal fetus after conception. The mechanisms are not understood fully in all cases but the range of factors which can lead to mental handicap is wide.

Infections. Maternal exposure to rubella (German measles) virus, particularly during the first trimester of pregnancy, puts the developing fetus at risk of the congenital rubella syndrome. The manifestations include congenital heart disease, deafness, blindness and mental handicap. Many other infections of the mother during pregnancy, in particular cytomegalovirus and toxoplasmosis, can cause mental handicap in the offspring. Congenital syphilis, acquired by the mother and passed to the fetus, has long been recognised as a cause of mental handicap as part of a general multisystem disorder. Infections acquired postnatally can also lead to mental handicap: for example, meningitis, encephalitis, malaria.

Alcohol intake in pregnancy. Mental handicap can arise from consumption of alcohol during pregnancy usually as part of the fetal alcohol syndrome (see also chapter 6).

Rhesus incompatibility. The problem of rhesus incompatibility and its prevention is discussed in chapter 6. The cerebral damage caused by jaundice (kernicterus) may result in cerebral palsy and mental handicap; though this condition is now largely preventable.

Exposure to radiation. Excessive use of diagnostic X-rays in pregnancy has, in the past, led to radiation being identified as a risk factor for mental handicap. This is not an important cause today and the use of ultrasound has in any case superseded X-rays as a diagnostic technique in pregnancy.

Perinatal factors. Two factors are of particular importance during the process of birth which may lead to injury of the brain and some degree of neurological impairment: hypoxia and birth injury. Hypoxia in the fetus may occur for a variety of reasons such as pre-eclamptic toxaemia, antepartum haemorrhage, anaesthetic complications, excessive sedation during labour, respiratory distress in the infant, pressure on the umbilical cord or prolonged labour. Trauma during delivery is particularly likely to occur with abnormal presentation of the fetus or with instrumental delivery. Fortunately, with modern obstetric care and the tendency towards early Caesarian section in difficult cases, birth trauma is probably less common today. Prematurity with low birth weight is strongly associated with the later development of mental handicap. It is unlikely, however, that the relationship is one of direct cause and effect but is probably explained by the fact that babies in this category are much more susceptible to adverse factors during delivery and afterwards. Indeed, intellectual impairment, epilepsy and cerebral palsy are sequelae of the same processes and problems.

Iodine deficiency. When considering mental handicap worldwide, iodine deficiency disease is an important cause of severe intellectual impairment. Other features may be associated, including the full syndrome of cretinism. In parts of the world where iodine is not present in sufficient quantities in water or in the diet, the solution is population based prevention strategies including dietary supplementation or injection (this lasts several years).

Neural tube defect. Mental handicap can be a feature of the group of disorders called neural tube defect which are described fully in chapter 6.

After birth. A wide variety of elements of the postnatal environment may lead to neurological impairment and mental handicap. In the early postnatal period hypoglycaemia is a serious problem which, if uncorrected, can cause convulsions and cerebral injury. Infectious diseases have already been discussed. Head injury, either accidental or deliberate (as part of child abuse), may have similar repercussions. One of the effects of excessive exposure to inorganic lead, either as a result of pica (ingestion) or environmental pollution, is varying degrees of intellectual impairment. There is no evidence of lead causing damage to a degree resulting in identified mental handicap but it probably does cause slight reduction in children's IQs at all levels of exposure.

General factors

Causes which are not associated with an underlying organic process can be considered in terms of the complex inter-relationships between genetic endowment, deprivation and educational underfunctioning. In general these factors are relevant to mild degrees of mental handicap.

At one time it was considered that the strong correlation between low social class and mild mental handicap (or mild intellectual impairment) was mainly genetic in origin. In other words, it was thought that there was a pool of people of low intelligence in the lower social classes who, by marrying and reproducing amongst their own kind, perpetuated the pool. This perspective based on a subcultural view of mental handicap is outmoded.

The number of people with IQ scores in the range 50–69 is a reflection of the statistical distribution of IQ within the population. Whether they are then labelled as intellectually impaired or mentally handicapped (in effect 'abnormal') is a socially-determined phenomenon.

Today, mild mental handicap is seen much more in terms of the processes which influence whether people with mild degrees of intellectual impairment or other characteristics are identified and labelled as mentally handicapped. This varies between localities, countries and societies. Factors which influence this are the structure and orientation of services, professional attitudes and training, employment and training practices, social and cultural expectations, family and kinship structures, as well as legislation in relation to health, welfare, education and employment.

PREVENTION OF MENTAL HANDICAP

As described in the section on the aetiology of mental handicap, some forms are potentially preventable. Preventive strategies can be grouped into three categories directed at processes before conception, processes during fetal life and birth, processes after birth.

Processes before conception

Health education campaigns aimed at reducing births in older women or lowering maternal age overall would reduce the frequency of Down's syndrome. The birth prevalence of a range of disorders could be reduced by minimising inherited disease in identified families by use of genetic counselling, screening and termination of pregnancy. Examples of causes of mental handicap which can be addressed by these kinds of strategies include: genetic counselling after one child (for example, translocation Down's syndrome), screening for carriers and preconceptual counselling (for example, Tay Sachs disease), population screening (for example, this may be possible for Fragile X syndrome in the near future). Other preventive measures directed at processes before conception include reduction of hazardous factors in the environment (such as drugs, chemical exposures and industrial radiation).

Processes during fetal life and birth

Preventive approaches at this stage include targeting the nutritional status of pregnant women, folate supplementation to avoid neural tube defects, and minimising harm to the fetus (reducing alcohol intake and smoking during pregnancy, measures to prevent rhesus haemolytic disease), screening to detect fetal abnormalities and termination of the affected pregnancies, as well as generally good obstetric and neonatal care.

Processes after birth

Preventive measures after birth include protection (as far as possible) against communicable diseases which can cause intellectual impairment, early recognition of problems such as hypothyroidism and phenylketonuria and strategies to reduce accidents and their impact.

SERVICES FOR PEOPLE WITH MENTAL HANDICAP

The philosophy of service provision for mentally handicapped children and adults must be based on a clear set of values which seeks to place individuals at the centre of a care process which regards their particular needs as paramount. A new organisation of services for mentally handicapped people (and other groups with special needs) to enable this needs assessment to take place, was created with the community care component of legislation contained in the NHS and Community Care Act 1990. This is described fully in chapter 4 as well as the chapters describing elderly people (chapter 8), and people with disability (chapter 5).

At its heart is a responsibility placed on all statutory and other agencies, under the lead of the social services department, to identify individuals (such as those who are mentally handicapped) with special needs and to design an appropriate service response to meet those needs whether it be a placement in the community, or in a residentially-based setting. All agencies must work together and all professionals must collaborate to provide appropriate care.

It is also important that service providers identify the needs of carers of mentally handicapped people and provide help and support to them. Running through the modern approach to care is the concept of normalisation in which, as far as possible, the mentally handicapped person is given the same rights and entitlements as other members of society. Some values and principles underlying service provision are shown in Table 7.10.

Living at home or in the community

Many children and adults with mental handicap can successfully live at home, only being admitted to residential or hospital care when serious problems develop with their health or with their behaviour.

Table 7.10: Principles of service delivery to mentally handicapped people

- Enable people, where possible, to live ordinary lives by using means which are common, accepted and valued in their local community and culture.
- Enhance the status of disabled people.
- Acknowledge and respect disabled people as individual human beings with their own needs, preferences, abilities and social networks.
- Work with disabled people, letting them retain where possible, the initiative, choice and direction of their own lives.
- No segregation from the rest of the community in housing, work, education or recreation.
- Special, easily accessible services to meet needs inadequately served by ordinary means.
- High professional standards in management, staffing and co-ordination of services.

Source: Fryers T. Public Health Approaches to Mental Retardation: Handicap due to Intellectual Impairment. In: Holland W W, Detels R, Knox E G (Eds). Oxford Textbook of Public Health (2nd Edition). Oxford: Oxford University Press, 1991.

Parents of a child with mental handicap will need a great deal of counselling as well as practical support to help them come to terms with the birth of an affected baby. Thereafter, as the child grows older, many will continue to require emotional support, advice and practical help including welfare benefits. The presence of a person with mental handicap can give rise to special problems in a family. Both day services and respite care provide some relief for parents. There are some schemes for placing carers in the family home to give parents an opportunity to get away. Aside from short-term care, support for a family can be given by a health visitor, a specially trained community nurse, social worker or voluntary worker. Usually this takes the form of advice and information about service availability. Families are often helped by being put in contact with other parents with similar problems. Practical assistance with transport for visiting or workload (for example, nappy service) is usually very valuable.

The provision of adequate and suitable housing can often ease the problems of helping with a mentally handicapped person. A frequently voiced concern amongst parents is the fate of the handicapped son or daughter when they die. The voluntary organisation MENCAP (Royal Society for Mentally Handicapped Children and Adults) attempts to meet part of the problem with its trustee scheme. Parents are encouraged to help their son or daughter move into residential care well before the parents become unable to cope but this is not easily achieved when there is an acute shortage of places.

Most health districts in England have at least one community mental handicap team. Such teams are made up of people from a variety of professional backgrounds but most have a social worker, a community mental handicap nurse, a psychiatrist or a psychologist and usually a therapist (physiotherapist, occupational therapist, or speech therapist).

Teams provide a domiciliary service to people with mental handicap and their families. Core team members make routine visits to clients' homes. They provide advice and assistance with current day-to-day problems, they advise on welfare benefits, arrange respite care and advise or assist with any problem behaviours.

They have an important role in coordinating domiciliary services and can also be helpful in breaking down organisational barriers which sometimes exist between agencies. On the other hand, they have to deal with issues relating to the blurring of professional boundaries whilst maintaining their own professional identities and at the same time, sharing their skills.

The range of services available to people with mental handicap who are no longer able to (or who do not) live in their family home is very wide and varies in type around the country. People with minor degrees of incapacity can often live in flats or houses with a small number of their peers. Such facilities may have warden assistance but in any case will usually be supported by a community mental handicap team.

Education of children

A key issue for families with a child with mental handicap is education. A child with mental handicap may attend an ordinary preschool playgroup or one for children similar to themselves. The latter facilities are very unevenly distributed throughout the country. A playgroup gives the child an opportunity of benefiting from contact with other children, as well as providing a period of relief to the parents.

A child with mental handicap may be admitted to a nursery class in an ordinary school. This is usually at the discretion of the head teacher and often for a trial period. Problems can arise because of lack of staff to cope with the extra requirement needed for a handicapped child.

The Education Act 1981 introduced the concept of 'special educational needs'. This replaced the notion of some children needing "special educational treatment", which came from the Education Act 1944.

A child has special educational needs if he or she has a learning difficulty which calls for special educational provision to be made for him or her.

A learning difficulty means that:

- A child has significantly greater difficulty in learning than the majority of children of the same age (moderate learning difficulty).
- A child has a disability which makes it impossible or difficult to use the educational facilities which are generally available to children of the same age (severe learning difficulty).

Children with mental handicap are therefore classified in the Education Act 1981 as having 'learning difficulties' and every local education authority must find ways of meeting their special educational needs. They must do this in mainstream schools if this is possible or, if not, in special schools.

Children with special educational needs can be exempted from some or all of the demands of the national curriculum, as laid down by the Education Reform Act 1988. The exemption from, or modification to, the national curriculum is detailed in the child's statement of special educational needs. This is a legal document which sets out the child's individual needs and the ways in which the local education authority will meet them.

Specialised provision is made within schools for children with severe learning difficulties and for those children with a profound intellectual handicap. These children often have severe physical and sensory disabilities in addition to their profound mental handicap.

A small number of children are educated in residential schools, some run by local education authorities but most run by the voluntary or the private sectors. The vast majority of children live at home and go to school on a daily basis. Transport is provided for them.

Most young people with severe learning difficulties remain at school until they are 19 years of age. An increasing number attend local colleges of further education where specialised courses are made available. Some young people attend special residential colleges, run either by the voluntary or the private sectors. Whichever type of college is chosen, the aim of the course is the same: a successful transition to adult life.

Youth training and employment training courses help many people with mental handicap to prepare for employment. Employment services, which help people find and keep work, are available in some parts of the country. Those who need to develop social and life skills before seeking employment are provided for by social services departments which run day services. These services are also available to those who do not wish to work or who are too disabled for work to be a realistic option.

It is recognised that the education of a child with mental handicap should start as early as possible. In some parts of the country peripatetic teachers visit the home and work with parents. Parents are encouraged to stimulate their children and teach them skills. A number of different schemes for use by parents in teaching their children are in operation in Britain.

One is the Portage Project (Bereweeke is roughly equivalent for older people), which was developed in the small town of Portage, Wisconsin, USA. The child is assessed by a home teacher using a developmental checklist. Parents are trained to teach skills in accordance with a set scheme. The project has the advantage that it does not require highly skilled teachers. After a short training course, health visitors and social workers can effectively work with the parents. Over 80% of preschool children who are severely mentally handicapped live at home with their parents and the most frequent professional visitors to the family are the health visitor and social worker. If this scheme is in operation, each child is usually visited weekly and each visit takes one to two hours. Developmental areas covered include socialisation, language, self help, cognitive and motor skills.

Education and training centres for adults

Centres, formerly called adult training centres, provide a place for mentally handicapped adults to go during the day-time. The main activity was light assembly work which was sub-contracted by local firms. The centres are now called special educational centres or resource centres, which more accurately reflects their purpose. Over the years the emphasis has switched to the development of social and personal skills, further education and work experience.

Whilst training centres remain part of the network of provision, there has also been a trend to encourage and support people with mental handicap to take paid employment within the general workforce where appropriate. The charitable organisation MENCAP, for example, runs a programme called PATHWAY which undertakes to prepare people for the workplace and assist with job placements.

Residential care

Local authorities now provide directly only about one third of non health service care. The type of residential care which can be provided by the local authority social services departments varies with the degree of social competence of the individual. The person may be placed with foster parents, in lodgings, in a home or a hostel specifically for mentally handicapped people or an unstaffed home or hostel supervised by supporting social work staff.

The typical local authority hostel of early community care developments had about 25 beds with attached staff accommodation. Such hostels are now often divided into smaller units and few new hostels of that type are being built.

There is a dearth of residential options for people with mental handicap living with their parents and too little respite residential care. Children do better with respite care, especially younger children. Both respite and long term residential care are often with families rather than in a local authority establishment.

The NHS and Community Care Act 1990 resulted in local authority social services departments reducing their involvement as providers of residential care. For people with mental handicap an increasingly common form of community accommodation is that provided by independent trusts. These are organisations consisting of several participating agencies, for example, a housing association, a health authority, a social services department and a voluntary organisation.

Voluntary organisations such as the MENCAP Homes Foundation, the Spastics Society and Barnardos also operate community housing. Many of these houses are ordinary dwellings in ordinary streets. Most of them are staffed during the day time and some will have a member of staff awake during the night. Others may have a member of staff sleeping in the house at night.

A popular method of providing housing is the 'core and cluster' model. This provides for a range of needs. It operates with a core house to accommodate the more dependent residents and most or all of the staff together with peripheral houses, not necessarily adjacent, but within reasonable proximity to the core house. The peripheral houses accommodate less dependent residents, and they can access the staff in the core house if they need any form of support.

Whilst the average home in the average street is where most people with mental handicap live and always have lived, there are those who disagree that this should be the only model. An alternative view is provided by the supporters of special villages and residential communities. RESCARE (The National Society for Mentally Handicapped People in Residential Care) supports larger settlements, especially for people who are severely handicapped. It is suggested that residential villages have the advantage of containing various sized residences, all with a domestic home-like atmosphere and at the same time ready access to a wide range of services. There is a view that people with severe mental handicap feel less isolated and more protected in a village setting than in the general community. Examples of village communities are those developed by the Camphill movement which was started in Scotland in the 1940s and has now spread to Europe and the United States. Other examples are the Home Farm Trust, which has village schemes in Kent, Devon and Yorkshire, and the Ravenswood Village in London.

A pragmatic case has been made in some parts of the country for the re-use of hospital sites for large settlements but with modern style accommodation. However, the geographic remoteness and the perceived stigma attached to those sites could militate against this.

The private sector has emerged as a major provider for community services for people with mental handicap. Many of these homes cater for rather large numbers of people and there is concern because they do not necessarily fit the ordinary life model.

Family placement schemes, where the mentally handicapped person lives with a family in a private household, have gained popularity during the 1990s.

Hospital provision

At the end of the 1960s, there were 7,400 children and 52,000 adults aged 16 years or older in hospitals for the mentally handicapped. The White Paper published in 1971 called 'Better Services for the Mentally Handicapped' envisaged that by the beginning of the 1990s, hospital beds for mentally handicapped people would be reduced to 33,000. In 1991, there were some 25,000 people in mental handicap hospitals. This reduction includes deaths as well as people who have moved to community living.

For some years, first admissions fell whilst re-admissions increased disproportionately, suggesting that while fewer people were admitted more of them were undertaken for special purposes, such as respite care. However, the provision of respite care in hospital has decreased and is now more commonly provided by the social services department or through family placement.

Different health authorities have adopted different approaches to the issue of closure. Probably the first hospital in England to have a formal closure programme was Darenth Park Hospital in Kent. Darenth Park was a fairly typical large (2,200 beds) isolated unit. The experiences which were part and parcel of its run down have guided the way for similar hospitals across the country. Some other mental handicap hospitals did not have formal closure plans and operated on the basis of ceasing to admit new patients and opportunistically moving others to community living where possible.

The issues associated with planning, organising and financing the resettlement of people into the community are only one part of planning for community services. There are many people with mental handicap who live with elderly parents and for whom provision will also eventually have to be made. Comprehensive community services must respond to where, how and with whom the person will live, how they wish to spend their time (work related and leisure related activities) and providing specialised services as necessary.

Clinical assessment, diagnosis and treatment, usually of behavioral problems, have historically been undertaken in the mental handicap hospitals. With the reduction in size of these hospitals and the desire of policy makers to develop services close to home, free standing community mental health centres, providing assessment and treatment units, are becoming increasingly common. Some believe that this type of clinical work should not be provided as a separate service but should be part of mainstream acute psychiatric care.

Challenging behaviour

Some people with mental handicap exhibit very disturbed behaviour. If the behaviour is such as to place the physical safety of the person or others in serious jeopardy or make impractical the use of community facilities, the term 'challenging behaviour' is applied. The disruptive behaviours are usually aggression and self-injury.

It has been estimated that 10–15 people with mental handicap per 100,000 of the total population demonstrate behaviours which present a serious challenge to current services. There is a view that people demonstrating seriously aggressive or self injurious behaviours should be cared for wherever possible by specialists visiting them in their own homes as that is the environment in which the behaviour has been manifest. Another view is that 'challenging behaviour units' should be planned for a health district or on a shared basis between several health districts. Such units can operate as part of an assessment and treatment unit.

Secure (forensic) units

People with a moderate or severe learning disability who have committed crimes (such as arson, assault, rape) may be admitted to one of the special hospitals or they may be admitted to a regional secure unit for treatment. It is a general view that this group should be treated in specialised units and not as part of the general forensic psychiatric services. The length of stay in these units is in the order of two years and problems often arise due to a shortage of half way houses or local authority hostels when patients are ready for discharge. Some secure units also admit people with challenging behaviours.

Voluntary organisations

There is a range of voluntary organisations solely or partly orientated towards the needs of people with a mental handicap. Many have a long tradition of providing care and support for this group. This can include the provision of residential accommodation (at the beginning of the 1990s there were over 11,000 places for people with mental handicap in registered private and voluntary homes in England) day nurseries and play groups, social clubs and recreational centres, holiday homes and outings and toy lending libraries. MENCAP is a national organisation with a network of independent local societies. It is exclusively concerned with people with mental handicap and their families. This society provides a wide range of advice and help. It also provides information, by way of leaflets and journals. MENCAP is responsible for some 300 residential homes and three training establishments for further education of school leavers with mental handicap. The society also has a trustee scheme which provides a visiting service for mentally handicapped people after the death of their parents. Through their Gateway Leisure Wing, they have 720 leisure clubs, providing access to ordinary leisure facilities for over 40,000 people with mental handicap, assisted by over 20,000 volunteers.

The organisation Values Into Action (formerly Campaign for Mental Handicap) is a body which works for the rights of people with mental handicap. It promotes new ideas about services through publications, a quarterly newsletter and conferences. An aim is to counter negative images and promote ones which are positive and valued. It submits evidence to government committees of enquiry and responds to reports and policy statements.

National Development Team for people with mental handicap

The National Development Team (NDT) was established in 1976 by the Secretary of State for Social Services. It is an independent advisory body and responds to invitations from health and local authorities to advise on aspects of their services to people with mental handicap and their families. It is not an inspectorate, but it is required to make public its written reports. From April 1992, the NDT became a not-for-profit voluntary agency registered under the Industrial and Provident Societies Act. Its stated mission is 'to promote, throughout the United Kingdom, valued opportunities for people with learning disabilities to develop, participate and contribute to our communities'. Its main function of advising statutory and independent agencies remains unchanged.

Advocacy

The desire to involve people with mental handicap in decisions about their own lives has resulted in a need for advocacy services. A system of citizen advocacy is one way of ensuring that handicapped people are personally represented. A citizen advocate is often a volunteer who has had some training for the role and who works on a one to one basis with the individual. Self advocacy is being promoted amongst disabled people themselves. An organisation called 'People First' has a particular interest in developing advocacy skills amongst people with mental handicap.

CONCLUSIONS

The mental health status of a population is an important component of its overall health, though difficult to conceptualise and measure. The two major categories of mental disorder (mental illness and mental handicap) are themselves bedeviled by conflicting terminology and definitions which have limited the extent to which their frequency within the population can be measured. However, by careful study design, including giving particular attention to defining terms and ascertaining cases, important information can be yielded on the pattern of mental illness and mental handicap in the population. This in turn can enable: ideas about disease causation to be generated, trends over time to be monitored and health needs assessments to be carried out.

Methods for the promotion of mental health and the prevention of mental illness in the population are not well developed. This is partly because of the complexity of describing mental health and partly because the aetiology of many mental illnesses has not yet been elucidated. In the field of mental handicap, the scope for prevention is greater and is likely to grow as techniques advance in antenatal detection and treatment of fetal abnormalities, as well as in genetic risk identification.

Services for people with mental illness and mental handicap must be wide ranging in nature. They must be characterised by team work at the level of the professionals providing the care and by strong collaboration and coordination at the level of the agencies organising the care. Increasingly, high quality care is seen as that provided in non-institutional surroundings, within or close to the community. Its hallmark is that the type of service should be based upon, and matched to, an assessment of the individual's needs.

8 Elderly people

INTRODUCTION

In this chapter, the terms 'the elderly' and 'older people' are used to refer to people aged either 65 years and over or 75 years and over depending upon the context. This is the only practical approach when many of the routinely available data as well as the organisation of services relate to these traditional age-defined cut-off points.

Chronological age is only a rough guide to the biological age of an individual. Examples can be cited of alert and active octogenarians as well as examples for those who have appeared to age prematurely. It has been suggested that we should think only in terms of biological age as measured by the abilities and performance of the individual. However, for most record keeping and administrative purposes, the convenient label of chronological age is used. However, there are strong arguments for regarding ageing in a different way. One such approach uses a social life cycle, comprising four Ages (Table 8.1). In this, the transition from the Second to the Third Ages may be entered for some people as late as 70 years (for example, the radio broadcaster who has continued to work and may even have fathered a second family) whilst for others the transition may be in their 50s (for example, the primary school headmistress who married young, has grown-up children and who decided to opt for early retirement as part of a restructuring of the teaching profession).

Table 8.1: The social life-cycle and ageing

First Age	The age of childhood and socialisation
Second Age	The age of paid work and family-raising
Third Age	The age of active, independent life beyond work and parenting
Fourth Age	The age of eventual dependence

Source: Midwinter E. The British Gas Report on attitudes to ageing. London: British Gas, 1991.

Even the terminology relating to old age is not straightforward. When older people themselves were asked to state preferences, they rejected terms such as 'older people' and 'elderly' as negative and perjorative and opted instead for 'senior citizens' and 'retired' (Table 8.2). Ironically, these are titles which have drawbacks when used to describe older people (rather than used by them). The former is often avoided by younger people as having a rather archaic ring to it whilst the latter is difficult to use with precision given the complex structure of the modern labour market.

In this chapter, the demographic origins of the present elderly population are described. So are the adverse physical, mental, social and financial factors which are frequent accompaniments of the ageing process. The spectrum of services available

Table 8.2: **How people aged 55 years and over said they would like to be addressed with advancing years**

Title preferred	Percentage of respondents
Senior Citizens	36
Retired	36
Elderly	5
Old age pensioner	5
Older people	4
Other	2
Nothing/not answered	12
Total	100

Source: Midwinter E. The British Gas Report on attitudes to ageing. London: British Gas, 1991.

to attempt to meet the problems of the elderly population is also examined. Some special health problems encountered by elderly people are dealt with in a separate section of the chapter.

Elderly people are an important group within the population, not just for those planning and providing health care but also in terms of social and other types of care and services. Many elderly people will remain fit and active into quite late old age but many will not. The onset of mental and physical frailty, the advent of chronic diseases (most of which occur more commonly in old age) lead many old people to have multiple, rather than single, reasons for needing help, support or care.

These considerations make it particularly important that a clear picture is built up of the health and social needs of the elderly population if the best kinds of services are to be developed to meet their needs. As with many other fields of care, no single measure or source of data can be relied upon to provide a comprehensive picture of the health and social status of an elderly population and the extent to which these translate into needs.

To describe the characteristics of the elderly population in the depth required to plan effectively to meet their needs, it is necessary to draw upon a wide range of sources of information. Even then, in many places, relevant information will not be routinely available. In such circumstances, it may be necessary to consider conducting local surveys of the elderly population.

DEMOGRAPHIC IMPLICATIONS OF AN AGEING POPULATION

Origins of Britain's elderly population

In the United Kingdom in 1901 there were 1.8 million people over the age of 65 years out of a population of 38.2 million, representing 4.7% of the total, and only half a million people 75 years and older, or 1.3% of the total population. By the beginning of the 1990s, the situation had changed dramatically: an estimated 15.7% of the population were aged 65 years and over, and 7% were aged 75 years and over.

It is a popular misconception that these historical changes in the elderly population have been due to advances in medical science, new drugs and high technology allowing older people to live longer. For the real reasons for the changes, it is necessary to look back to the turn of the century. At that time, there was a marked improvement in infant and child mortality which coincided with one of the periodic increases in birth rates. Hence, more children were born and more survived to provide the present elderly population. The lower fertility levels associated with modern industrialised countries have served to increase the elderly as a proportion of the total population.

Changes in life expectancy have occurred for all ages during the present century, but the most marked have been the increase in expectation of life at birth (Figure 8.1). A male child born in 1901 could expect on average to live a further 46 years, whereas a male child born at the beginning of the 1990s could expect on average a further 73 years of life. Even greater improvements have occurred in females. Expectation of life for a girl born in 1901 was an average of 49 further years of life. By the beginning of the 1990s, it had become 78 years (Figure 8.1).

This greater improvement in survival for women is a result of a complex relationship between behavioural, social, environmental, economic and genetically linked factors. The excess male mortality can be largely accounted for by higher

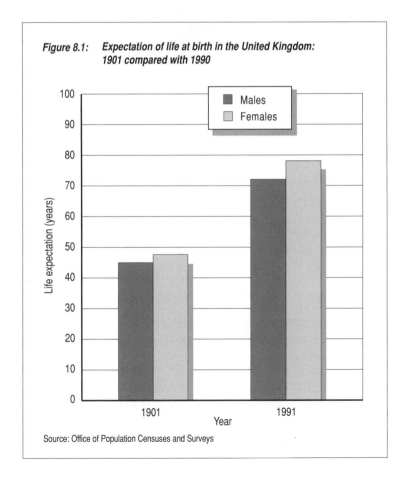

Figure 8.1: Expectation of life at birth in the United Kingdom: 1901 compared with 1990

Source: Office of Population Censuses and Surveys

mortality from coronary heart disease, carcinoma of the bronchus, cirrhosis of the liver and fatal accidents.

Although there is evidence that the gap in mortality between the two sexes may now be narrowing slightly, the sex composition of the elderly population, particularly in the oldest age groups has implications for the provision of services. There is a large population of elderly women who have out-lived their husbands (Figure 8.2) and who are beset by the range of medical and social problems associated with old age without the usual first-line of support, the spouse.

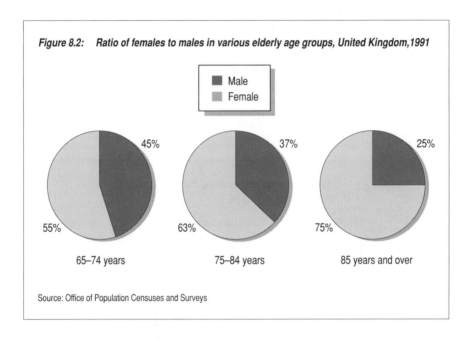

Figure 8.2:   Ratio of females to males in various elderly age groups, United Kingdom, 1991

■ Male
■ Female

45%   37%   25%

55%   63%   75%

65–74 years   75–84 years   85 years and over

Source: Office of Population Censuses and Surveys

The change in expectation of life at birth in the first part of the century has not been fully explained, but includes factors such as improvement in living standards, public hygiene, nutrition and the emergence of qualified midwives. It was certainly well before the advent of advanced therapeutic procedures.

Life expectancy for people who have already lived to the middle and later years of their lives has also increased during the present century. For example, a woman aged 60 years in 1901 lived an average of 15 further years. At the beginning of the 1990s, the comparable figure was 22 years. These changes over time in life expectancy at different ages are shown in Figure 8.3. Expectation of life at birth varies between industrialised countries with Japanese women currently predicted to have the greatest life expectancy at birth (Figure 8.4). There have also been differential gains in life expectancy between countries over the last thirty years. The percentage of people who die at certain ages has changed substantially over the last hundred years with deaths occurring later now than they did in the past. The postponement of deaths is even more marked in a country like Japan where many more people survive into very old age.

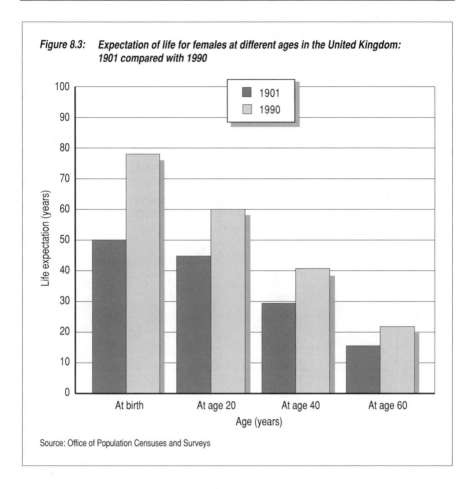

Figure 8.3:   Expectation of life for females at different ages in the United Kingdom: 1901 compared with 1990

Source: Office of Population Censuses and Surveys

The overall changes in the age-structure of the population are reflected in the shape of the so called 'population pyramids' (Figure 8.5). At the turn of the century, the age structure of the population of Britain plotted graphically, did indeed resemble a pyramid, with large numbers of young people at its base and very few elderly people at its peak. In this respect, it resembled present day developing countries which also have predominantly young populations with the proportion of elderly people being some 4–5%. The present day age structure of Britain's population causes the graph to look more like a box than a pyramid, with a relative shrinking in the numbers of young people and a larger proportion of elderly people.

Whilst in many developing countries, the numbers of elderly people occupy a relatively small proportion of the total population, the annual growth in numbers of older people in these countries is exceeding that of their developed counterparts. Population ageing is thus becoming an issue for the World population as well as for developed countries like Britain, other parts of Western Europe, the United States and Japan.

The speed with which the population ages in different countries has varied. Japan, for example, has taken only 26 years for the proportion of its population

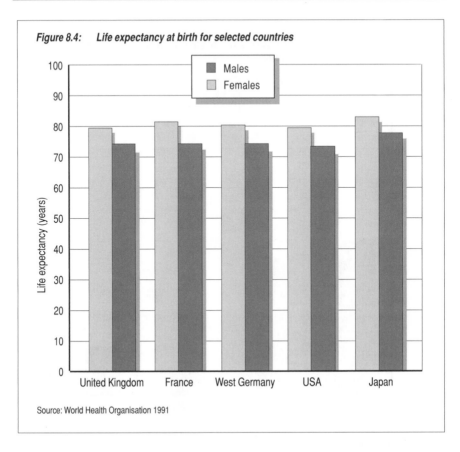

Figure 8.4:   Life expectancy at birth for selected countries

Source: World Health Organisation 1991

aged 65 years to move from seven per cent to 14% compared with over 80 years for Sweden and over 100 years for France (Figure 8.6).

Whilst the major changes in the age structure of the population of Britain this century have been due to changes in birth rates and improvements in expectation of life, more recently, additional ageing of the population has been produced by falling mortality rates in old age. When a population is already ageing but has relatively low fertility and low mortality rates, changes in death rates in the older age groups are the major determinant of further population ageing.

Demographic and social factors affecting informal support for the elderly

Much of the care and support given to elderly people in the population is still provided informally by their children or other relatives. In considering the needs of the elderly population it is important, therefore, to take account of the size of the pool of potential informal carers. A broad indication is provided by comparing the extent to which the numbers of elderly people within a society are balanced by those in adult age groups prior to conventional retirement age. Table 8.3 shows that, for a number of industrialised countries, the so-called age dependency ratio will increase over the next few decades. In the United Kingdom, for example, this will mean that whilst at the beginning of the 1990s there were 23 people aged 65 years for every 100 people aged between 15 and 64 years, by the year 2030, 31 over 65 year olds will be present in the population for every 100 younger adults.

These projected changes represent marked further ageing of the population. However, the aged dependency ratio is an index which can only give a general

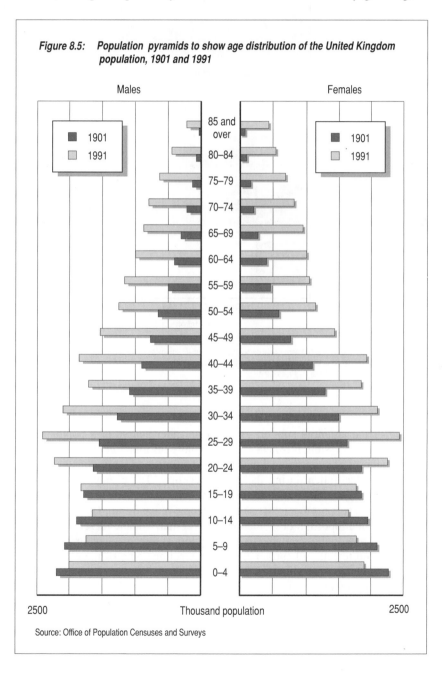

Figure 8.5: *Population pyramids to show age distribution of the United Kingdom population, 1901 and 1991*

Males   Females

1901
1991

1901
1991

85 and over
80–84
75–79
70–74
65–69
60–64
55–59
50–54
45–49
40–44
35–39
30–34
25–29
20–24
15–19
10–14
5–9
0–4

2500   Thousand population   2500

Source: Office of Population Censuses and Surveys

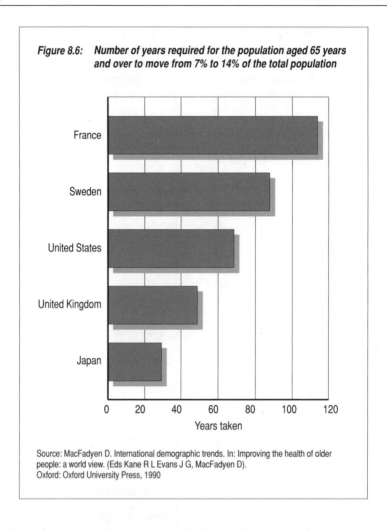

Figure 8.6: *Number of years required for the population aged 65 years and over to move from 7% to 14% of the total population*

Source: MacFadyen D. International demographic trends. In: Improving the health of older people: a world view. (Eds Kane R L Evans J G, MacFadyen D). Oxford: Oxford University Press, 1990

indication of the potential support available to older people in a population. To obtain a fuller impression, it is necessary to explore information on family size and structure, patterns of geographical mobility and attitudes to family life.

Family size has fallen during the present century. The change away from the Victorian tendency to have large families, has meant that there are fewer children available to give support to parents as they become old and frail. However, in more recent times, the proportion of women who never married, and therefore would not have children potentially available to give support as they grow older has declined and is projected to fall still further thus counteracting some of the earlier trends. The extent to which very elderly women are likely to have no surviving children (and hence less potential source of support) is also projected to fall. These higher marriage rates mean that more women will have the potential support of a spouse and one or more children.

Such demographic considerations do not, of course, give any indication as to what level and type of support from children actually materialises when the elderly

Table 8.3: *Aged dependency ratios in countries of the Organisation for Economic Cooperation and Development (OECD)*

	Year				
	1990	*2000*	*2010*	*2020*	*2030*
United Kingdom	23.0	22.3	22.3	25.5	31.1
France	20.9	23.3	24.5	30.6	35.8
Germany (West)	22.3	25.4	30.6	33.5	43.6
Italy	20.1	22.6	25.7	29.3	35.3
USA	18.5	18.2	18.8	25.0	31.7
Japan	16.2	22.6	29.5	33.6	31.9
Average for all members of OECD	19.4	20.8	22.9	27.6	33.3

Source: Organisation for Economic Co-operation and Development, Ageing Populations: The Social Policy Implications, Paris 1988.
* The "aged dependency ratio" is defined as the population aged 65 years and over, as a percentage of the population aged 15–64 years (the population of working age).
Source: The health of elderly people: an epidemiological overview. London: HMSO, 1992.

parent needs it. Other factors relating to marriage and family building have potential implications for the informal support available to people as they grow old. If, for example, there were more marriages in which both partners agree not to have children (perhaps to enable the woman to pursue a full career) there would be implications for future generations of older people. Moreover, the increased divorce rate which has been such a feature of the last thirty years in Britain, will also have an impact. Firstly, divorced elderly people who have not remarried will not have the support of a spouse when they begin to develop the problems associated with old age. Secondly, younger people who become divorced (whether or not they remarry) will have more complex family relationships which may weaken their capacity or commitment to provide tangible support to their elderly parents when it is needed.

Increased geographical mobility also affects the pool of potential supporters of elderly people. The direct effect of this on the availability of informal care for elderly people is difficult to judge as improved transport now makes travel more straightforward. However, making the not unreasonable assumption that mobility is likely to be greater for those under 65 years of age than for those above it, it is quite possible that the effect of this change will be to reduce the level of informal care available when compared with previous decades.

It is difficult fully to discern the implications of all these factors on the actual support given to elderly people. However, of equal importance to the numerical assessment of potential supporters in the light of socio-demographic changes of the kind described above, is the actual response made by grown-up children and other relatives of old people when they do need help. Many men and women who are in their middle years of life, with dependent children of their own, will at some time be faced with the problem of how to respond when one or more of their surviving elderly parents or parents-in-law becomes too frail, too ill, or simply too lonely to maintain an independent way of life. Sometimes, this will be precipitated by the sudden death of the spouse of one of the elderly people concerned but more often it will be a situation which builds up gradually.

Depending on the extent of need of the old person, the type of support provided by families varies enormously, ranging from a regular telephone call from a son or daughter, to periodic or regular visits, to the elderly person actually taking up residence with their children and grandchildren.

The way in which such situations are resolved depends upon a complex interaction of factors including: geographical proximity of the families; the nature of the housing of the elderly person and of the family; the quality of family relationships; the attitude of the elderly person towards independent living and financial considerations. There are as yet few available data to describe the pattern of this informal network of care and support to elderly people.

Future population changes and implications

The immediacy of the problems encountered by the elderly population is highlighted by a simple demographic fact, older people are not a homogeneous

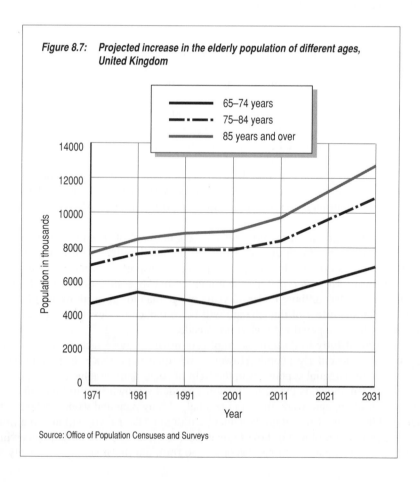

Figure 8.7:   Projected increase in the elderly population of different ages,
               United Kingdom

— 65–74 years
—·—· 75–84 years
— 85 years and over

Source: Office of Population Censuses and Surveys

group. Although the predicted increase in the younger elderly is quite modest, a much greater increase will occur amongst the very elderly (Figure 8.7).

It is well known that older people make much heavier demands on health and social services than do young adults. The most elderly make the heaviest demands of all. The very elderly also tend to be proportionally highly represented in the most intensive forms of non-home based care such as hospital inpatient care. In addition to their having the highest rate of hospital admission, this group also have a much longer average duration of stay in such care when compared to other sections of the elderly population.

Thus, overshadowing the more subtle factors which determine the need for care within the elderly population are some stark and simple facts. During the remainder of the 1990s and well into the next century, there will be an inexorable increase in the numbers of people in Britain who are in the oldest age groups. These are the people who are the frailest, sickest, poorest and more likely to be living on their own.

DEATH, DISEASE AND LOSS OF FUNCTION

One of the characteristics of any ageing organism is that the older it becomes the greater is the risk of impairment, disease or death. In most organisms, including man, the risk of death fluctuates during the early years of life before beginning to rise progressively with time.

Ageing is related to disease in three main ways:

(1) Altered response to disease – some diseases are overcome less easily when they occur in elderly people than in younger people, for example, pneumonia, fractures.
(2) Diseases associated with ageing – some diseases are so closely associated with ageing that they occur to some extent in all individuals as they age. The best example of this is arteriosclerosis.
(3) Increased risk with ageing – many diseases, although not exclusive to ageing individuals, occur much more commonly when old age is reached. Examples of this are many of the common neoplasms.

The hallmark of the occurrence of disease in older people is the presence of multiple pathology. Elderly people rarely suffer from a single disease, but several chronic degenerative processes. Some surface for the first time in old age, others are carried over from middle age. In addition to multiple pathology, there are other

Table 8.4: Properties of illness in old age with implications for medical care

- Multiple pathology
- Non-specific presentation of disease
- Rapid deterioration if untreated
- High incidence of complications of disease and treatment
- Need for rehabilitation
- Importance of environmental factors

Source: Evans J G. How are the elderly different? In: Improving the health of older people: a world view. (Eds Kane R L, Evans J G, MacFadyen D). Oxford: Oxford University Press, 1990.

properties of ill health in old age which are important when designing medical care responses (Table 8.4). Older people often display impaired adaptability to disease so that their health problems manifest themselves in different ways, making them difficult to diagnose. Rapid deterioration and a relatively high incidence of complications are also features of disease in old age. The importance of rehabilitation services in recovery is much more important amongst the elderly than it is in younger age groups. So is the environment in which care is provided.

When considering the additional years of life resulting from greater expectation of life at various ages, the importance lies not just in the extension *per se* but also in the degree of illness and incapacity experienced in these later years. The presence of impairment, disability and handicap increases markedly with advancing years.

The assessment of the types of diseases experienced by an elderly population has a place in assessing its health status but this approach is not appropriate on its own. It is particularly relevant to consider the way in which pathological processes manifest themselves by interfering with the old person's level of functioning (in relation, for example, to particular aspects of self-care). The activities which have been considered in the context of limitation of function are broad and include: those activities concerned with self-care (for example, washing, dressing, eating and using the toilet); walking and other movements; mobility in the wider sense (for example, the ability to move from house to shops), the performance of socially-allocated roles and self-determination.

Data on activities of daily living amongst the elderly are mostly available through surveys of local populations. These can be invaluable in assessing the needs of older people in a locality and planning the response of services. Some national data on self-care tasks are available on a sample basis from the General Household Survey and show the strong relationship between increasing age with loss of independence in such functions (Figure 8.8).

It is likely that information on functional capacity will become a predominant feature in assessing the needs of elderly populations. Such data have many attractions but in particular they provide a measure which is of value at the individual care level. Defining, for example, the help an elderly woman requires against an assessment of her ability to wash, dress, cook and go out to the shops is of relevance to most caring professionals. It provides moreover, a focus for a multidisciplinary approach to care. In addition, assessments of functional capacity provide a common currency which enables the aggregation of data to population level; so that it is possible, for example, to describe the proportion of a local elderly population with incontinence of urine and organise an appropriate service response.

The use of a functional capacity perspective of elderly people's needs has led to the formulation of the concept of active life expectancy. It separates the years of relatively healthy life from those characterised by disability, major illness or dependency. One of the aims of public health is not just to enable more people to live into late old age but to 'compress morbidity' so that active life expectancy is as close as possible to the number of years lived *per se*.

SOCIAL AND ECONOMIC FACTORS

Two of the major factors which affect the material and psychological wellbeing of an elderly person are the loss of employment (and hence income and status) and the loss through death of the companionship of husband, wife or peers.

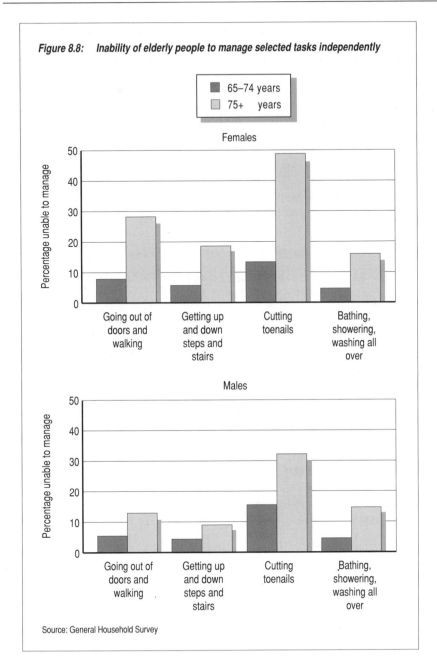

Figure 8.8: *Inability of elderly people to manage selected tasks independently*

Source: General Household Survey

Elderly people's social networks are a vital aspect of the assessment of their need for care as they grow older. It does not, of course, automatically follow that an elderly person living alone is socially isolated. It does raise, however, the importance of the nature of social contacts (as opposed to their number) in the lives of elderly people. For most elderly people, their main social contacts are either with those with whom they live or with relatives outside their home. The potential impact of social and demographic changes related to these issues was discussed in the previous section. Much less is known about the extent to which other societal changes have influenced elderly people's own perceptions of the importance of social networks. For example, an old person living alone in an inner city area who enjoys regular social contact with relatives and friends may be so fearful of personal attack that she would much rather be resident in a sheltered housing scheme than remain in her own home any longer.

Changes in the position of elderly people in society are also closely related to the economic effects of growing old. Figure 8.9 shows that retired people, mainly dependent on state pension, are disproportionately represented in the low income groups of one man, one woman households. State pensions and other welfare benefits provide the main source of income for elderly people.

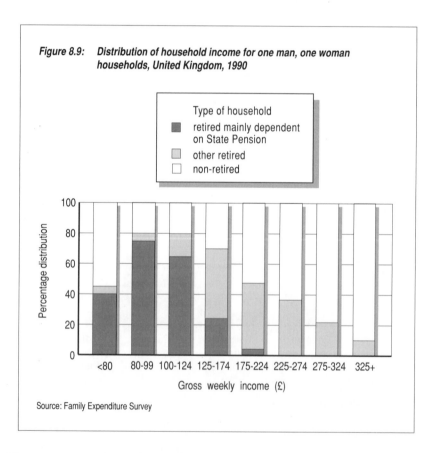

Figure 8.9: *Distribution of household income for one man, one woman households, United Kingdom, 1990*

Type of household
- retired mainly dependent on State Pension
- other retired
- non-retired

Source: Family Expenditure Survey

However, comparison of standards of living for the elderly with those of the younger age groups in society on the basis of income alone is complicated by the fact that younger adults have considerable outgoings. A key issue may well be the distribution of income among the over 65s. There is evidence that this distribution has been widening considerably over the last two decades with major differences in standard of living between those dependent upon state benefit for their income and the smaller number with other income such as investments and occupational pensions.

There is a growing problem of isolation amongst elderly people, particularly in the inner-city areas from which the young have migrated. Loneliness can be a major factor in many of the problems of the elderly. It can cause apathy and lack of interest. It can lead to problems such as malnutrition, hypothermia, and general self-neglect.

Most industrialised countries have an enforced retirement age, usually 60 or 65 years of age. Aside from the economic considerations, loss of employment can have profound effects on the elderly person. Many people's lifestyle and leisure pursuits are determined by their occupation and after retirement it is necessary to structure life differently. Equally important is the link between employment and self-image. For some people the latter can fall dramatically after retirement. Many people are retiring earlier than they did in the past and living for a great many more years. The use of this time will become an increasingly important consideration for society as more and more people enter life post-retirement.

ELDERLY PEOPLE IN ETHNIC MINORITY·GROUPS

Ethnic minority communities now make up a substantial proportion of Britain's population, particularly in certain conurbations. Their relatively young age-structure reflects a high birth rate (in some groups), and the waves of immigration which occurred in the 1960s and early 1970s and (for those who came from Afro-Caribbean countries) in earlier years still.

Whilst the numbers of older people belonging to ethnic minority groups are as yet small compared to the indigenous elderly, their numbers will increase as the structure of the minority populations begins to resemble that of the majority.

Relatively little information is available on the health of older people in the ethnic minority populations and it is important not to fall into stereotypic assumptions about the needs of these elderly populations. For example, it is widely believed that old age is a greatly revered state in some ethnic minority communities within Britain. Hence it is assumed that an elderly person will enjoy the warmth, support and care of an extended family, so that little attention should be given by statutory services to meeting the needs of this group of elderly people.

Whilst this may be the ideal shared by people in some ethnic minority communities themselves, patterns of geographical mobility and other factors will mean that it is unlikely always to be realised. Contrasts between this cultural ideal and the social reality may give rise to problems for elderly people belonging to ethnic minority groups as well as leading to false assumptions amongst those responsible for providing services.

Nevertheless, a population survey of the health and social status of elderly 'Asians' in Leicestershire (described as an example of a public health investigation in Chapter 2) is one of the few to provide objective data on need amongst the ethnic minority elderly in Britain.

It showed similar levels of incapacity to the indigenous population, but a greater direct involvement with the extended family. Wider social contact was seriously limited, however, by lack of literacy and language skills which may also limit contact with the helping agencies in the health and social care arena.

Any consideration of the needs of elderly people belonging to ethnic minority groups must acknowledge the sometimes promulgated view that to take policy initiatives could represent positive discrimination which is unfair to the majority of the elderly population. This argument runs counter to one of the main values of the Welfare State which is to identify sensitively and fairly, groups of the population which have particular needs and to try to meet them. In responding to the needs of older people from ethnic minority communities it will be especially important for health services to ensure that they are aware of and work with varying cultural norms. Knowledge of and sensitivity to issues such as diet, religious practice and observance and the role of the older person in his or her own community will be of particular significance.

SOME SPECIAL HEALTH PROBLEMS OF THE ELDERLY

Hypothermia

There is a danger of hypothermia in the elderly, particularly during the winter months. Accidental hypothermia is said to be present if a deep body (core) temperature falls to below 35°C. The term 'accidental' is used to distinguish this type of hypothermia from that which might be induced deliberately for therapeutic purposes. The diagnosis of hypothermia must be confirmed with a special low-reading thermometer inserted rectally. Such instruments are becoming an increasingly common part of the equipment of doctors and nurses working in the community.

It is estimated that 3–4% of people aged 65 years and over who are admitted to hospital have a core body temperature below 35°C. Over 90% of cases of accidental hypothermia occur indoors.

The elderly person with hypothermia does not usually shiver or complain of being cold because of an impaired perception of temperature change. However, the skin is pale and cold to the touch and consciousness is clouded leading to drowsiness, disordered thought and speech. Coma is more likely the lower the body temperature. Movement and reflexes are sluggish. Speech may be slurred and the hearing and respiratory rates are slow and characteristic changes in an electrocardiograph may be present. The blood pressure may also fall. Some patients with hypothermia may become agitated and restless and if tranquillisers are prescribed this can complicate their serious condition.

Fatality amongst patients with hypothermia is high. Treatment, usually in hospital, consists of gradual rewarming (if conducted too rapidly this may be fatal) and other supportive measures, such as administration of oxygen, intravenous fluids, and broad-spectrum antibiotics.

The main causes of accidental hypothermia are defective thermo-regulatory mechanisms (a consequence of ageing) and exposure to cold through low environmental temperature. Other factors such as immobility due to general infirmity, mental impairment, strokes, falls, effects of medicines, certain illness (for example, infections, endocrine disorders) may be superimposed.

A programme of prevention is the most effective answer to hypothermia. Living accommodation should be reviewed to ensure that there is a high enough indoor temperature. This can be maintained by a combination of heating, draught reduction and insulation measures. In addition, the old person should be encouraged to move around to increase body heat by metabolic activity and to ensure adequate nutrition and clothing, especially in advanced age. Financial support for heating as well as health education are the main strategies. In addition, all health and social care professionals and informal carers should be made aware of, and be vigilant for, the danger signs of hypothermia, especially in cold weather. It is also valuable to ensure a basic knowledge of those issues amongst members of the general public coming into regular contact with older people (for example, milkmen, postmen).

Falls and other accidents

Death rates amongst elderly people as a result of accidents in the home are more common than those amongst children. Falls are the most important single cause of these accidents, the remainder resulting from poisoning, fires, suffocation and other causes.

Falls

The propensity of older people to fall over has long been recognised. Many falls in the elderly will produce no injuries. However, partly because of the increased fragility of bones in old age, a fracture is a common outcome of a fall. Fracture of the neck of the femur is a particularly serious example which can result from seemingly quite trivial falls. Even with a modern approach of immediate operation (to pin the fracture or replace the hip joint) and early mobilisation, fatality can still be as high as 25%. A less serious fracture, such as Colles' fracture of the wrist, may still be a considerable handicap for an elderly woman attempting to cook her meals and do her housework with an arm immobilised in plaster.

The causes of falls (see Table 8.5) have been classified into:

(a) Trips or accidental falls, which account for more than one third of all falls in the elderly. There is a decline in the proportion of falls due to this cause in the very elderly, possibly because of their decreased mobility, combined with the growing importance of other causes.
(b) Drop attacks, which are sudden falls (without warning), not the result of a trip, in which consciousness is retained throughout. The precise mechanism is not clear although it is thought to be due to a momentary reduction in the flow of the blood through the vertebral artery.
(c) Giddiness is a less common cause of falls possibly because the slow development of an attack allows the elderly person to grab hold of something or to sit down. Giddiness is, however, a more important cause of falls amongst the very old. There are very many reasons why giddiness can occur such as hypertension, cardiac insufficiency, transient attacks or side effects of therapy.
(d) Loss of balance may also be caused by a variety of factors, perhaps disorder of the labyrinthine apparatus.

All cases of falls in the elderly should be investigated to determine whether there is any underlying correctable pathology present, but the main strategy is prevention. Much can be done to prevent falls in the home by simple measures such as minimising the use of stairs and steps, attending to loose stair rods, uneven carpets and dangling flex and providing adequate lighting. The elderly person's vision and hearing should be tested and, if necessary, spectacles and hearing aids

Table 8.5:   Causes of falls in a sample of elderly women

	Falls (%)	
	Age Group (years)	
Cause	65–74 (n=77)	75+ (n=113)
Tripping	37	22
Drop attacks	14	12
Giddiness	6	16
Loss of balance	10	9

Source: Exton-Smith A N. Functional consequences of ageing. In: Care of the Elderly: Meeting the Challenge of Dependency. London: Royal Society of Medicine, 1977.

supplied. Ensuring the wearing of proper footwear rather than loosely fitting carpet slippers is another important preventive measure. Careful use of medications, particularly hypnotics and tranquillisers, in the very elderly is also very important. Such health educative measures may be introduced by health visitors, social workers and general practitioners if they are in regular contact.

Urinary incontinence

Urinary incontinence is a common problem in the elderly. It is perhaps the most embarrassing, distressing and ultimately humiliating sequel to old age. Moreover, its onset is often the reason why the elderly person is judged as no longer fit to remain in his or her home, rejected in a family or friend's home or considered an unsuitable candidate for certain forms of residential care.

The causes of urinary incontinence are many and may arise from local factors, for example, bladder neck obstruction (most often due to prostatic enlargement), stress incontinence (usually due to weakening of pelvic floor musculature following childbirth), urinary tract infections or general factors. General factors in the elderly which may lead to incontinence are often multiple and not clear cut. A common reason for urinary incontinence is loss of inhibition of need to void when the bladder is partly full. This mainly occurs at night and is associated with early brain failure. Emotional upsets resulting from bereavement, accidents or illnesses can give rise to incontinence of either a transient or permanent nature. Confusion arising from organic cerebral disease (including stroke) or side effects of sedatives or psychotropic drugs can also lead to incontinence. Other drugs such as rapidly acting diuretics may also contribute. Incontinence may be a feature of limitation of mobility so that the elderly person is unable to reach the toilet in time to avoid an accident.

In order for continence of urine to be maintained five conditions need to be fulfilled (Table 8.6). Approaches to management need to identify which of these factors is contributing to the loss of continence in the individual concerned and to address the problem.

Table 8.6:   Factors necessary to maintain urinary continence

- Adequate function of the lower urinary tract to store and empty urine
- Adequate cognitive function to recognise the need to urinate and to find the appropriate place
- Adequate physical mobility and dexterity to get to a toilet and use it
- Motivation to be continent
- Absence of environmental barriers to continence

Source: Ouslander J G. The efficiency of continence treatment. In: Improving the health of older people: a world view. (Eds Kane R L, Evans J G, MacFadyen D). Oxford: Oxford University Press, 1990.

The cornerstone of management of urinary incontinence in the elderly is making a correct diagnosis of the cause together with a sympathetic and understanding attitude on the part of the professionals. It cannot be over-emphasised that the presence of incontinence is a deeply emotional issue both for the elderly people who have it and relatives, friends and neighbours who are in contact with them. Incontinence is seldom the result of a single underlying cause and all efforts should be made to carry out a full investigation.

In some cases operative treatment of an enlarged prostate or gynaecological disorder, treatment of an underlying urinary tract infection, or review of a long-standing drug regime may solve the problem. Aside from these measures, probably the most important step in treating urinary incontinence is bladder training. For incontinent patients already in an institutional setting, episodes of incontinence are recorded on a fluid chart, and nursing staff ensure regular toileting of the patient to re-educate the bladder. Such bladder training may be supplemented by physio-therapy in the form of exercise for the pelvic floor muscles. Despite such measures some will continue to experience episodes of incontinence.

In the community, for patients who have problems with mobility, the provision of bedpans or other suitable receptacles in the home may be helpful, as may the provision of a commode or chemical closet in the bedroom or living room when the toilet is some distance away. If incontinence still cannot be controlled with these measures, a number of steps may be taken to provide protection and increased comfort for the elderly incontinent patient. Stigma is still attached to the idea of the catheter in the minds of many health professionals, who often regard its use as an abject failure of management. This is quite unjustified. The modern disposable in-dwelling urinary catheter is of value in carefully selected cases. Whilst the likelihood of urinary infection is high, this will seldom lead to systemic infections. And, with careful management involving catheter changes and bladder washouts performed regularly by a district nurse in the home, the elderly person with intractable incontinence can enjoy freedom quite impossible without it. In the male, other appliances may be fitted to the penis to avoid the use of an in-dwelling catheter. Usually these are in the form of a condom-type sheath surrounding the penis with the urine collecting in a bag strapped to the inside of the leg. Surgical treatment to create artificial sphincters is increasingly being used in younger age groups to treat incontinence. In the elderly its use is limited to carefully selected cases but this may change in the future as technologies advance.

A wide variety of support is possible for elderly people with incontinence who are living in the community. In many parts of the country, specialised continence advisers, often with a nursing background visit old people and make assessments as well as providing help to those whose problem has been diagnosed. The use of specialised underclothes and pads are a particularly important part of a support strategy once specific interventions have been tried or as an accompaniment to other therapies. The range of available products is quite wide and make use of disposable pads with highly absorbent materials.

Nutrition in old age

The diagnosis of malnutrition in old people is difficult because there are often co-existing medical conditions and there is considerable lack of knowledge of changes which accompany the ageing process. The clinical manifestations are usually non-specific and laboratory investigations are only of limited value.

Malnutrition in the elderly arises from a combination of social and medical factors. The medical factors can include, for example, poor dentition, partial gastrectomy and mental illness. Malnutrition is also associated with those who have lost interest in preparing food because they are housebound, have been recently bereaved or are living alone.

The diets of those who are malnourished will usually be of a poor quality with lower mean intakes of animal protein, vitamins C and D and nicotinic acid. In the case of those who are housebound, lack of sunshine may add to the problems of shortage of vitamin D.

The factors which may influence nutrition in the elderly are wide-ranging, complex and inter-related (see Figure 8.10). Meals-on-wheels can be called on to deal with problems of malnutrition, but informal help with shopping and preparing meals can be invaluable, as can help with transport to luncheon clubs when these are available.

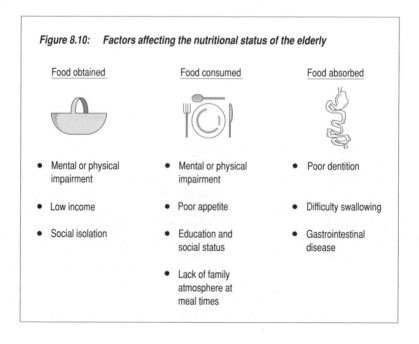

Figure 8.10:   Factors affecting the nutritional status of the elderly

Food obtained	Food consumed	Food absorbed
• Mental or physical impairment	• Mental or physical impairment	• Poor dentition
• Low income	• Poor appetite	• Difficulty swallowing
• Social isolation	• Education and social status	• Gastrointestinal disease
	• Lack of family atmosphere at meal times	

Mental illness in elderly people

Mental illness in the elderly can take many different forms. Some degree of depression is the commonest disorder and affects approximately 15% of the population aged 65 years and over. In addition to the causes of the disease amongst younger people, depression amongst elderly people can be precipitated by any of the major life-events which are common in this age group: for example, the loss of a spouse, retirement, or the onset of physical illness associated with pain. The manifestations of depression can be quite wide-ranging and include: apathy, social withdrawal, neglect of personal appearance, tearfulness, sleep disorders, loss of appetite and suicide. Although for many old people, the episode of depression may resolve with professional help, in others the condition becomes chronic.

Another serious mental illness of later old age is dementia, a disorder of brain functioning which leads to deterioration in the capacity of the mind affecting areas such as memory, decision-making, understanding and the use of language to communicate with others. Old people with dementia can also have disturbances of normal behaviour which lead them to wander, sleep irregularly and fitfully, and to exhibit disruptive and anti-social behaviour. Another practical aspect of the effect of dementia on elderly people is the extent to which they are able to care for themselves. Progressive loss of function in this respect is an important feature of the disease. Dementia varies in the way in which it affects the mental, physical and social functioning of any individual elderly person but it is capable of affecting all such areas of functioning (Table 8.7).

Table 8.7:   Practical features of dementia

Progressive impairment of intellectual functioning

- Memory problems
- Loss of sense of time
- Loss of sense of where or who they are
- Speech difficulties

Personality and behavioural changes

- Neglect of personal care and hygiene
- Incontinence
- Emotional lability
- Loss of social inhibitions

Minor degrees of memory impairment and temporary confusion may not necessarily threaten an old person's capacity to maintain an independent existence in the community. However, more severe and sustained problems of this kind, especially when coupled with disturbed or erratic behaviour and an inability to perform basic activities of daily living, will lead rapidly to a state of dependency.

Dementia affects around five per cent of people aged 65 years and over whilst closer to 20% of over-85s will exhibit some signs of it. Dementia is of two main types. The first and most common is Alzheimer's disease, in which there are permanent changes in the brain characterised by loss and severe abnormalities of nerve cells and their processes. In particular, nerve cells which produce important chemical substances for brain activities are lost. Alzheimer's disease accounts for about half of all cases of dementia amongst the over-65s. Dementia is much less common in middle-age and early old-age but, when it does occur here, Alzheimer's disease is commonly found. The second type of dementia is associated with disease of the arteries of the brain causing death of small or large areas of brain tissue, so called multi-infarct dementia.

Aside from these two main types of dementia, there are other less common forms including, Huntingdon's chorea, Parkinson's disease and Creutzfeld–Jacob disease. In addition, the symptoms and signs of dementia can be produced by vitamin B-12 deficiency, brain tumours, thyroid disease and chronic alcoholism. Some of these less common forms of dementia are treatable but where Alzheimer's disease or multi-infarct dementia are the underlying pathologies, treatment is not effective and clinical management is aimed at containing and ameliorating the effects of the disease.

As the population ages still further, the estimated number of people with dementia will increase sharply (Table 8.8). This has major implications for service provision.

Table 8.8:   Prediction of the number of people with dementia in the United Kingdom

Year	Age group (years)			
	40–64	65–79	80 and over	Total 40 and over
1991	14,670	196,280	387,600	598,550
2001	16,049	194,748	449,200	659,997
2011	17,977	198,740	487,200	703,917
2021	17,261	240,480	495,000	752,741

Source: Alzheimer's Disease Society. Caring for Dementia: Today and tomorrow. London: Alzheimer's Disease Society, 1992.

Other groups of elderly people with mental illness are important in terms of their need for services. Many of those with psychotic illnesses such as schizophrenia have grown old within large, old-style psychiatric hospitals. With the policy of phasing out such long-stay institutional type facilities these patients have particular needs which must be matched by appropriate community services if they are to leave what has effectively become their home over many years. Amongst elderly people admitted to hospital for treatment of acute medical, surgical or orthopaedic conditions, so-called 'confusion' (more properly 'delirium') is not uncommon. Many cases can be managed clinically if identified at an early stage and underlying factors treated.

SERVICES FOR THE ELDERLY

It often surprises people to learn that the majority of elderly people are able to lead an independent existence in their own home.

However, with advancing age and the impact of the negative forces of old age, this independence is less easily maintained. When elderly people are no longer able to manage on their own, a wide range of services are available to provide help, support and advice.

The promotion of health in old age

The promotion of health through health education, disease prevention and health protection can have an impact in old age. Examples of health promotion programmes targeted at the elderly include the detection and treatment of hypertension, smoking cessation, exercise, healthy eating and weight control. A wider perspective on the promotion of health would also include programmes which prepare older people psychologically for retirement and which address their social welfare in ways which prevent problems and crises occurring.

Primary and community care

The majority of elderly people will continue to live in the community either with their spouse, with their children or other members of their family or, increasingly as they grow older, alone. For some considerable time, the central objective of policy for care of the aged in the United Kingdom, has been to enable elderly people to remain in the community for as long as possible. For most old people, their ability to reside in their own home is a potent symbol of autonomy, independence and self-determination.

The nature of services provided in the community is critical in determining successful outcomes of care for old people who do have needs. For example, district nurses, home helps and health visitors are vital professionals whose input to the care of housebound old people can help to convert their tenuous hold on independent living into a well-supported daily routine enhanced by social contacts. Similarly, the availability of day and respite care backed up by good transport to provide widespread access can be another key ingredient of support for the vulnerable elderly. Services which are available on a 24 hour, seven day a week basis to provide, for example, night nursing, toileting, bathing or sitting services will often make the difference between a hospital or residential care admission and sustaining an old person with a reasonable quality of life at home.

The primary health care team composed of different professional disciplines and organised around the local general practice is a cornerstone in the care of the elderly. It is well known that many elderly people who are ill or incapacitated do not seek out medical help. A primary health care team can organise itself in such a way that some of this need is ascertained and problems are recognised early. The general practitioner's contract of employment requires a regular check of all over 75 year olds registered with the practice. Given the multiplicity of health and social care needs an older person can have, it is important that general practitioners are both well informed about, and have an influence upon, the range of supportive services. General practitioners have a duty to advise their patients on the availability of social as well as health care.

Whether organised around the general practice as part of the primary health care team directly, or based within a community health service unit, or located within a hospital's management structure (as an outreach function), health professionals other than doctors are also an essential element of the network of health care delivered to elderly people in the community.

Although the health visitor is mainly concerned with the youngest age groups, a proportion of her case load may be taken up with the elderly. Her training equips her to detect early signs of disease and disability and to take the necessary action to ameliorate these conditions. A knowledge of the complex network of services available can enable her to play a part in obtaining the assistance which an elderly person may require.

Community nurses also have a major role in caring for the elderly. Of all the patients treated at home by nurses in Britain, almost half are elderly. Increasingly, in many parts of the country, although overall responsibility remains in the hands of a qualified nurse, nursing auxiliaries assist with some duties such as bathing, washing hair, cutting toe-nails and generally performing home nursing tasks. Other health professionals working in the community, such as chiropodists and dieticians, are also part of the care team supporting old people.

Specialist nursing services such as community psychiatric nurses, (for example, for elderly people with severe depression or dementia) or palliative care nurses (for example, for elderly people with end stage cancer) are a valuable adjunct to these general community services.

New legislation contained in the NHS and Community Care Act 1990 (see Chapter 4), which was implemented in full from April 1993, requires a combined approach to the assessment of need, led by the social services department, in which all agencies and professional disciplines collaborate. On the basis of such assessments a care manager will be appointed (normally from the social services department but possibly from the health service if the individual requires mainly health care). He or she will take the lead in ensuring the services identified by the assessment are delivered. This role will include the commissioning of the social care components of the individual's care package.

Professionals delivering such forms of service to elderly people in their own homes can include social workers and home helps. The latter group, if their traditional role is extended, can be particularly valuable in maintaining a frail or incapacitated elderly person at home. Many social services departments have developed their home help services into home care services based around a much wider range of tasks being provided in response to individual need than was previously the case. In some parts of the country, the potential for a joint health and social care approach to domiciliary care for older people is being examined via the provision of domiciliary workers who undertake both the functions of district nurse auxiliaries and local authority home care workers. This model has particular merit in meeting individual need across the health-social care divide.

Other services delivered to the home and which are also an important component in the network of support, include meals-on-wheels and home laundry facilities.

Day centres, lunch and recreational clubs

Many old people will attend a day centre or be a member of a club (often organised by a voluntary organisation or in some places by a church). Such facilities are places where elderly people can interact with their peers and with staff. They can help to counteract loneliness and social isolation. A hot meal is often provided midday and helps to meet the overall nutritional needs of the elderly people concerned. Day centres like these can also help to relieve some of the burden of care for informal carers and allow them time and space to unwind, to go shopping or to get on with household tasks.

Respite care

Respite care can be of major importance in allowing dependent older people to remain in their own homes. Whilst the term respite care implies a single form of care service, this is increasingly incorrect. Currently there are a variety of models of respite care which are designed to meet a range of individual needs. There is still a clear role for the health service in providing hospital inpatient respite care and for the provision of such care in residential homes but there is an increasing recognition that respite care does not have to cause individuals to leave their homes. Given the importance of familiar surroundings to many older people (and especially those with mental illnesses of old age such as dementia) models of respite care involving care workers looking after the person in their own home are becoming more common.

Voluntary organisations

In Britain, voluntary organisations have traditionally played a vital role in the care of elderly people in the community. Whilst their role will vary according to the philosophy and infrastructure of the organisation concerned, it will invariably include raising public awareness of the issues involved as well as providing information to elderly people and their carers. Many voluntary organisations will additionally have a service provision role which can encompass the delivery of specialist advice on state financial benefit entitlements, the running of day care centres, counselling, advice, and home visiting.

Caring for carers

Understanding the full spectrum of care needs of the elderly requires an understanding of the needs of those who look after elderly people, many of whom are themselves elderly. Carers must be given practical support, as partners with professionals in giving care. This should also be based on an assessment of their individual needs separate from their dependants, in order that conflicts of needs can be identified and wherever possible reconciled. Above all, they should have access to high quality, up-to-date information about the availability of facilities, services, rights and entitlements. They must also be recognised as having needs of their own. There might be a need for counselling and emotional support, for training in particular aspects of disease management, or a need for more rest through provision of better day or respite care for the elderly person, and in some cases treatment for physical problems such as back pain. Much of this work is anticipatory, to prevent a breakdown of the caring relationship.

Elderly people with continuing care needs who cannot manage at home

Sometimes, even with a high level of support from services it is just not feasible or humane to allow old people to remain at home. Through multiagency assessment, the social services department is the lead agency which commissions care for them. The choice of care will be from within the range of facilities in a locality which is best suited to their needs. Sometimes, for example, this would be a private nursing or residential home, sometimes residential care provided by the local authority. For a small group of highly dependent people, the health service will need to continue to provide consultant-led hospital inpatient care.

For elderly people whose conditions are too severe for them to continue in their own homes, even with support services, there has been a growing realisation of the importance of the nature of the institutional environment and regime of long-stay accommodation. The term 'institution' itself is increasingly unfavourably regarded because it has become synonymous with the negative features of long-stay facilities which it is sought to eliminate. Places where the interior fabric is drab and decaying, furnishing is uniform, where there is a permanent smell of urine and privacy is limited, coupled with regimes which are organised and regimented to facilitate the tasks of the staff rather than the needs of the individual resident or patient, can be destructive. This lack of self determination encourages an apathy and indifference amongst people with special or long-term care needs which may lead not only to poor quality of life but to poor outcome of care. Such long-stay institutions are also often characterised by poor staff morale, high turnover and problems with recruitment.

There is a broad range of facilities available for elderly people who require long-term care and support who cannot manage within their own homes. The health service continues to provide what are often called 'long-stay geriatric beds', which usually cater for moderate to heavily dependent elderly people who require nursing care. The local authority social services department provides places in homes for the elderly, aimed particularly at those frail elderly people who are not heavily physically or mentally incapacitated (often still called Part III accommodation after the relevant part of the National Assistance Act 1948). The private sector provides places in private nursing homes as well as in rest or residential homes; the not-for-profit and voluntary sectors also provide some residential and nursing home care.

There are two major groups of elderly people who require these forms of continuing care: those who need care for considerable parts of a 24 hour period from staff with nursing training and those who need staff to give help or assistance in carrying out some of the activities of daily living such as washing, dressing, getting to the toilet and feeding themselves.

In the past, these types of care have been regarded as discrete entities, developed to a level within the population determined by the agencies which control them and with admission and care policies which were similarly individual agency orientated. The advent of the changes to the organisation and funding of community care, implemented in full from April 1993, have helped to achieve a greater degree of integration. Under these arrangements Community Care Plans, produced jointly between health authorities and social services departments, must ensure that the decisions of each agency are co-ordinated in order that the population's needs determine the quantity of the various forms of continuing care commissioned. At the level of the individual elderly person, the system of multi-disciplinary assessment aims to ensure that he or she receives the form of continuing care most suited to their needs.

The aim of all facilities which care for elderly people should be to allow the old person to have maximum dignity and self-determination. Whilst in practice the daily routine for elderly patients or residents can often seem dull and monotonous, there is much that can be done to ensure that the regime does not develop the adverse features of an institution. Elderly people in continuing care facilities should not spend extended periods of the day bedridden or chairfast unless their condition dictates that this must be so. Elderly people should receive personalised care and should not be subjected to set regimes in relation to toileting, bathing or feeding. Each continuing care facility should pursue a personalised clothing scheme to encourage the maintenance of self-respect and individuality. Elderly people should be encouraged to bring as many of their personal possessions with them as is feasible.

The elderly person's environment should provide a sense of security and cheerfulness. Therefore, floors should be safe to walk on and appropriate furniture, including a wide variety of chairs, provided. The layout and furnishing of the hospital or home should be designed to avoid confusion, particularly important for the elderly with dementia. Decoration should be in a non-institutional manner with soft furnishings and colour schemes homely in appearance. The communal rooms should be arranged to allow each resident to pursue their own hobbies and interests. With positive attention to building design, environment, regimes, individual care plans and staff training, adverse factors of institutional life can be reversed (Table 8.9).

Table 8.9: Longer term care for old people with dementia: some quality features

- Emphasis on personalised care, retention of personal possessions and own washing and bathing facilities
- Preservation of choice
- Domestic routines established for the benefit of elderly residents rather than for administrative convenience
- Right to privacy respected
- Well designed, modern environment decorated in a non-institutional manner

Hospital based services

A central part of a comprehensive system of care for the elderly is the capacity to provide specialist assessment and treatment for elderly people with acute medical problems.

Elderly people with acute illnesses present a particular challenge for the service seeking to provide the most effective clinical management of their condition and to maximise their level of independence. Elderly people will often have several problems co-existing which require skilful assessment and treatment, but their functional capacity (in terms of factors such as mobility and continence) will be equally as influential in determining both recovery and future living status. Moreover, the acute presentation will often bring to light issues of family and social support which have previously not been addressed but which require resolution as part of the care plan.

Inpatient care

The appropriate organisation of acute medical care to provide prompt and accurate assessment, treatment and rehabilitation, and ultimately a return to the community or other care facility, has been the focus of attention over the past ten years. Much of this has centred on what kind of hospital bed the elderly person with an acute illness should be admitted to and what the relationship should be between geriatric medicine and general medicine as specialties of clinical practice. It is now widely acknowledged that care of the acutely ill elderly person is best provided within a bed in a general hospital setting where there is access to the full range of diagnostic and therapeutic facilities.

A number of models of hospital care for acutely ill elderly people have evolved and these tend to take one of three main forms.

Age defined approach. In some localities, all patients above a certain age (usually 75 years and over) are admitted to a specialist geriatric service. This model of care has attractions in that it is easily understood by general practitioners and it provides a ward environment and care team especially geared to the needs of the elderly. It has the disadvantage inherent in the differences between chronological and biological ageing. With a cut-off point which is chronologically-based, say at 70 or 75 years, the 66 year old with problems of biological old age (such as stroke) will miss out on the assessment and rehabilitation skills of the geriatric team.

Integrated approach. An alternative model of service is one in which all acutely ill elderly people are admitted to an acute medical ward which deals with other age groups and are cared for by a group of physicians. Although one or more of these physicians will have special expertise in the care of the elderly, he or she will also participate in the care of the young age groups.

This has the advantage that all medical staff are in touch with medical care across all age groups and it enables more scope in the use of beds. However, there can be difficulties. Patients may be spread around the hospital, be subject to different ward routines and there can be problems in getting nursing staff to take a common approach with a split across different wards. Moreover, there is a danger that the 'urgent' will always take priority over the 'important' (for example, the younger person with a myocardial infarction rather than the elderly person with a stroke).

Needs based approach. Some hospitals run a model of care in which there are separate departments of geriatric and general medicine but the decision about which team takes care of the patient is governed by his or her care needs.

This has the advantage that patients are selected at the time of admission according to whether they will benefit from the assessment and rehabilitation skills of the geriatric team. Patients with more straightforward medical problems (even though they are elderly) will be admitted under the care of the general medical team. The success of this model of care depends upon very close collaboration between the two departments. Where this does not exist, the approach can lose much of its attraction and effectiveness.

It is not appropriate to think of a single model of practice for the whole service. Those securing services for the needs of their elderly population will be concerned to know about the organisation of acute medical care for elderly people within each local hospital.

It is the success in achieving recovery rather than the response to illness *per se* which is the real test of the quality of hospital services. This is only partly dependent on the medical input. It also crucially depends on access to non-medical advice and support from groups such as occupational therapists or physiotherapists. The role, too, of social workers in ensuring discharge is co-ordinated with support services is vital.

The nature of services for the treatment of non-emergency problems of the elderly within the acute care sector is also of great importance. Many elderly people's lives are impaired by the presence of conditions which are potentially correctable. For example, many elderly women with chronic pain and severe limitation of movement caused by osteoarthrosis of the hip could have their level of independence and quality of life immediately improved by a hip joint replacement. Similarly, the lives of old people with very poor eyesight due to cataracts can be transformed by a simple operation.

Specialist hospital facilities for elderly people with mental illness are increasingly being provided by a Consultant in the Psychiatry of Old Age supported by a specialist multidisciplinary team working from a district general hospital with outreach facilities.

Day hospital and outpatient facilities

Much of the initial assessment of elderly people with physical or mental illness is undertaken on an outpatient basis or by the consultant or other members of the hospital team visiting the old person's home at the request of the general practitioner. The inappropriate use of hospital beds can also be avoided by the provision of adequate day hospital care. The day hospital now has a firmly established place in most hospital services for the elderly. Day hospitals usually operate five days per week with patients generally arriving early morning and departing mid- to late afternoon, having had their midday meal at the hospital. The day hospital is often situated close to or within a hospital which has inpatient facilities for the elderly. The emphasis in day hospitals is on active treatment and rehabilitation with multidisciplinary team work involving professionals such as nurses, physiotherapists, occupational therapists and speech therapists.

The day hospital also permits earlier discharge from a hospital bed so that rehabilitation takes place alongside reintegration into the community, and thus the risks of relapse and re-admission are reduced. As with day centres, the day hospital can be an invaluable aid to carers in providing a respite from care (this is especially so for the most dependent elderly people).

Housing

There is little doubt that adequate and properly designed housing is the foundation upon which medical and social services for the elderly should be built. Over half of elderly people in Britain are owner-occupiers. If they are to continue to remain in the community, then their dwelling places must be adapted to meet their special needs. This can be achieved by the renovation or adaptation of existing houses or by providing specialised dwellings of the kind which are often described as sheltered housing.

Sheltered housing is provided by local authorities, by private organisations and by housing associations. Some specialised housing for the elderly is warden controlled. Essentially, the warden acts a a friendly neighbour and keeps regular contact by personal visits, encouraging the elderly resident to contact him or her by means of some communication apparatus, for example, buzzer, bell or two-way speaking system. The warden does not provide a personal service such as cooking, cleaning or shopping, but can obtain help when necessary by providing a point of contact through which health and social services can be delivered. Sheltered housing is an important form of provision which allows frail, elderly people to continue to live in the community. Without such a protected environment, in which they can maintain supervised independence, they would probably be unable to cope, and the only recourse would be towards hospital or residential care.

The size of the specialised dwelling sectors is of key importance and there is no doubt that during the decade up to the beginning of the 1990s, it did not keep pace with the growth of need in the frail elderly population.

Compulsory admission

Powers exist under the National Assistance Act 1948 for the local authority to arrange compulsory removal to hospital or other institution of a person who is unwilling to go voluntarily from their own home. A person can be removed if he or she is suffering from grave chronic disease or if through being aged, infirm or physically incapacitated he or she is living in insanitary conditions and unable to care for himself or herself, and/or does not receive from others, proper care and attention. Details of the procedure are laid down in Section 47 of the National Assistance Act 1948. A 'proper officer' (usually a public health doctor) and another registered medical practitioner (usually the patient's general practitioner) must certify that such removal is in the interests of the patient or that it would prevent injury to the health of, or serious nuisance to, other people. The next step is for an application to be made to a Magistrate's Court and for the patient to be given seven days' notice.

In 1951 an incident exposed a weakness in the procedure and highlighted the need for more immediate intervention. An elderly lady in Yorkshire fell in her house, refused to go into hospital and rejected other help. She lay on her floor for the statutory seven days watched by officials powerless to act. Her pressure sores became infected and she subsequently died from tetanus. The local Member of Parliament was appalled by the affair and introduced a Private Members Bill which became the National Assistance (Amendment) Act 1951 which introduced an emergency procedure permitting the two doctors mentioned above to make an application to a magistrate for the patient to be removed to a place of care for a period of three weeks.

CONCLUSIONS

Old age can be a time of continuing participation in the life of the community and of personal fulfilment. With ever advancing years, however, the need for support for old people who become frail, ill, incapacitated or socially isolated becomes increasingly important. The key to this process is identifying and assessing individual need and then organising an appropriate response. In some cases, this will come from statutory services. In other cases, the voluntary or private sector will have a part to play. Much, if not the majority, of the care provided to old people is given by informal carers (families and friends) and this must be recognised by all care agencies. Practical and emotional support for such carers is a vital part of the infrastructure of support for elderly people themselves and it is important that old people and their carers are fully involved as part of the care process.

If these services work well, many old people with problems will be able to remain in the community, well supported, close to family and friends. Throughout, however, emphasis must be placed on setting and maintaining high standards of care, whether this is to be provided in the community, in a hospital or in a residential care facility.

In these ways, quality of life and dignity for people in the final years of their lives will be sustained.

9 Communicable diseases and parasites

INTRODUCTION

Communicable diseases regularly feature as topics in newspaper headlines. Food related illness frequently captures media attention and is one of the main ways in which the general public is made aware of communicable diseases as a phenomenon. In the late 1980s and early 1990s a series of food hygiene issues received media coverage for weeks at a time – salmonella and eggs, listeria and soft cheeses, botulism and hazelnut yoghurt, and bovine spongiform encephalopathy in cattle, to name the most prominent. In addition to food related problems, conditions such as legionnaires' disease, cryptosporidiosis and the acquired immune deficiency syndrome have also emerged as important public health problems.

Although deaths from communicable diseases in Britain are relatively rare now compared with the last century, they do still occur. It is only necessary to recall the small number of children who die each year from meningococcal infection to realise that micro-organisms continue to contribute to the toll of human misery. In developing countries, communicable diseases are still an important cause of premature death. Combatting communicable diseases depends upon surveillance, preventive measures, and, where appropriate, outbreak investigation and the institution of control measures. This chapter describes the principles of surveillance and control of communicable diseases, defines some of the terms in common use, briefly outlines the services to deal with infectious conditions and reviews the legal framework.

SURVEILLANCE OF COMMUNICABLE DISEASES

A pre-requisite for detecting outbreaks of communicable disease is to have a mechanism in place which draws attention to their existence.

Surveillance is the systematic collection, collation, and analysis of data and dissemination of the results so that appropriate control measures can be taken. In communicable diseases, this information is needed to monitor disease trends, identify epidemics or outbreaks and evaluate prevention and control programmes. A number of systems, both formal and informal, exists to enable information about communicable disease occurrences in the population to be gathered and analysed (Figure 9.1).

A legal duty rests on all registered medical practitioners, who are attending people suspected of having certain specified infectious diseases (Table 9.1), to notify the names and addresses of these patients. Notifications in England and Wales are made to the Proper Officer of the local authority (local authorities are required to appoint such officers to ensure the proper discharge of their functions). They are required to submit this information to the Office of Population Censuses

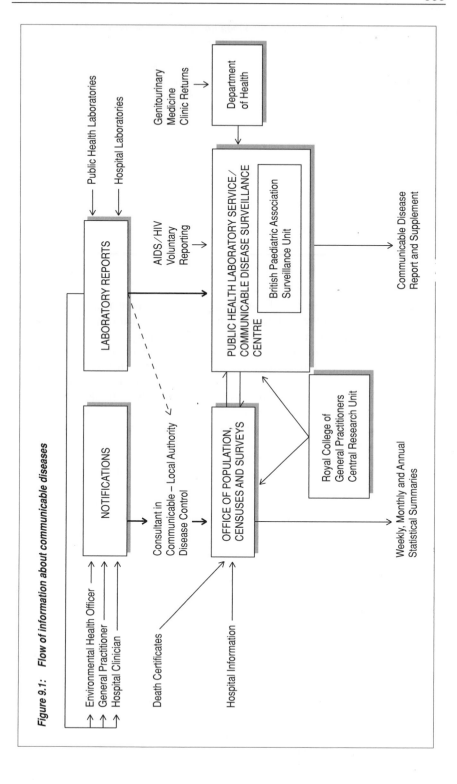

Figure 9.1: Flow of information about communicable diseases

Table 9.1:   Communicable diseases notifiable in England and Wales

Anthrax	Plague
Cholera	Acute poliomyelitis
Diphtheria	Acute encephalitis
Dysentery	Relapsing fever
Rabies	Rubella
Food poisoning	Scarlet fever
Leprosy	Smallpox
Leptospirosis	Tetanus
Malaria	Tuberculosis (all forms)
Measles	Typhoid fever
Mumps	Typhus fever
Meningitis	Viral haemorrhagic fevers
Meningococcal septicaemia	Viral hepatitis
Ophthalmia neonatorum	Whooping cough
Paratyphoid fever	Yellow fever

and Surveys (OPCS) which produces weekly statistical summaries. In addition to the weekly returns, the Proper Officers submit returns at quarterly intervals which enables corrections to be made to the data gathered weekly.

In Scotland and Northern Ireland notifications are sent to the Chief Administrative Medical Officer (CAMO) of the appropriate Health Board.

Unfortunately, the effectiveness of this system is variable because there is a serious degree of under notification of these statutorily notifiable diseases by medical practitioners. This is compounded by the fact that the list of notifiable diseases contains conditions which rarely occur in this country but which appear by international agreement.

The other major source of epidemiological information is reports of positive laboratory isolates which laboratories make to the Public Health Laboratory Service Communicable Disease Surveillance Centre (CDSC). Laboratories include the Public Health Laboratories, hospital departments of microbiology and virology, and a small number of private laboratories. In addition, there are specialist reference laboratories which undertake detailed diagnostic work in relation to particular organisms or sources of infection. Information from them is also collated by the Communicable Disease Surveillance Centre (it collects information from active surveillance systems, for example, the British Paediatric Surveillance Unit).

The special confidential reporting system for HIV infection and AIDS has been mentioned in chapter 3. In addition, genito urinary medicine clinics make returns directly to the Department of Health on a quarterly and annual basis about the incidence of sexually transmitted diseases.

In England and Wales a sentinel scheme for reporting disease in general practice, under the auspices of the Royal College of General Practitioners (RCGP), includes some communicable diseases. Returns from a number of selected spotter practices are made on a weekly basis to the College's Research Unit. The sentinel practice scheme involves some sixty general practices covering approximately 425,000 patients. In Scotland there is a much larger system involving 124 general practices collecting information about almost 700,000 patients.

In England and Wales information is fed back by OPCS which publishes data about communicable diseases on a weekly, quarterly and annual basis, and by the Communicable Disease Surveillance Centre which also publishes reports weekly and quarterly containing details of isolates derived from hospital laboratories and the Public Health Laboratory Service. In Scotland a weekly report is produced by the Communicable Diseases (Scotland) Unit, in addition to data published by the Registrar General in Scotland.

In addition to these usual routes, the consultant in communicable disease control (the role of this post is described later in this chapter) may glean information about previously unsuspected cases of communicable diseases from death notifications.

Informal communications between the consultant in communicable disease control and colleagues are of paramount importance. A telephone call from a general practitioner, practice nurse, microbiologist, environmental health officer, or school nurse yields rapid information and these links should be nurtured.

In an attempt to speed up the passage of information between clinicians, laboratories and the consultant in communicable disease control some health authorities have now installed computer networks linked directly by electronic communication.

INVESTIGATION OF COMMUNICABLE DISEASE OCCURRENCES

The accounts of individual communicable diseases given later in this chapter will illustrate the importance of thoroughly investigating people with symptoms suggestive of an infectious cause. In this way, the specific organism responsible can be identified (wherever possible), the most effective treatment instituted and other potential cases or contacts can be traced (if appropriate for disease control). The rapid identification of organisms which cause illness is also essential for good surveillance of communicable diseases in the population to enable control measures to be instituted.

It cannot be over-emphasised that the key to successful communicable disease control in the population is prevention. However, when cases occur, either singly, in small or in large numbers, the situation should be approached from the viewpoint that current preventive or control measures have failed. Everything possible should be learned from such occurrences. In this way, control measures can be strengthened so that new incidents or outbreaks can often be ended rapidly to minimise the numbers of people affected.

Whilst the circumstances of communicable disease occurrences will differ in practice, a number of general principles apply when approaching an investigation. The most common reason for starting an investigation is because of an outbreak. Whatever the circumstances, the aims must be to act quickly, to establish clear operational principles and to perform a sound investigation.

How problems come to light

The way in which occurrences of communicable diseases prompt investigation varies. With good surveillance systems, a sudden upsurge in the incidence of a particular disease, clustering of several cases in a certain geographical area or the occurrence of one or two cases of a very rare disease, will be rapidly detected and could be the starting point for further study. Some incidents will come to light in other ways. For example, a call for help may be received from an hotel after a large number of guests have developed vomiting and diarrhoea. Similarly, enquiries from the media may be made to a health authority's press office after a large number of people in a locality have reported being ill. A publication by a research team may draw attention to the unusually high incidence of a particular disease or a previously unrecognised causation.

Steps in an investigation

Broadly, investigation of an outbreak involves three tasks. These are to describe the incident, analyse the data and give public health advice. Information needs to be collected which describes the outbreak, (i.e. the nature and timing of the illness, where people acquired the disease, and the characteristics of the affected people). This descriptive information often yields clues to the source of an infection and its means of spread thereby allowing early intervention. When the source is not readily apparent a more detailed analytical approach needs to be undertaken. This will often involve comparing the food intakes of people who became ill with those who did not. A variety of statistical techniques are used in such analyses. The results help to draw out inferences concerning transmission and exposure to disease.

The logical sequence of action in investigating an outbreak or epidemic is outlined in Figure 9.2. The first requirement is to confirm the existence of an epidemic and to verify the diagnosis. This involves the collection of as much

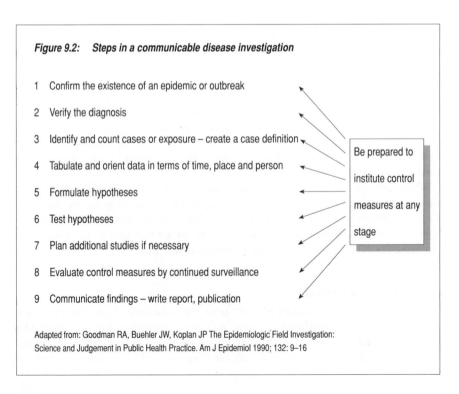

Figure 9.2:   Steps in a communicable disease investigation

1   Confirm the existence of an epidemic or outbreak

2   Verify the diagnosis

3   Identify and count cases or exposure – create a case definition

4   Tabulate and orient data in terms of time, place and person

5   Formulate hypotheses

6   Test hypotheses

7   Plan additional studies if necessary

8   Evaluate control measures by continued surveillance

9   Communicate findings – write report, publication

Be prepared to institute control measures at any stage

Adapted from: Goodman RA, Buehler JW, Koplan JP The Epidemiologic Field Investigation:
Science and Judgement in Public Health Practice. Am J Epidemiol 1990; 132: 9–16

information as possible about the disease and its characteristics. Information also needs to be assembled about the expected level of such an infection under normal circumstances, and about the population who are primarily affected. This preliminary exercise will help to determine the extent of any subsequent investigation and the urgency with which it is carried out.

It is important to involve microbiological experts at a very early stage once the decision to proceed with an investigation has been made. The microbiologist can ensure that the most appropriate arrangements are made for the collection and rapid processing of specimens.

Environmental health officers of local authorities play a key part in the investigation process, particularly of food borne outbreaks. Their areas of expertise include inspection of premises, knowledge about food hygiene and food preparation, collection of environmental and food samples for microbiological testing, and education of, for example, food handlers.

The next step requires the identification of the number of people affected and what they have been exposed to. In order to do this, a working case definition must be created. It is surprising how often this step is overlooked, but without it, highly misleading conclusions can be drawn from an investigation. For example, in an outbreak of food borne illness in which people have presented with symptoms of vomiting, are people who report feelings of nausea to be counted as cases or not? In outbreaks of illnesses with ill-defined symptoms several case definitions may be used to test an association between illness and exposure, but great care must be taken to ensure that whichever case definition is used it is rigorously adhered to.

Case finding methods will vary according to the severity or importance of the suspected disease and the setting in which the outbreak or epidemic has occurred. In a hospital outbreak, there is likely to be a clearly identifiable risk group, however, for the community this is likely to be far more complex. Cases are usually obtained either by finding other people who were exposed to the probable risk factor (for example, people on an affected flight) or by contacting local doctors or hospitals. For diseases which do not have a clear presentation (for example, atypical pneumonia) extensive checking of possible cases, which may be recorded under a different diagnosis, on a local surveillance system or in clinical notes will need to be undertaken. This ensures that case ascertainment is as comprehensive as possible.

Care is required in choosing appropriate controls if either a case control or a cohort study is undertaken. This reduces the risk of inadvertent biases. A discussion of the use of controls in studies of chronic diseases is contained in chapter 2.

The precise method of gathering information from cases and controls will again depend upon the incident being investigated. With a group of tourists who are leaving shortly for their next travel destination the chosen method may be a simple listing of case details along one side of a grid and exposures down the other side. On the other hand, where there is less urgency the chosen method may be administration of a detailed, carefully constructed questionnaire. Whichever method is chosen, it is important that the interviewers ask questions in the same way so that one group of people is not prompted to remember more details than others, thus introducing an element of bias.

Once data have been collected they are arranged in terms of time, place, and person, in the same descriptive epidemiological terms which are described in chapter 2. When graphs of the occurrence of cases over time (an epidemic curve) are plotted it is frequently possible to distinguish different types of epidemic such as a common or point source (Figure 9.3) or person to person transmission (Figure 9.4). In the former there is a rapid upsurge to a peak and then a rapid fall-off. With the latter, the curve is much less steep and the period over which people develop symptoms is much longer as secondary cases appear.

Plotting data geographically can often provide a clue to the source of an infectious agent or the nature of exposure. This has proved particularly useful in determining the source of *Legionella pneumophila* in outbreaks of Legionnaires' disease.

Arranging data in terms of patient characteristics, such as age, sex or occupation may point to a particular risk group or mode of spread.

By this time, the investigators may have a very good idea about the organism responsible, its source and mode of spread. It is still necessary, however, to determine the most likely exposure which caused disease. It is at this stage that hypotheses are formulated and those concerning causation are then tested by using appropriate statistical techniques. When investigating outbreaks of food borne illness it is usual to compare exposure to different foodstuffs in those who developed illness and in those who did not. This is illustrated in the following example of an outbreak of food borne illness amongst hotels guests in Brighton. The results of the investigation are shown in Table 9.2.

An outbreak of gastrointestinal symptoms occurred amongst a party of 136 elderly people who stayed in an hotel over the six day Christmas period. Sixty-eight people were ill. The authorities were notified about the outbreak after the guests had left.

A guest list was obtained. The guests were contacted and a standard questionnaire administered to them asking them about foods eaten and about symptoms. Stool samples were obtained from the 68 guests who had symptoms and from the nine food handlers on duty over the Christmas period. The hotel kitchen was inspected and information obtained about food handling practices, food supplies and cooking methods. Samples of food were taken but little remained from batches used over the period concerned.

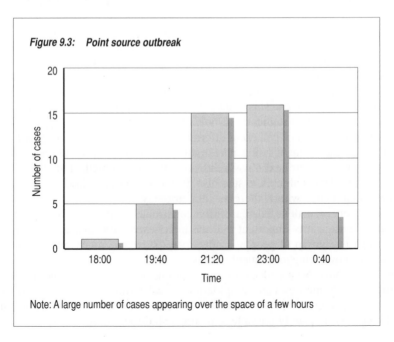

Figure 9.3:   Point source outbreak

Note: A large number of cases appearing over the space of a few hours

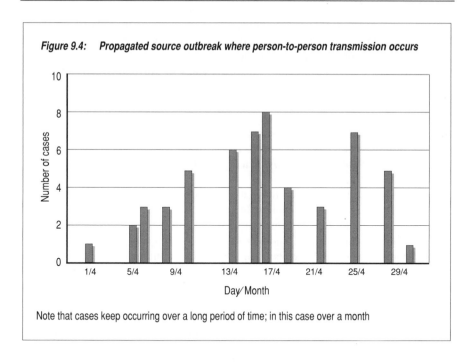

Figure 9.4:   Propagated source outbreak where person-to-person transmission occurs

Note that cases keep occurring over a long period of time; in this case over a month

Analysis of the food items revealed three which showed an independent, statistically significant association with the illness: chocolate mousse, lemon mousse and creme caramel (Table 9.2). All had been made with fresh eggs. The preparation of the mousse involved the heating of raw egg yolks over a low heat for two minutes. The creme caramel was baked in the oven for half an hour. *Salmonella enteritidis* was isolated from the stools of 29 of the 68 cases. A high proportion of these were submitted to phage typing and found to be *phage type 4*. Stool samples from food handlers were negative. No organisms were grown from the food samples which were taken. Kitchen practices were found to be good.

The investigators concluded that it was probable that the organism responsible for the outbreak was introduced into the kitchen via the eggs in the dishes containing raw eggs.

The report described is an excellent example of a practical investigation of a communicable disease outbreak. It should be noted that controls were members of

Table 9.2:   An investigation of an outbreak of Salmonella enteritidis associated with the consumption of egg dishes

Food	Cases		Controls	
	Ate	Did not eat	Ate	Did not eat
Chocolate mousse	66	2	21	14
Lemon mousse	60	4	25	12
Creme caramel	55	9	24	13

Source: Franks C R, Harding B H, Jeffrey P A, Iverson A M, Thom B T. Communicable Disease Report 1990; 90/47.
[Note: People who were unsure of what they ate are excluded from the analysis]

the same hotel party. Some investigations would require controls to be chosen from other sources. Investigators also conclude the probability of the cause being eggs. Investigations establish associations; deciding whether the association is causal or otherwise is a separate process. The same rules of attributing causality apply in communicable disease investigation as in chronic disease investigation (see chapter 2).

In outbreak investigation generally, having identified the probable source, it is important to revisit the facts and ask the following question: does the hypothesis fit with the natural history of the disease in question? The clinical, laboratory and epidemiological results should provide a logical, biologically plausible explanation of the events which have taken place.

At this stage the investigation may be complete or the decision may be taken to conduct additional systematic studies. In any event communicating the findings of an outbreak investigation is extremely important and the final report should contain details of the investigation, the findings and any recommendations.

Once control measures have been implemented, continuing surveillance must be put in place to monitor their effects.

Instigating control measures

The question of when to instigate control measures during a communicable disease investigation can be very difficult. There are no general rules to guide the handling of individual situations. However, it is important both to investigate quickly using sound methodologies and have the best possible information available when taking such decisions. When in doubt, the balance should always lie with protection of the public.

Organisation and management of an investigation

Most investigations will involve teamwork so that coordinating the various team members is an integral part of the investigation. The composition of a team will depend upon the disease under investigation.

An important point to bear in mind, particularly when dealing with a larger outbreak, is the relationship with the media. Possibly because of a fear of sensationalism by the local press, radio and television, many health professionals are apprehensive about having contact with the media. A single spokesperson should be appointed who is acceptable to both health and local authorities and should be available to the media at appointed times only. If either authority has a press officer he or she might be the right person to act as a spokesperson although members of the press often prefer to discuss such matters with a person who is medically qualified. In any case, it is essential that factual information is reported in an unbiased way. Reporters are quick to realise when relevant information is being withheld. They will not expect personal details about patients to be divulged but, otherwise, experience shows that a more accurate report is much more likely to result where the fullest possible information is released to the media. It is wrong to regard the media as a nuisance. Indeed, if good relations are established, particularly with local press, radio and television, this contact can be a great asset, helping, for example, to trace contacts or give health education advice.

ORGANISATION OF SERVICES

Communicable diseases do not respect administrative boundaries and efforts to prevent, control and treat communicable diseases depend upon input from Local Government, the National Health Service, the Public Health Laboratory Service and Central Government.

Local Government

Local authorities are empowered to take action in relation to the control of notifiable diseases within their boundaries. They are required to appoint a proper officer for this function who is usually a public health physician nominated from within the district health authority to provide medical advice relating to communicable disease control. The person concerned is usually the district health authority's Consultant in Communicable Disease Control (CCDC), sometimes it is the authority's Director of Public Health or another consultant in Public Health Medicine who also has other duties within the district health authority's department of public health medicine. The role of public health doctor in the National Health Service is described more fully in chapter 3.

The local authority department concerned with communicable disease control is the Environmental Health Department, led by a Chief Environmental Health Officer. These departments have a wide range of duties which include the registration and investigation of food premises, investigating outbreaks of communicable diseases, monitoring and dealing with other environmental hazards and responding to concerns and enquiries from the public about environmental food quality and communicable disease matters.

Health Authority Services

In addition to the formal communicable disease control responsibilities, health authorities have an important role in promoting health, preventing disease, and securing care to meet the population's needs. Thus, surveillance of communicable diseases, the identification of particular problems and the use of preventive measures such as immunisation programmes are key roles for health authorities.

The health service also has responsibilities for the treatment and care of people with illnesses caused by communicable diseases and parasites. The general practitioner, with the support of the primary care team, is the person who treats the majority of cases of communicable diseases in the community. Only serious cases or those with complications are admitted to hospital. The fall in the incidence of infectious diseases over the years has led to fewer hospital beds being required for treatment. Many general hospitals are able to provide only limited isolation facilities but specialist advice and care is provided by Infectious Diseases Physicians as necessary.

Each major hospital or group of hospitals has a Hospital Control of Infection Committee consisting of senior professional staff. The committee meets at regular intervals and keeps problems in relation to infection in the hospital under review. The day to day work is carried out by an Infection Control Officer, usually a microbiologist on the hospital staff, and a full time Control of Infection Sister. They carry out regular checks on the level of infection (for example, in operating theatres) and deal with outbreaks when they do occur. Reports are made at regular intervals to the committee.

In addition, there is a district Control of Infection Committee whose objective is to provide management support to the Consultant in Communicable Disease Control and ensure interprofessional cooperation within the district.

It should be noted that although both health and local authorities provide an infectious disease control service, neither has a statutory duty to do so. Local authorities are generally believed to be responsible for infectious disease control and, indeed, they do have powers to exercise certain control measures. However, they have no legal requirement to provide a service. Similarly, although health authorities have statutory duties which includes promotion of health, prevention and treatment of disease, they do not have a statutory duty to provide a communicable control disease service.

The Public Health Laboratory Service

The Public Health Laboratory Service was originally established as an emergency service to deal with problems anticipated in World War II, since when, it has proved to be so useful that it was established permanently. It is administered by the Secretary of State for Health through an appointed board whose headquarters and specialist laboratories are at Collindale in London. There are 52 Public Health Laboratories in different parts of the country. Most are in hospitals and take part in the hospital diagnostic microbiology service. They also work closely with the district health authorities and local authority environmental health departments to provide microbiological investigation of communicable disease outbreaks, food and drink products, drinking water quality and routine samples of other material. Local laboratories can refer particular cases to the reference laboratories.

In 1977, the Public Health Laboratory Service established a Communicable Disease Surveillance Centre to make available advice and assistance to Public Health Physicians and others involved in the investigation and control of communicable disease. The Communicable Disease Surveillance Centre is situated in London at the headquarters of the Public Health Laboratory Service with an outpost in Wales. These centres maintain surveillance on the occurrence of communicable disease in England and Wales. The members of staff of the centres also play an important part in educational programmes concerned with the control of infectious diseases. The Communicable Disease (Scotland) Unit (CD(S)U) has provided similar functions since 1969.

Department of Health

The Department of Health has overall responsibility for national policy matters in relation to communicable diseases, for example:

- ensuring that adequate and suitable hospital accommodation is available for communicable disease cases;
- supervision of immunisation levels, not just at the time of outbreaks;
- maintaining international communication networks on communicable diseases matters.

The Chief Medical Officer for England is the Government's principal adviser on communicable disease matters. The Chief Medical Officers for the other United Kingdom countries advise their Ministers directly (although in practice efforts are made to ensure that advice is consistent between the Chief Medical Officers). In turn, the Chief Medical Officer will seek advice from a wide range of sources including experts within and outside the Department of Health and from the Director of the Public Health Laboratory Service (and specialists on his staff).

It is important to remember that the Chief Medical Officer advises Government as a whole and not just the Department of Health. Hence, other relevant departments, for example, the Ministry of Agriculture, Fisheries and Foods or the Department of the Environment may seek or receive advice from the Chief Medical Officer.

LEGISLATION

A considerable amount of legislation exists which relates to the control of the spread of communicable diseases. For half a century, this legislation has been added to and amended as knowledge has advanced and new hazards have been identified. Most of it is enforceable by local authorities although in practice the courts are kept as a last resort and persuasion and education are mainly used.

GENERAL PRINCIPLES OF COMMUNICABLE DISEASE CONTROL

When describing the spread of an infection and its control, three aspects should be considered. These are source, mode of transmission and susceptible recipient (Figure 9.5).

The source

This is the person, animal, object or substance from which an infectious agent is transmitted to a host.

Most communicable diseases in Britain are caused by either bacteria or viruses, and some of these pathogens have man as their sole host. There are numerous exceptions. The Salmonella group of organisms have reservoirs in many domestic and wild animals. Other examples are brucellosis in cattle and rabies in foxes. Viruses multiply only in living cells and never in inanimate substances. Certain fungi may cause infection but most, such as monilia (thrush), are mild and not life threatening except in circumstances where immunity is impaired. Medical parasitology includes the study of pathogenic protozoa, worms and insects. The first two groups often have reservoirs in wild or domestic animals, sometimes with insect vectors and complex life cycles involving several hosts.

Mode of transmission

There are three main mechanisms through which infection can enter the body.

Direct transmission involves the direct transfer of micro-organisms to the skin or mucous membranes by touching, biting, kissing or sexual intercourse. Diseases which spread in this way include scabies (touching), rabies (biting), glandular fever (kissing) and syphilis (sexual intercourse). Droplets spread onto the conjunctiva or

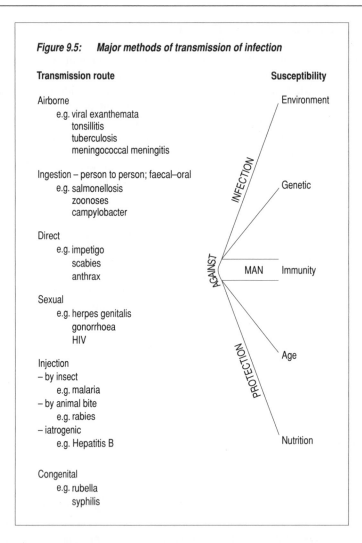

Figure 9.5:   Major methods of transmission of infection

Transmission route   **Susceptibility**

Airborne
    e.g. viral exanthemata
        tonsillitis
        tuberculosis
        meningococcal meningitis

Ingestion – person to person; faecal–oral
    e.g. salmonellosis
        zoonoses
        campylobacter

Direct
    e.g. impetigo
        scabies
        anthrax

Sexual
    e.g. herpes genitalis
        gonorrhoea
        HIV

Injection
– by insect
    e.g. malaria
– by animal bite
    e.g. rabies
– iatrogenic
    e.g. Hepatitis B

Congenital
    e.g. rubella
        syphilis

Environment

Genetic

MAN   Immunity

Age

Nutrition

INFECTION

AGAINST

PROTECTION

other mucous membranes by coughing or sneezing also counts as direct transmission.

Indirect transmission involves an intermediate stage between the source of infection and the individual. The infection may be vehicle-borne for example, by infected food, water, soiled clothing or toys, or vector-borne by insects. Vehicle-borne infections include food poisoning, whilst malaria is vector-borne.

Airborne transmission involves inhaling aerosols containing micro-organisms. It is different from direct transmission by droplets because the particles are much smaller. They can penetrate therefore right down to the alveoli of the lungs and be retained there. The micro-organisms in the aerosols can remain suspended in the air for a long time. Legionnaires' disease is a good example of an infection due to airborne transmission.

Some infections spread from pregnant mothers to their babies via the placenta, for example, rubella.

Measures directed at the route of transmission are key control measures for many communicable diseases. For example, typhoid and cholera may be controlled by the efficient disposal of sewage and the supply of uncontaminated drinking water.

Susceptible recipient

Whether a person develops an infectious disease after contact with any given causal agent is governed by a number of factors such as the virulence and dose of the organism; previous exposure to the organism conferring immunity; the age of the individual (babies up to six months have natural immunity to some infections from their mothers); the nutritional state of the person; the presence of other diseases and whether the individual is receiving immunosuppressive therapy.

DEFINITIONS

It is important to understand the common terminology associated with communicable diseases and parasitology.

Communicable diseases. Synonymous with 'infectious diseases' and sometimes referred to as 'contagious diseases', communicable diseases are caused by a living organism and transmitted from person to person or from animal or bird to man either directly or indirectly.

Epidemic. An epidemic is an increase in the frequency of occurrence of a disease in a population above its baseline level for a specified period of time.

Endemic. An endemic disease is one which is constantly present in a given geographical area, although it may temporarily increase its incidence to become an epidemic.

Pandemic. An epidemic of world-wide proportions.

Sporadic. A term used when cases of communicable diseases are not found to be linked to each other.

Exotic disease. An infectious condition which is not usually found in Britain but may be imported from overseas.

Incubation period. The time which elapses between the person becoming infected and the appearance of the first symptoms. Its length is mainly determined by the nature of the infecting organism but it is also influenced to some extent by the dose of the organism, the route of entry into the body and the susceptibility of the host.

Primary case. The first case which occurs in an outbreak, also referred to as the index case.

Subclinical or unapparent infection. An infection by an agent which gives rise to no reported symptoms or signs in the host.

Carriers. People who intermittently or continuously harbour infective organisms without suffering the clinical manifestations of the disease. People who excrete the organisms only occasionally are referred to as intermittent carriers. Convalescent carriers are those who remain infective even after recovering from the illness and the term chronic carrier is applied if this condition persists over months or years. Typhoid carriers may excrete the organism for years usually because *Salmonella typhi* has infected the gallbladder. Some infections are carried by people who give no history of illness caused by the agent. This healthy carrier state occurs in diphtheria.

Exotoxins. Toxins (poisons) produced by bacteria which pass into the tissues of the body. Examples of organisms which produce toxins resulting in illness are diphtheria and tetanus.

Endotoxins. Types of toxins liberated only when the bacterial cell wall is broken and are important in causing shock.

Disinfection. The killing of an infectious agent outside the body by direct application of a chemical substance or by physical means such as heat. Concurrent disinfection is the application of disinfective measures to discharges, or excreta from the patient, as they occur. Terminal disinfection is the use of disinfective measures after the recovery or removal of the patient. It usually applies to rooms and furniture but is seldom necessary because thorough cleansing and good ventilation are equally effective.

Disinfestation. The removal or destruction of insects, their ova or larvae associated with an individual, his clothing or premises. It also applies to the destruction or removal of rodents.

Reservoir of infection. Any animal, insect, plant or inanimate substance (for example, foodstuff) in which an infectious agent dwells and from which it is capable of being transmitted to a susceptible host.

Droplet infection. Infection caused by a projection of small droplets from the nose or mouth due to sneezing, coughing, talking or exhaling. The range of spread is usually limited to a few feet.

Airborne infection. This is due to the formation of droplet nuclei by evaporation; the particles are small and can be widely dispersed.

Nosocomial infection. An infection occurring in patients or staff which originated within the hospital or other institution.

Medical parasitology. Although many viruses, bacteria and fungi which cause disease in a strictly biological sense are parasites, it is customary to restrict the term medical parasitology to that branch of medicine which deals with those parasites living in or on man which are members of the animal kingdom. They fall into three main groups: protozoa (single cell organisms); helminths (worms); and arthropods (insects).

Zoonoses. Communicable diseases which are transmitted to man from animals.

Hosts. Animals (including man) which give support to and provide a living environment for an infectious agent. Some parasites pass through their stages of development in different hosts.

Definitive or primary host. One in which the parasite reaches maturity or passes through its sexual stage.

Intermediate or secondary host. One in which the parasite is in its larval or asexual stage

Obligatory parasites. Parasites which cannot survive outside the host.

Facultative parasites. Parasites which are capable of an independent existence outside the host.

Pathogenic parasites. Parasites which cause disease.

Commensals. Parasites which cause no harm to the host and one or both may gain benefit. If both gain benefit the state is symbiosis.

Ectoparasites. These parasites live only on the surface of the host's body and are usually insects.

Endoparasites. These parasites live only inside the host's body; examples are worms and many protozoa.

Insect vector. An insect which carries the disease agent either mechanically (on its feet or other parts of its body) or within its body so that the agent is transmitted to the person being infected either by saliva (when the insect bites) or by faeces (deposited on the skin).

INDIVIDUAL COMMUNICABLE DISEASES

Any classification of communicable diseases is necessarily arbitrary. No matter what system is used, some diseases will fit into more than one category. Therefore, in this next section of the chapter, infections which could be placed in more than one category are described in detail once only, but cross-referenced where necessary. Not all the infections described are notifiable, but in order to keep up-to-date with this rapidly changing field, the important, emerging non-notifiable diseases are also discussed.

The main features of some of the important infectious conditions which may be encountered in Britain are also described in this section.

GASTROINTESTINAL INFECTIONS INCLUDING FOOD BORNE ILLNESS

Examples of diseases which can be transmitted by food are discussed throughout this chapter. This particular section deals with the specific causes of food borne illness (sometimes called food poisoning) which result in the acute onset of symptoms, predominantly vomiting and/or diarrhoea.

The causal agents which are responsible for food borne illness are bacterial (these will be considered in detail in this section), viral and relatively infrequently other substances (for example, heavy metal, mushroom and shellfish toxins).

In Britain reported food borne illness caused by infectious agents showed a major upsurge during the 1980s, increasing approximately four times between the start of that decade and the beginning of the 1990s.

This may have reflected an increased tendency on the part of the public to seek help when they had symptoms related to food poisoning or an increased tendency of medical practitioners to investigate and report cases which presented to them. In addition, major changes have occurred in people's eating habits. With more women working outside the home, and the development of a more leisure-orientated society, there is a greater tendency for people not to cook at home. Despite these possible changes in reporting, the underlying trend in food poisoning is of a marked increase in cases.

Salmonella infections

There are some 2,000 Salmonella serotypes which can cause illness in man. In Britain, the reported occurrence of Salmonella food borne infections has increased sharply in the last decade to the beginning of the 1990s (Figure 9.6). Whilst part of the increase is due to increased awareness, and hence greater reporting, it is nevertheless a matter of great public health concern.

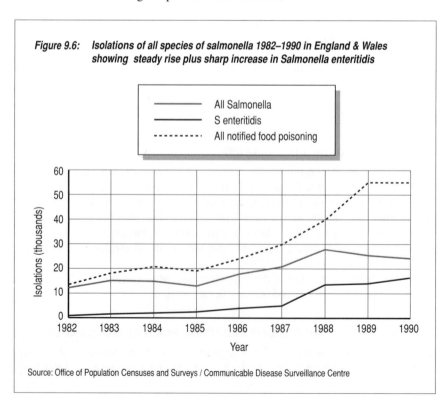

Figure 9.6:   *Isolations of all species of salmonella 1982–1990 in England & Wales showing steady rise plus sharp increase in Salmonella enteritidis*

All Salmonella
S enteritidis
All notified food poisoning

Isolations (thousands)

Year

Source: Office of Population Censuses and Surveys / Communicable Disease Surveillance Centre

One of the principal Salmonella organisms associated with illness in Britain is *Salmonella enteritidis*. Illnesses due to this one organism showed a very large increase in Britain since the mid-1980s. Illnesses caused by Salmonella organisms in food vary in severity. Common symptoms include fever, headache, abdominal pain, diarrhoea and vomiting. Illness usually lasts between one and seven days. However, infections can be fatal, particularly in the elderly or the very young.

Foodstuffs commonly implicated in outbreaks of Salmonella infection include undercooked poultry, pre-cooked meats, eggs (particularly dishes prepared with raw eggs), milk and milk products.

Clostridium botulinum infections

Toxin produced by the organism *Clostridium botulinum*, (a gram-positive, anaerobic bacillus which produces spores that are very resistant to destruction by heat) is the cause of an uncommon but potentially fatal illness called botulism. The toxin affects the nervous system and can cause double vision, respiratory (and more generalised) paralysis in addition to vomiting and diarrhoea.

Classically, the illness is associated with the toxin accumulating in anaerobic conditions (for example, during home bottling or canning of vegetables) but it also occurs with smoked or preserved meats and fish. In the United States, outbreaks of botulism in infants have been associated with contamination of honey by spores of *Clostridium botulinum*, subsequent multiplication of the organism within the intestine and toxin formation (this is an unusual mechanism of acquiring botulism compared with primary ingestion of the toxin). In Britain, cases of botulism have been associated with diverse foodstuffs (Table 9.3). The time between ingestion of the toxin and the onset of symptoms is typically between five and 36 hours but can occur as early as three hours or as late as eight days.

Treatment involves the administration of antitoxin and intensive care, including respiratory support. If such care is instituted promptly and effectively then the case

Table 9.3: Botulism in food in the United Kingdom

Year	Cases	(Deaths)	Implicated food
1922	8	(8)	Duck paste
1932	2	(1)	Rabbit and pigeon broth
1934	1	(0)	Jugged hare
1935	5?	(4?)	Vegetarian nut brawn
1935	1	(1)	Minced meat pie
1947	5	(1)	Macaroni cheese
1955	2	(0)	Pickled fish from Mauritius
1978	4	(2)	Canned salmon from USA
1987	1	(0)	Kosher airline meal
1989	27	(1)	Hazelnut yoghurt

Source: Gilbert R J, Rodhouse J C, Haugh C A. Anaerobes and Food Poisoning. In Clinical and Molecular Aspects of Anaerobes. Borriello SP (ed) Petersfield, England: Wrightson Biomedical Publishing Ltd, 1990.

fatality rate can be reduced. Some people will still die from what is a very serious food borne illness.

Bacillus cereus infections

Bacillus cereus is an aerobic gram-positive bacillus which produces spores and is widely found in nature (for example, in soil and dust).

It produces two main types of illness both of which are self-limiting, almost always leading to a full recovery within a day or so. The first, called the *diarrhoeal type* usually takes longer for symptoms to appear (between eight and 16 hours) and gives rise to severe abdominal pain and profuse diarrhoea (often there is no vomiting). It arises from an enterotoxin which the organism releases into the bowel following infection. The second main presentation of *Bacillus cereus* infection, called the *emetic type* presents with sudden onset of vomiting relatively early (one to six hours) after ingestion of the suspected foodstuff. It is caused by a toxin produced by the organism and accumulated in the contaminated foodstuff prior to ingestion. Diarrhoea is much less common with this presentation.

The diarrhoeal type infection is associated with foods such as cornflour, sauces, soups and meat dishes which have been insufficiently heated. The emetic type infection is classically associated with rice which has been cooked, stored and reheated later (some people for example have contracted this form of *Bacillus cereus* infection after eating a Chinese take-away).

Campylobacter infections

The importance of campylobacter as a cause of gastroenteritis has been recognised relatively recently with the development of improved laboratory techniques for diagnosis. *Campylobacter jejuni* is a gram-negative vibrio-like organism. *Campylobacter coli* is a similar organism which also causes illness in humans.

Between two and 11 days after ingesting the suspected foodstuff, or water, Campylobacter infections result in a range of symptoms but characteristically blood stained diarrhoea occurs. This can be alarming for those concerned (and often results in hospital admission) but usually it subsides and the person affected makes a full recovery.

The source of the organism is probably the gastro-intestinal tract of poultry, cattle and pets. The mode of transmission is usually by food (for example, undercooked poultry), milk or contaminated water. Cases have occurred after drinking milk which has been pecked on the doorstep by wild birds (such as jackdaws).

Staphylococcus aureus infections

Staphylococcus aureus is a very commonly occurring gram-positive coccus which causes a range of infections including superficial skin infections (for example, boils) and wound infections following surgical operations. It is a cause of food borne illness by virtue of the production of a toxin (for example, after it has accumulated in a foodstuff following contamination by a food handler with an infected finger).

Ingestion of the contaminated foodstuff results in sudden onset (usually within one to six hours) of abdominal pain, vomiting and diarrhoea.

Foods commonly incriminated include those left at room temperature for the organism to multiply, for example, cakes, trifles, sandwiches, cold meats. Outbreaks are frequent in the summer when salad lunches and cold buffets are served out of doors, in marquees or pavilions at fetes, weddings or sporting events.

Clostridium perfringens infections

An illness with sudden onset of vomiting, abdominal pain, nausea and diarrhoea (but not usually fever) anything between eight to 24 hours after ingestion of a suspected foodstuff is characteristic of infection with *Clostridium perfringens* (an anaerobic, gram-positive bacillus) which produces spores and is widely distributed in nature (soil and the gut of animals).

It typically occurs when poultry or meat dishes are inadequately cooked in the first place or re-heated. The spores change into vegetative form and grow rapidly if the cooling process is slow or multiply further during re-warming. The organism then produces a toxin when in the intestine. The illness usually lasts about 24 hours and is very seldom fatal (except occasionally in the elderly).

Yersinia infections

Yersinia enterocolitica is a small gram-negative bacillus which is found amongst wild and farm animals (particularly pigs), in water and sewage.

It produces an illness with abdominal pain, diarrhoea and fever which is seen most commonly in children. The clinical picture can closely mimic acute appendicitis or mesenteric adenitis. Erythema nodosum can occur as a complication in up to one third of adults who acquire infection.

The most common routes of transmission are contaminated milk or water or various foodstuffs. Another species of Yersinia, *Yersinia pestis*, whose reservoir is rodents, causes plague. Although a scourge of the past, it no longer occurs in Britain though it is still found in some parts of the world.

Cryptosporidiosis

Cryptosporidium is a protozoan organism with a parasitic life cycle which causes illness after the ingestion of the oocystic stage. It is a relatively commonly reported cause of diarrhoeal illness and usually produces watery diarrhoea which can last up to ten days, or much longer in immunocompromised patients. Water borne transmission can occur and this was the subject of recommendations made by an expert committee (the Badenoch report) which reviewed the risks from domestic water supplies. The organism is spread to humans from infected animals but then can be transmitted from person to person. Contact with farm animals associated with poor personal hygiene is a cause. One outbreak which occurred in Britain resulted from a party of schoolchildren visiting a farm and being encouraged to taste animal foodstuffs. Specific control measures for this disease are still being evolved but the general measures described at the end of this section are relevant.

Escherichia coli infections

Escherichia coli (E. coli) is a gram-negative bacillus which is frequently found in the intestine of humans and animals. *E. coli* organisms are usually classified into four broad groups in each of which there are many serotypes. *Enteropathic E. coli (EPEC)* cause outbreaks of diarrhoea in infants and are a particular problem when they occur in hospital neonatal or paediatric wards.

Enteroinvasive E. coli (EIEC) are very similar in their modes of infection to Shigella bacteria and occur in sporadic cases and outbreaks in similar circumstances to the latter.

Enterotoxigenic E. coli (ETEC) produce toxins and watery diarrhoea rather like that which occurs in cholera. They are a common cause of diarrhoeal illness amongst infants in tropical countries and in adults visiting tropical countries. They are one of the causes of traveller's diarrhoea and are acquired by contaminated food and water.

Verocytotoxin producing E. coli (VTEC) are a group of *E. coli* organisms which also produce toxin similar to shigella. This results in a spectrum of illness ranging from profuse diarrhoea to bloody diarrhoea. Some cases are complicated by the development of the haemolytic uraemic syndrome. This usually affects children and may necessitate them undergoing renal dialysis. A particular sero group of VTEC E. coli, *E. coli 0157* has been responsible for a number of reports of this type of illness in Britain. An upsurge has also occurred in North America where the mode of transmission has been through infected milk and beef products.

Listeriosis

Listeria (more correctly 'listeriosis') made headline news in Britain during the late 1980s when it was one of a number of food hygiene issues which aroused public concern and which led to urgent Government action. The causative organism is a gram-positive bacillus, *Listeria monocytogenes*, which is widely distributed in nature. The organism can grow at temperatures as low as those maintained in refrigerators, which is unusual for a microorganism. It is usually transmitted to man via foodstuffs such as soft cheese, milk, pâté, cold meats, and cook-chill recipe dishes. It is mainly a danger to people whose immune system is impaired or to very young, the very old and pregnant women. It is an important cause of neonatal septicaemia and meningitis and can spread from mother to fetus either *in utero* or through direct contact with mother's infected genital tract. Listeria infection in pregnant women may also cause abortion.

Non-bacterial toxins

In addition to the many food borne illnesses caused by toxins produced by bacteria, some toxins can be ingested in foods which do not result from bacterial sources (Table 9.4).

The prevention and control of food borne illness

A major reduction in the occurrence of food borne illness could be achieved if well established control measures were rigorously applied.

Table 9.4: **Some causes of non-bacterial food poisoning**

Toxin	Source	Comments
Muscarine	Amanita pantherina Amanita muscaria	Toxin found in two of the more common poisonous fungi which can easily be eaten in error. Incubation period < 6 hours. Symptoms include diarrhoea, vomiting, abdominal pain, sweating, twitching, diplopia and convulsions.
Amanitine	Amanita phalloides ("death cap")	Incubation period 6–24 hours. Symptoms include diarrhoea and vomiting, abdominal pain, jaundice and acute renal failure. Mortality 50–90%.
Solanine	Solanum tuberosum (potatoes)	Incubation period is a few hours. Leads to headache, fever, abdominal pain, diarrhoea and vomiting. The alkaloid toxin is water soluble so peeling and soaking potatoes before cooking alleviates the problem.
Scombrotoxin	Scombroid fish – tuna and mackerel. Also pilchards, herring	An increased histamine level in the fish leads to facial flushing, urticarial rash, nausea, diarrhoea and vomiting. Incubation period usually within 1–2 hours.
Ciguatera fish poisoning	Toxin produced by dinoflagellates and accumulates within flesh of fish which feed on them	Incubation period usually within 1–2 hours. Causes nausea, diarrhoea, paraesthesia of mouth and feet, weakness of legs. Seen increasingly because of tendency to holiday in exotic locations. Barracuda is one of the fish implicated.
Paralytic shellfish poisoning	Toxin produced by dinoflagellates which are eaten by shellfish. Toxin does not harm the shellfish but accumulates in the flesh.	Incubation period 30 minutes to 12 hours. Symptoms include circumoral paraesthesiae, numbness of limbs, incoordination, dizziness, drowsiness. In extreme cases may cause respiratory muscle paralysis. Has been a problem in the last few years off the north-eastern coast of Britain.
Tetramine*	Red whelks	Incubation period often less than 1 hour. Causes headache, dizziness, diplopia, incoordination and drowsiness.
Nicotinic acid	Along with ascorbic acid added to minced beef to keep it pink.	Dose-related incubation period. Causes rash and tingling of face and extremities.

Source: Christie A B (1987). Infectious Diseases. Churchill Livingstone: London. (except * which is additional material).

In practice this means enforcing safeguards and taking preventive action at all points in the food chain from the rearing of animals which are to be consumed by humans, to the process of food production, storage and distribution, its points of sale and preparation for eating.

There are control measures which are particular to individual organisms described in this section but the majority of measures are common to all.

Good animal husbandry, careful attention to the content of animal foodstuffs, the raising of Salmonella free flocks of poultry, high standards of slaughterhouse hygiene and a range of other measures are essential steps in ensuring that, when food and drinks are consumed, they are free of harmful microorganisms and their toxins.

It is also important to ensure that strict control measures operate during the manufacture of food. Increasingly food in Britain is bought in processed form. Whether this is as joints of meat or poultry, canned or frozen products or more elaborate heat and serve recipe dishes, measures to prevent food borne illness must be built in at all stages of the production process.

This has implications for design and building materials used in food processing plants, the type of equipment used and how it is maintained, heat and other treatments given to various types of food, the type and content of packaging materials, operating practices for and training of staff, inspection and quality control procedures. Many of the same considerations apply to storage and distribution chains which should maintain the food in a hygienic condition in the interval between it leaving the production plant and reaching the shop, supermarket or catering outlet.

Enormous expenditure and extensive research and development takes place in these aspects of food technology, particularly by the major producers and suppliers.

Food hygiene and safety are an integral part of the food industry but the fact that there is such a large number of producers and suppliers, and the fact that even a small lapse can lead to a serious outbreak of food borne illness, means that the task is one of constant vigilance and improvement of standards.

The storage, handling and preparation of food in the home, in institutions (such as hospitals, schools), in restaurants, cafes and other catering outlets is a vital issue for the prevention and control of food borne illness. This will be evident from the accounts of individual causes of food poisoning earlier in this section of the chapter.

The following are the main principles and practices which are important:

- Maintenance of high standards of personal hygiene by those handling food (for example, washing hands before and after handling food, between stages of preparation and after going to the toilet).
- Separation of raw meat (which should always be regarded as potentially contaminated) from cooked meat and other foodstuffs. Avoidance of cross-infection by using separate cutting tools and other utensils.
- Adoption of recommended standards in the design and layout of food preparation areas and kitchens.
- Keeping kitchen utensils, chopping boards and worktops clean. Cleaning again between stages of preparation and not using the same utensils and surfaces for preparation of raw and cooked food.
- Avoidance of transference of infection from the nose and throat by the fingers to food. Where all cuts and sores occur, ensuring that they are covered.
- Exclusion of people with symptoms of food poisoning and symptomless carriers from food handling.
- Attention to the temperature of storage. Fridges and freezers should be kept at the correct temperatures: below 4 degrees centigrade and below −18 degrees centigrade respectively. Thermometers should always be in place to check

temperatures. Foods should not be maintained at room temperature for any length of time. High risk foods should be held in the temperature danger zone (5°C to 63°C) for the shortest possible time. Cold foods (for example, salads, cream cakes) should be kept refrigerated and hot foods (for example, casseroles, meat dishes) should be kept hot (not warm). Frozen food, especially poultry, must be completely defrosted before cooking and, if possible, eaten immediately.

- Special care should be taken when cooking food for later use and when re-heating it. Cooling should be undertaken quickly using small quantities. Re-heating should not be undertaken more than once and should take place quickly and thoroughly.
- Shoppers should take chilled or frozen food home quickly and store it in the fridge or freezer rather than letting it stand in the car or office. It is good practice to use cool boxes, especially in the summer.
- Food should be allowed to stand for the recommended periods of time before serving after microwave cooking.
- Pets should be kept out of, and pests and insects should be eliminated from, food storage, display and preparation areas.

Ensuring proper adherence to these measures in all situations in which food is stored, prepared and served is clearly a major and difficult task. In the commercial context it requires that senior management is fully committed to food hygiene and safety and that all relevant staff are effectively trained and qualified. With the kind of transient workforces which exist in the catering and hotel industries this requires special effort. In addition, environmental health officers play a key role in education and in protecting the public.

Careful preparation of food in the home is just as important as it is for large scale catering concerns. Even if foodstuffs are contaminated when they are bought, the measures listed above can be taken in the home to ensure that micro-organisms do not cause illness either directly or through being spread to other foods.

It is essential that the public also receives information on specific issues, for example, about the risks of home bottling of vegetables and botulism (described earlier). The public needs also to be given specific advice on food borne illness from time to time. For example, because of the risks of Salmonella transmission, current Government advice to the general public is not to eat raw eggs. To pregnant women, to the very young, to the elderly and to the sick the advice is that eggs should be cooked until the white and the yolk are hard before they are eaten.

The law relating to food borne illness

In addition to general legislation relating to communicable diseases, specific pieces of legislation relating to food hygiene and safety are an important element of the range of control measures for food borne illness.

The Report of the Committee on the Microbiological Safety of Food (Chairman: Sir Mark Richmond) provided the basis for the Food Safety Act 1990, a pivotal piece of legislation.

The Food Safety Act 1990 is intended to span the spectrum of food production, processing, distribution, preparation and sale to ensure high standards of quality control and safety. It also places particular emphasis on consumers both in terms of protecting and ensuring that they receive information about food as an entitlement.

Under the Act and its associated regulations, it is a requirement that all food premises should be registered as a food business. This provides local authorities with a register upon which to enforce the law and carry out inspections. It is an offence to operate in food premises other than those which are registered. It is also an offence to provide food injurious to health (penalties involve large fines and possible imprisonment).

Regulations associated with the Act relating to the *Training of Food Handlers* have had far reaching implications for the food and catering industries, laying down requirements for mandatory training and certified training courses.

An important aspect of the Food Safety Act 1990 is that it is enabling legislation. It allows Government to bring in secondary legislation at any time to deal with problems as they arise. Changes in the law are being harmonised with European Community directives. A range of other legislation introduced at the beginning of the 1990s targeted the animal end of the food chain.

OTHER INFECTIVE CAUSES OF VOMITING AND DIARRHOEA

Illnesses characterised by vomiting, diarrhoea and associated symptoms are common in the population but not all are food borne. Many are transmitted from person to person by the faecal-oral route or by droplets. Some of the organisms which can be transmitted in this way can also be food borne.

This section of the chapter describes organisms which cause illness mainly through person to person spread, though the fact that they are not described in the previous section does not mean that some of them cannot also be spread by ingestion of food contaminated with the organism.

Viruses

A variety of viruses regularly cause diarrhoea and vomiting. A spectrum of gastro-intestinal symptoms in which viruses have been implicated has been recognised for many years and referred to as winter or summer vomiting depending on its season of onset. Characteristics of viral gastroenteritis are that symptoms are sometimes severe but shortlived, lasting up to 24 hours and the incubation period is usually fairly short. Fatalities are rare but can occur in the elderly and the very young. Viruses are much more difficult to identify from specimens like faeces than are bacteria and are only present at the beginning of the acute stage of the illness so that reported cases undoubtedly grossly under-represent the true size of the problem.

The fact that people do not always present to medical care for these self-limiting illnesses, the fact that general pracititoners treat symptomatically and do not collect samples, and the fact that viruses are difficult to isolate from human and food specimens means that their frequency in the population and other aspects of their epidemiology are not well understood.

Rotaviruses are RNA viruses which cause vomiting, diarrhoea and fever, mainly amongst children under five years of age. Adults are less frequently affected. *Adenoviruses* cause similar symptoms.

Another group of viruses which cause symptoms of diarrhoea and vomiting are the so called *'small round viruses'*, of which the most well known is, perhaps, the

Norwalk Virus. Small round viruses are probably responsible for up to one third of non-bacterial outbreaks of gastroenteritis. Sewage pollution of shellfish is an important means of food-borne spread.

Dysentery: bacillary

Causal agent

Shigella is a group of gram-negative bacilli of which there are four species: *Shigella sonnei* which accounts for the great majority of cases of dysentery occurring in Britain; *Shigella flexneri* only an occasional cause of infection in Britain but found most frequently in hospitals for the mentally ill or mentally handicapped; *Shigella boydii* and *Shigella dysenteriae* very seldom the cause of dysentery in Britain.

Frequency and distribution

The disease has a worldwide distribution. In Britain there are several thousand notifications each year. Outbreaks of sonnei dysentery are often associated with day and residential nurseries, nursery schools and infant schools as well as mental illness and mental handicap hospitals.

Identification

There are many mild cases of this disease whilst others have few or no symptoms. When the full clinical picture occurs it is typified by diarrhoea of acute onset (with mucus, blood and pus in more severe cases), abdominal pain and fever.

The laboratory diagnosis of Shigella infection is made by isolation of the organisms from the faeces. This applies to acute cases as well as chronic carriers.

Incubation period

Usually two to three days but can vary between one and seven days.

Infectivity period

Patients are highly infectious during the acute stage of the illness and continue to excrete the organism for about four weeks after recovery. In a minority of cases, a chronic carrier state may develop.

Reservoir

Man.

Mode of transmission

By the faecal-oral route either directly or indirectly. The direct method is probably quite common. Young children carry the infection on their hands and pass it to other children or members of the family. Indirect transmission by ingestion of contaminated food or drink is also quite common.

Control measures

In an established case, standard precautions should be instituted, including care in the handling of excreta from the patient. Bacteriological screening of well contacts is usually not necessary unless the contacts are food handlers or work in the health care field. General preventive measures include hand washing after using the toilet, the use of disposable paper towels, regular cleaning of lavatory door handles and seats and extra precautions in the preparation of food. Food handlers with bacillary dysentery should be excluded from work until three negative specimens have been obtained. In the event of an outbreak in a day nursery, all new admissions should cease and all infected children should be excluded. Three negative specimens are required before affected children may be re-admitted. Once an outbreak is established in an infants school or nursery it is difficult to control the spread of sonnei dysentery even with the measures recommended. General environmental measures are less important in Britain but include adequate disposal of sewage and the control of fly populations.

Dysentery: amoebic

Causal agent

Entamoeba histolytica, a protozoan which can become a cyst with a tough resistant membrane. In the human intestine it can emerge from the cyst in its active form and cause symptoms.

Frequency and distribution

Most common in the tropics and sub-tropics. Most of the cases occurring in Britain each year are people who have contracted the disease in an endemic area overseas. A small proportion, possibly 2% of the population, are carriers.

Identification

There is a spectrum of severity with many people remaining asymptomatic whilst others proceed to ulceration of the bowel and hepatic involvement. The classical clinical picture of amoebic dysentery is abdominal pain and recurrent attacks of diarrhoea containing blood or mucus. There are periods of remission and the cycle may continue for years. From this primary colonic site, in a small proportion of cases, the infection can spread to involve other organs (most often the liver). It is important to exclude amoebic dysentery when making the diagnosis of ulcerative colitis. The diagnosis is made by observing large amoebae containing red blood cells on microscopic examination of specimens of faeces. Tests on sera are available but are positive in only a proportion of cases and, most importantly, do not identify the carrier state.

Incubation period

Variable, most often two to four weeks, but can extend to months.

Infectivity period

Cysts may be passed in the faeces for many years.

Reservoir

Man is the sole reservoir either as symptomless excreter or with the chronic disease.

Mode of transmission

The infection is transmitted by the cysts by faecal-oral spread. The usual vehicle is contaminated water or food, especially salads and raw fruit.

Control measures

Provided proper precautions are taken in nursing the patient no isolation is necessary nor is there any need for surveillance of contacts except to ensure that fellow travellers have not contracted the disease. The maintenance of good standards of personal hygiene and the exclusion of cases and carriers from food handling are important in preventing this disease, as is the provision of a pure water supply and an adequate sewage disposal system.

Enteric fever

Causal agents

Salmonella typhi (typhoid fever), *Salmonella paratyphi* types A, B and C (paratyphoid fever). These are gram-negative rods identical in appearance and only distinguished by different reactions in laboratory tests. An enteric fever-like illness can also be caused by other members of the salmonella family which usually cause gastro-enteritis.

Frequency and distribution

The diseases occur in all parts of the world but endemic typhoid and paratyphoid has been virtually eliminated from North Western Europe, North America and Australasia. Imported disease is, however, still common. The majority (approximately 90%) of the few hundred cases of typhoid in Britain each year are contracted abroad, although cases of typhoid and occasional outbreaks have occurred indigenously. Similarly most of the 100 or so notified cases of paratyphoid fever in Britain are contracted abroad.

Identification

The clinical picture of typhoid fever varies. Symptoms can include: pyrexia, headache, anorexia and constipation more often than diarrhoea. A classical rose spot rash may appear on the trunk and enlargement of the spleen may also occur. Rarely intestinal ulceration and perforation may occur. Paratyphoid fever has similar but milder symptomatology with a lower fatality rate. Clinical symptoms depend on the dose of the organism and a much larger dose is required to cause paratyphoid fever than typhoid fever. Sub-clinical cases of paratyphoid fever also occur. The laboratory diagnosis of the enteric fevers is made by isolating the organisms from blood culture (which is usually positive in the first week of illness) or from culture of faeces or urine (usually in the second and third weeks of the illness). Antibodies can be detected from the second week (Widal test) and a sharply rising titre in serial samples of sera confirms the diagnosis.

Incubation period

For typhoid fever this is usually 10–14 days but can vary from one to three weeks depending on the dose of organism. Paratyphoid infections have a shorter incubation period.

Infectivity period

For as long as the person excretes the organism, usually from the early stages of the illness until some weeks or even months after recovery.

Reservoir

Man. Usually the organism is found in the faeces but also can occur in the urine. Up to 5% of typhoid fever cases become permanent carriers. A permanent residue of infection is the gall bladder and in extremely persistent carrier states where antibiotic therapy has failed surgical intervention to remove it may be considered.

Mode of transmission

The mode of transmission of infection *par excellence* is by food and drink which have been contaminated by faeces of the case or carrier. Particularly implicated are those substances on which the organism can multiply: pastries, meat, milk, milk products, ice cream, raw fruit and vegetables. Direct or indirect contact with a case or carrier is another possible means of spread but is much less common. Impure water supplies have also been responsible for typhoid outbreaks.

Control measures

Cases should be isolated and particular care should be taken when handling the patient's urine and faeces. Contacts should be traced, kept under surveillance for three weeks and investigated if symptoms occur. If the contacts are food handlers or work with vulnerable groups of people (for example, health care workers) they should be excluded from work during this period. If the infection is traced to a food source, then a search should be made amongst the food handlers to identify the carrier. Special care must be taken to ensure that the recovered case does not return to food handling until clear of infection and many experts recommend that patients who have had typhoid should never again handle food. The same approach should be taken with employees of water companies. Education of ex-patients about the risks of contaminating food is important. Monovalent typhoid vaccine gives around 70% protection to travellers to areas where typhoid is endemic but it is important that travellers are aware of the risks and take precautions with their choice of food and do not drink local tap water. Other environmental control measures include adequate sewage disposal, the provision of a pure water supply and the control of flies and rodents. The public should be educated to high standards in food handling and particular care should be taken when dealing with milk and shellfish.

Cholera

Causal agent

Vibrio cholerae, a slightly curved and twisted (comma shaped), motile, aerobic gram-negative rod. The 01 serogroup includes two bio-types cholerae: classical and El Tor. Both produce illnesses which are indistinguishable but they differ in laboratory haemolysis tests.

Frequency and distribution

During the last several hundred years, classical cholera has been endemic in the basins of the rivers Ganges and Brahmaputra, from which it has spread repeatedly as pandemics to many countries of the world. Fatality rates have been high especially amongst the poor. A pandemic of the El Tor variant started in Indonesia in the 1960s and reached Western Europe. Britain has been virtually free of cholera during the present century except for the occasional imported case.

Evidence of the devastating effects which epidemics of the disease can still have in many parts of the World are seen from time to time on the television screens of the West when there are natural disasters (floods, earthquakes) or war. In such circumstances, sanitation can break down as people are displaced from their houses into makeshift and overcrowded camps. Cholera outbreaks then occur, often associated with huge loss of life, especially in the very young.

Identification

The characteristic clinical features of cholera are very severe diarrhoea with copious watery stools ('rice water') accompanied by vomiting and rapid dehydration. The latter causes death in a high proportion of untreated cases. The organism may be identified in cultures from specimens of vomit, faeces or in rectal swabs. A rise in antibody titre in paired samples of sera is helpful in confirming the diagnosis.

Incubation period

Usually one to three days, although may be up to five days.

Infectivity period

The organism is excreted during the illness and for a few days after recovery. The carrier state is uncommon and usually lasts only a few months, in contrast to typhoid fever.

Reservoir

Man is the only known mammalian host, although recent observations from America and Australia suggest that environmental reservoirs might exist.

Mode of transmission

Mainly by faeces contaminated water but also by food and flies. Direct spread from cases, carriers or contaminated objects is very much less important. Gastric acid acts as a protector against infection.

Control measures

Acutely ill patients require hospital treatment with careful management to replace lost fluids and electrolytes but strict isolation is unnecessary. Surveillance of contacts is important and their stools should be examined for *Vibrio cholerae* for five days following the last exposure. Vaccination gives low protection and short lived immunity and is therefore of limited value. People travelling to areas where cholera is known to be present should take precautions with drinking water, salads and other uncooked foods. The main environmental control measures are the protection of water supplies and supervision of disposal of sewage. Health education of food handlers and measures to protect food against flies are also important. In a country with modern water supply and sewage disposal systems, cholera is of almost no public health importance (aside from recognising occasional imported cases).

RESPIRATORY INFECTIONS

A number of organisms described in this chapter cause respiratory infections. Acute upper respiratory infections are still the commonest manifestation of illness caused by communicable disease in the population of Britain. They range from colds, coughs, ear infections and bronchitis, to pneumonia. A wide range of organisms are responsible, most of them viruses. Although such illnesses occur throughout the year, most display a marked seasonal variation. Some common examples are: viruses causing the common cold (for example, rhinoviruses, myxoviruses, picornaviruses, coronaviruses); viruses causing sore throats (for example, ECHO virus, Coxsackie virus, adenoviruses); the Epstein-Barr virus which causes infectious mononucleosis (also called glandular fever); the respiratory syncytial virus which causes coughs, ear and chest infections; parainfluenza viruses which cause croup in children and other respiratory infections.

There are no satisfactory control measures for this group of infections and action is directed at minimising the complications of the clinical syndrome by prompt diagnosis, symptomatic treatment and treatment of complications.

Streptococcal infections

Causal agent

Streptococci are gram-positive, spherical in shape and tend to form chains when they grow. An important feature which determines their classification is whether or not they produce haemolysis when grown on a medium containing red blood cells (beta-haemolytic streptococci); only partial or incomplete haemolysis (alpha-haemolytic streptococci) or no haemolysis at all. A further classification is made on the basis of antigenic differences in the components of the cell wall. On this basis beta-haemolytic streptococci are divided into a number of serological groups (A to O).

Beta-haemolytic group A streptococci are the most important human pathogen and often cause sore throats and tonsillitis. *Scarlet fever* is now, fortunately, an infrequent complication. More rarely the organism can result in a number of other infections: erysipelas, impetigo, puerperal fever or bacterial endocarditis. After a delay of several weeks, infection with the beta-haemolytic Group A streptococcus may result in acute nephritis, or rheumatic fever. These delayed manifestations are probably hypersensitivity reactions and not infections. They were much more common in the past but it is possible that they will again become problematic if virulence of the causative organism changes.

Haemolytic streptococci also cause other infections. Groups A, B and G cause several thousand cases of bacteraemia each year in Britain. The infection occurs in all age groups but is particularly serious when it occurs in babies, especially premature babies. Much less commonly, the same groups of organism cause bacterial meningitis. Again all age groups are affected but the disease is a particular problem in neonates.

Frequency and distribution

The disease occurs in most parts of the world but is more common in temperate zones.

Identification

Streptococcal throats are characterised by sudden onset of sore throat, fever and inflamed tonsils, with exudate and enlarged lymph glands. The tongue has a strawberry-like appearance in the early stages of the disease. The main differential diagnosis is with viral infections of the upper-respiratory tract. If, in addition, an erythematous rash appears several days later scarlet fever is likely. At the beginning of the century this disease was a major cause of death of children but is now a milder, treatable illness. The more serious complications: bacteraemia, nephritis, meningitis, endocarditis, rheumatic fever are identified by the clinical manifestations characteristic of these conditions. It can usually be cultured from throat swabs, where the beta-haemolytic streptococcus will be seen surrounded by its characteristic zone of haemolysis. Blood cultures are taken where bacteraemia is suspected. Rising serum antibody titres may be helpful in aiding diagnosis.

Incubation period

Two to three days.

Infectivity period

Most patients cease to be infective twenty-four hours after the treatment with antibiotics, although in some, persistent carrier state may develop.

Reservoir

Man.

Mode of transmission

Direct contact, droplet spread and via articles freshly contaminated with nasopharyngeal secretions. Airborne spread is unlikely as the streptococcus does not resist drying well. In the past, outbreaks have occurred through infected milk.

Control measures

Isolation of the case is probably unnecessary because the patient becomes non-infective shortly after treatment is started but it is usual to keep close contacts under surveillance for a few days to see if they develop the disease. In closed communities of children, prophylactic antibodies should be considered and in hospitals, children with streptococcal sore throat should be separated from other patients.

Pneumonia is a common cause of death amongst elderly people and those with suppressed immune systems. A wide range of organisms can be responsible.

It is much less common in younger, previously healthy people. When it does occur in such circumstances, the common organisms are Pneumococcus which may cause classical lobar pneumonia. *Mycoplasma pneumoniae* also can cause pneumonia but is also much more commonly responsible for milder respiratory illnesses. In Britain it tends to occur in small winter epidemics every four years or so.

Legionnaires' disease

Causal agent

The illness derived its name from 183 cases of pneumonia which occurred amongst nearly 4,000 delegates attending an American Legion convention in Philadelphia in July 1976. The episode attracted wide publicity, particularly in view of the 15% fatality rate and it was intensely investigated. Many agents were suggested as being responsible for the outbreak, some of them fanciful, but it was eventually established that the disease was caused by a small gram-negative bacillus (named *Legionella pneumophila*), previously unrecognised, which was isolated from the water in the air-conditioning system in the hotel. Since then, over 30 species of *Legionella* have been identified and more than a dozen serogroups of *Legionella Pneumophila*.

Frequency and distribution

Between two and three hundred cases occur in England and Wales each year, mostly sporadic or in small groups. About one third of affected people acquire the infection abroad. A number of larger outbreaks have occurred.

An outbreak in which 101 people developed Legionnaires' disease (28 died from it) was associated with a hospital cooling tower in Stafford in 1985. The subsequent Committee of Inquiry made recommendations which form part of present policy to control the disease. Another outbreak affecting over 90 people in central London in 1988 was associated with a British Broadcasting Corporation (BBC) building.

Identification

The disease is commonest in adults and whilst anyone can acquire the infection, those who smoke heavily, or who have a chronic disease appear to be at higher risk.

Early symptoms are non-specific with fever, malaise, myalgia, headache and often diarrhoea. As the illness progresses the patient develops a high fever and non-productive cough which becomes productive. Chest signs are often unimpressive and not in-keeping with the marked changes observed on chest X-ray. The overall case fatality rate in patients admitted to hospital is about 15 per cent. In addition to history and clinical features, diagnosis is made by culture of the organism from secretions, serological testing and more sophisticated tests carried out in specialist reference laboratories to which samples may be sent.

Incubation period

Usually between two and ten days but may be as long as 18 days.

Infectivity period

Person-to-person spread has not been demonstrated.

Reservoir

The bacterium is widely distributed in nature and often found in soil and water. Although not usually found in mains water supplies, it may become established in hot water systems in large buildings such as hotels, hospitals and office blocks. Surveys have shown that the organism is commonly present in systems of such buildings. The likelihood of this is increased by stagnation and temperatures between 20°C and 45°C. Water cooled air conditioning systems and the towers associated with them are another common source of the organism.

Mode of transmission

The presence of *Legionella pneumophila* does not usually lead to an outbreak of Legionnaires' disease. Nevertheless, the main route of infection when it does occur, seems to be via inhalation of contaminated aerosols from cooling towers or from shower-heads.

Control measures

Since Legionnaires' disease was first recognised and since the larger outbreaks which have occurred in Britain, a wide range of regulatory and standard setting guidance has been put in place. This will continue to be updated as research into the organism and the disease continues. The key to control lies in preventive measures taken by those involved in the design, operation, supervision and maintenance of water systems and cooling systems, particularly in large buildings. Detailed codes of practice are available, much of them of a highly technical nature. Important aspects include regular inspection, cleaning and disinfection as well as careful temperature regulation.

Because of the specialised nature of the control measures, various expert committees have been created to advise Government and other bodies on codes of practice and other measures necessary to prevent and control the disease.

A rare non-pneumonic infection with *Legionella pneumophila* also occurs: so called 'Pontiac Fever'. It has a much shorter incubation period (five to 66 hours) and, although the attack rate is much higher (approximately 95% in outbreaks compared with 0.1–5% for Legionnaires' disease), it is a much less severe illness from which patients recover spontaneously in about two to five days.

Influenza

Causal agent

Influenza viruses, of which three types have been identified. Epidemics are caused by types A and B. Type C is less common and associated with sporadic cases.

Frequency and distribution

It is worldwide in its occurrence. The very high fatality rate of the pandemic of 1918–19 (as many as 20 million people are estimated to have died) is thought to have been due to poor nutrition following World War I but it may have resulted from a virus of enhanced virulence. Later pandemics caused by different strains of the Type A influenza virus – the 'Asian' influenza pandemic of 1957–58 and the 'Hong Kong' influenza pandemic of 1968–69 – produced milder illnesses, but large numbers of fatalities occurred particularly in susceptible groups such as the elderly. Although sporadic cases are reported, large or small epidemics are the usual mode of occurrence. They occur with a regular periodicity of about three to four years and peak occurrences are in the winter months. Mortality is mainly confined to elderly people but the excess deaths from all causes which occur in the population at the time of an influenza epidemic can be very substantial.

Identification

The clinical picture is of sudden onset of headache, fever, muscle pains and respiratory symptoms which may be followed by secondary bacterial infection. Respiratory infections are often labelled as 'flu' when they are not in fact truly caused by the influenza virus. Indeed, the kind of upper respiratory symptoms which occur with the common cold are not a feature of influenza. In the early stages of the illness, the virus may be grown in culture from throat or nasal swabs. An increasing level of antibody in paired sera at 10 to 14 day intervals may assist in making the diagnosis. A rare but important complication in children (usually with influenza B) is the development of Reye's syndrome which affects the liver and the central nervous system and occurs if a child has been given salicylates (aspirin) to reduce his or her temperature. The use of aspirin in children, particularly those under 12 years is not therefore recommended.

Incubation period

This is short, usually one to four days.

Infectivity period

It is a highly infectious disease particularly during the early period of the illness. Adults are infectious for the first three to five days after clinical onset, and children a little longer, until about seven days.

Reservoir

Man, although identical type A viruses have been isolated from horses, birds and swine. Hence it has been suggested that changes in the genetic structure may arise from animal reservoirs or are mixtures of human and animal strains. Types B and C have been isolated only from man.

Mode of transmission

Droplet and airborne spread and directly by objects contaminated with fresh secretions from the nasopharynx.

Control measures

There is little value in isolating cases because of the large number of cases which occur in epidemics. Active immunisation with the influenza vaccine is usually reserved for people at special risk such as the elderly and those with cardio-respiratory problems. The Chief Medical Officer issues guidance each autumn about the prevailing influenza strains. Immunisation is around 70% – 80% effective in giving protection to healthy young adults. It is less effective in the elderly. Although it does not necessarily prevent infection, immunisation modifies the severity of the illness. Regular changes in the antigenic profile of the virus mean that the vaccine components have to be reviewed each year.

Tuberculosis

Causal agents

Mycobacterium tuberculosis: human type; *Mycobacterium bovis:* bovine type.

Frequency and distribution

Tuberculosis is endemic in most countries of the world. In Britain, there has been a dramatic decline in the number of notifications and deaths from tuberculosis during the present century. A concurrent decline in other infectious conditions means that tuberculosis remains an important endemic infectious disease. At the beginning of the 1990s there was a worrying worldwide resurgence of the disease, in part linked to the growing number of susceptible people with AIDS.

The disease is a particular problem in immigrants in Britain, especially those of Asian origin, where it has a much higher reported incidence than in the indigenous population (notifications of respiratory tuberculosis approximately thirty times higher; non-respiratory tuberculosis approximately eighty times higher). Other risk groups include homeless people and those whose immunity is suppressed. For example, in the summer of 1990, nine cases of tuberculosis occurred amongst children on the oncology ward of the Royal Liverpool Children's Hospital.

Identification

The primary infection in childhood usually occurs without noticeable symptoms. It is overcome with the body's natural defence mechanisms. The lesion becomes inactive, the person recovers and acquires tuberculin sensitivity and a degree of resistance. In a small proportion of children, progressive primary pulmonary tuberculosis may ensue. Rarely, a miliary form occurs in which the infection is widely disseminated through the body in the blood stream, producing a serious illness in which there may be meningeal involvement. In the adult, pulmonary tuberculosis is the most important form of the disease and is a major source of infection for other members of the population. There is a clinical spectrum of severity but many cases may present only with a persistent, productive cough. Other symptoms include lassitude, fever, loss of weight and haemoptysis. It is a chronic condition in which there is gradual erosion of the lung tissue with exacerbations and remissions. Diagnosis is confirmed by a chest X-ray and bacteriological examination of sputum. The adult disease is considered by many authorities to result from reactivation of lesions which have lain dormant since primary infection. A proportion of infections will also occur through first infection taking place in adult life, but the relative frequencies of such cases is not known.

Non-respiratory tuberculosis is also of importance, particularly in the Asian population, and may affect most systems of the body. Particularly common sites are the bones and joints, the genito-urinary tract and the lymph nodes (typically the cervical glands).

Incubation period

From the time of exposure to development of a primary lesion can take from one to three months, as demonstrated by a strongly positive tuberculin reaction. The development of secondary lesions may take years but the risk is highest within the first two years of infection.

Infectivity period

The case is infectious as long as viable tubercle bacilli are produced in sputum. However, the degree of infectivity depends on the virulence of the organism, the closeness of contacts, the personal behaviour of the sputum-positive individual and the degree of immunity of the exposed person.

Reservoir

Man for the human type and cattle for the bovine type.

Mode of transmission

Droplets spread from an infected person; indirect spread is not thought to be important. Bovine tuberculosis is usually spread from drinking unpasteurised milk from infected cows. All cattle in Britain are now in tuberculosis-free herds.

Control measures

Strict isolation of the case in hospital is no longer necessary because an appropriate chemotherapy quickly renders the organisms which are coughed up non-viable. They may be demonstrated though in the sputum on staining for several weeks after the commencement of antimicrobial therapy. Although outpatient treatment is the normal approach, inpatient hospital treatment may be indicated for certain clinical or social reasons. All contacts of the patients should be traced and screened using tuberculin testing and/or chest X-ray if necessary.

People who have or have had tuberculosis show a skin reaction to protein from the tubercle bacillus (tuberculin). This is administered either as a single measured dose injected intradermally (the Mantoux test) or in the form of small multiple punctures of the skin (the Heaf test). In each case, the skin reaction is assessed after a specified period of time. The degree of reaction to the test is the basis for a decision on further action. Strong reactors should be referred to a chest clinic for further investigation. BCG vaccination should be offered to negative reactors as follows, the infants of tuberculous parents; contacts of open cases; in some parts of the country immigrants and their babies; nurses and doctors who are at special risk of exposure to infection; laboratory workers likely to deal with sputum; schoolchildren aged between 11 and 13 years. In some parts of the country this last indication has been abandoned because it was felt to be uneconomical in the light of the falling incidence of tuberculosis. However, a recent increasing trend might necessitate revision of this decision. Pre-employment chest X-rays are recommended for special groups for their own protection and for those with whom they may associate, such as teachers, nurses, doctors and special occupational groups already mentioned. Repeated routine X-ray examinations are no longer recommended. There have been examples of outbreaks of tuberculosis arising in children where the source of infection has been a teacher with tuberculosis. Mass radiography which played a large part in reducing tuberculosis in the past is no longer regarded as economic for use with the public at large.

Screening of new immigrants to Britain should also be carried out. Now that all the dairy herds in Britain are tuberculosis-free and over 90% of milk is pasteurised, the risks from bovine infection have become very much less.

INFECTIONS FOR WHICH COMPREHENSIVE IMMUNISATION PROGRAMMES ARE AVAILABLE

An important way of combating certain infectious diseases is through the childhood immunisation programme. This section describes those infections for which large scale immunisation is available (Table 9.5). Tuberculosis is covered in the respiratory diseases section and *Haemophilius influenzae* type B in the section on meningitis.

Measles

Causal agent

The Measles virus is a paramyxovirus.

Frequency and distribution

Measles occurs in all parts of the World. In developed countries it is usually a mild disease with a low mortality rate but in developing countries, with poorly nourished inhabitants, childhood mortality can be 10% or more. Until the introduction of mass measles vaccination few people in Britain reached adult life without having had the disease. The use of the vaccine has also altered the previous classical two-

Table 9.5: **Childhood immunisation schedule in operation from October 1992**

Age	Vaccine	Comment
2 months	Diphtheria, Pertussis, Tetanus (DPT) Oral Polio Vaccine (OPV) *Haemophilus influenzae* b (Hib)	Killed Live-attenuated Killed
3 months	DPT OPV Hib	
4 months	DPT OPV Hib	
12–24 months	Measles/Mumps/Rubella (MMR) (+ Hib if not previously given)	Live-attenuated
5 years (school entry)	DT OPV (+ MMR if not previously given)	
10–14 years	Rubella	Live-attenuated For girls not previously given MMR
	BCG (Bacille Calmette-Guerain)	Live-attenuated Given to tuberculin negative children. Some authorities no longer give it routinely.
15–19 years (school leaving)	OPV Tetanus	

yearly epidemic but the number of notifications continues to be substantial (13,302 in 1990).

Identification

The virus produces a prodromal illness with upper respiratory symptoms, pyrexia and spots (Koplik spots) on the buccal mucosa. Classically the maculopapular rash appears on the fourth day of the illness but this is variable. The blotchy rash starts on the face and spreads over the body. Secondary bacterial infection of the respiratory tract and otitis media are common complications, encephalitis is rare. A very rare complication is sub-acute sclerosing panencephalitis which develops late (approximately seven years after infection) and results in death within a few months. The frequency of cases proceeding to complications has remained unchanged since the introduction of the vaccination programme. The diagnosis is usually made purely on clinical grounds but a rising antibody titre is also indicative.

Incubation period

Seven to fourteen days, usually ten days.

Infectivity period

This is a very infectious illness particularly in the prodromal phase and the patient is infectious for four to five days after the appearance of the rash.

Reservoir

Man only.

Mode of transmission

Droplet spread and directly by objects freshly contaminated by secretions from the nasopharynx.

Control measures

Immunisation offers the only real protection. The advent of a combined vaccine (mumps, measles and rubella) in Britain in late 1988, coupled with targets to achieve high uptake in the population, gives hope that measles will be greatly reduced or even eradicated in the near future. Great results have been achieved in other countries, notably the United States of America, where immunisation levels against measles of 97% have been the reason for the successful control of the disease.

Pertussis (whooping cough)

Causal agent

Bordetella pertussis a small ovoid, gram-negative coccobacillus which is difficult to culture and grows only on special media.

Frequency and distribution

This occurs throughout the world. Epidemics of whooping cough tended to occur every four years but since the early 1950s when pertussis vaccine was introduced, their size has progressively lessened. An epidemic occurred in 1978 and was a probable consequence of the reduction in the uptake of pertussis vaccination. Although the occurrence of the disease was at a generally lower level in the 1980s, periodic up-swings have occurred, including one at the beginning of the 1990s, leading to strengthened measures to achieve fuller immunisation uptake.

Identification

The disease begins with a slow onset of an irritating cough which progresses to paroxysmal attacks over a period of a few weeks and lasts for up to two months. The coughing attacks are accompanied by 'whooping' and vomiting. Pulmonary atelectasis and bronchopneumonia are common complications during the paroxysmal phase. Persisting low-grade infection encourages the development of chronic lung damage, bronchiectasis, but fortunately this has become a rare occurrence. Convulsions may occur in infants. Fatality rates are highest in children under six months. It can be difficult to diagnose and depends on the history given by the mother. Similar clinical syndromes can be produced by viral respiratory infections. Organisms can be cultured from carefully taken pernasal swabs if there is no delay in getting them to a laboratory, although the organism is isolated in less than half the swabs taken.

Incubation period
Usually seven to 14 days.

Infectivity period
The patient is highly infectious during the catarrhal stages of the illness and for about three weeks after the onset of paroxysmal coughing. If treated with antibiotics, however, the infectivity period only lasts for about five days after the onset of therapy.

Reservoir
Man.

Mode of transmission
Mainly droplet spread but also indirectly from objects contaminated by fresh discharges from the upper respiratory tract.

Control measures
The main control measure is prevention through the use of pertussis vaccine which is a key element of the childhood vaccination programme in Britain (the course of three doses is given at two, three and four months of age in combination with diphtheria and tetanus vaccines). Population control requires vaccine uptake in excess of 90%. Rates in Britain have fallen below this level, in part reflecting parental concern about the safety of earlier vaccines and litigation brought on the basis of allegations of neurological damage caused by them. Although modern vaccines are regarded as extremely safe, research is continuing to create even safer ones.

The major concern is the protection of unimmunised and therefore susceptible infants, although the introduction of an immunisation schedule starting at two months of age should help to alleviate this problem. Although it is often advised that babies should be excluded from infected children such a measure is rarely, if ever, successful. There is an argument for protecting a vulnerable baby with a two week course of antibiotics to stop them developing the infection. The child with the disease should be treated at the same time since erythromycin rapidly eliminates the organism, although it has little effect on the clinical course unless given in the catarrhal phase of the disease. Cleansing and disinfection of articles soiled with upper respiratory discharges is advisable as is the use of disposable tissues and handkerchiefs.

Poliomyelitis

Causal agent
Poliovirus (three serological types) belongs to the enteroviruses. Type 1 is the most virulent, most commonly causes epidemics and is most often isolated from paralytic cases.

Frequency and distribution

The disease is still endemic in many countries of the world but effective vaccination programmes have reduced its incidence dramatically. In Britain, sporadic cases have occurred during the last decade. The majority were in unvaccinated children under the age of five years. In 1992 public attention focused on the cases of two fathers who, unimmunised themselves, were infected by their recently immunised infants. This reinforces the fact that parents' immunisation status should be checked and they should be offered immunisation at the same time as their babies if necessary.

Identification

Many people who are infected with the virus remain asymptomatic whilst some develop an acute pyrexial illness in which the person affected may have a fever accompanied by headache, stiffness of the neck and gastro-intestinal upset. A minority of patients develop paralysis through involvement of the motor neurones. The diagnosis is essentially clinical but suspected cases should be investigated by attempting to culture viruses from the patient's faeces.

Incubation period

Commonly seven to 14 days, although it has been as short as three days and as long as 35 days.

Infectivity period

Poliovirus can appear in throat secretions as quickly as 36 hours after infection and in faeces about three days after infection. The virus is excreted in the faeces for three to six weeks or more although it can be isolated from the throat for only about a week after onset.

Reservoir

Man.

Mode of transmission

The faecal-oral route is the major mode of transmission especially in areas of poor sanitation. In areas of good sanitation spread by direct contact with pharyngeal secretions becomes much more significant.

Control measures

Isolation of the case is essential and contacts should be given booster doses of vaccine immediately. This is one of the few diseases where mass vaccination of all possible contacts in the neighbourhood is recommended as a control procedure in outbreak situations. In areas with modern sewage disposal systems environmental measures should not be needed. Poliomyelitis has virtually been eradicated in the population of Britain by the maintenance of high levels of immunisation in the population, based upon a comprehensive childhood immunisation programme. In some developing countries, where sanitation is poor and immunisation of the population unsatisfactory, paralytic poliomyelitis occurs more commonly. Britain's immunisation programme is based upon a live attenuated virus vaccine administered orally. It is safe and very effective but very rarely it can cause the disease. For this reason, the live attenuated vaccine should not be used in people who are immunocompromised.

Rubella

Causal agent

The rubella virus is a member of the Togaviridae family of viruses.

Frequency and distribution

It has a worldwide distribution and is endemic in Britain with periodic epidemics in children. It tends to show winter and spring peaks.

Identification

The virus produces a mild febrile illness with upper respiratory symptoms, a fine macular rash, enlargement of the posterior cervical and occipital glands. The disease is easily confused with other viral infections and in many cases is subclinical. Its public health importance lies in the risk of the congenital rubella syndrome which affects infants whose mothers had the disease during the first trimester of pregnancy. Defects are rare in women infected after the 20th week of pregnancy. At birth the infant can have a variety of defects which include cataracts, deafness, mental retardation and cardiac abnormalities. In some cases these are mild and not detected for some years after birth at which stage it is too late to make a definitive diagnosis. Rising antibody titre can be demonstrated in paired sera with 10–14 day intervals during the 2–4 weeks following infection and specific immunoglobin detected for a month or so.

Incubation period

Fourteen to 21 days, usually 17 to 18 days.

Infectivity period

A highly infectious disease: the patient is infectious a week before and a week after the appearance of the rash. Babies affected by congenital rubella may shed the virus for months.

Reservoir

Man.

Mode of transmission

Mainly by direct contact with droplets and respiratory secretions.

Control measures

Pregnant women should avoid contact with cases of rubella, but any pregnant woman who is in contact should undergo serological screening. Until recently, the main control measure was a vigorous vaccination programme of schoolgirls between 11 and 13 years of age and women of reproductive age having no antibodies (sero-negative). It is important to remember that there is a risk in giving the vaccine in the early stages of pregnancy, hence its use is not recommended when there is a possibility of the woman being pregnant, although no cases of congenital rubella have so far arisen by this means.

The main thrust to control the disease in the population of Britain changed in 1988 with the introduction of a new immunisation policy to add to the existing policy. The live attenuated rubella vaccine is now combined with mumps and measles as part of MMR (mumps, measles, rubella) vaccine given to all children at around 18 months of age or at school entry if not previously given. Until high levels of immunity have been achieved, for the foreseeable future it will be important to continue the policy of ensuring that teenage girls and women approaching the child bearing years are immunised. Staff working with pregnant women should also be vaccinated (for example, nursing staff, medical students, ambulance personnel).

Diphtheria

Causal agent

Corynebacterium diphtheriae is a slender, gram-positive rod. The organism produces a powerful exotoxin.

Frequency and distribution

The disease has a worldwide distribution but is more common in temperate climates. Since the 1960s, Britain has seen only sporadic cases or limited outbreaks largely due to the success of the immunisation policy in childhood. The disease is seen in Britain in imported cases from time to time.

Identification

The disease is an acute upper respiratory tract infection which may affect the tonsils, pharynx, larynx or nostrils and, very occasionally, the skin. The characteristic feature is the presence of a greyish membrane in the throat firmly attached and surrounded by inflammation with enlarged cervical lymph glands. The main hazards (which may cause death particularly in the untreated case) are local obstruction of the respiratory passages (by the membrane) and the effects of the exotoxin on the myocardium and on the peripheral nervous system (most seriously leading to paralysis of the respiratory muscles). Throat or nose swabs are taken from the suspected case, carrier or contact and the organism is identified after culture on a suitable medium. Once isolated, the corynebacterium should be tested for toxigenicity by injection into guinea pigs or by *in vitro* diffusion techniques. Serum antitoxin levels may further assist in diagnosis. Treatment and control measures should be taken without waiting for laboratory confirmation.

Incubation period

Two to five days, occasionally a little longer.

Infectivity

Cases are seldom infectious beyond four weeks, especially with effective treatment but, rarely, a chronic carrier can shed organisms for six months or more.

Reservoir

Man alone.

Mode of transmission

Direct contact with another human case or carrier, usually by the airborne route, may be spread by discharges, or by fomites (inanimate objects).

Control measures

The person infected is isolated and treated with antitoxin and suitable antibiotic therapy. Close contacts should have nose and throat swabs taken and be kept under surveillance for seven days. The non-immune are immunised with the toxoid and some authorities believe that prophylactic antibiotics are also of value. Nose and throat swabs may identify carriers who are then also isolated and treated with antibiotics until the carrier state no longer exists. Articles that have been in close contact with the patient should be disinfected especially those which may have been contaminated with nasal or oral secretions. Immunisation is an important control measure so non-immunised children should be given a full course at once and others a booster dose. If immunisation levels fall, there would be a risk that diphtheria might once again occur in epidemic form, particularly as a result of the infection being imported from parts of the world where it is still common. The key control measure is the maintenance of a high level of immunity in the child population by means of an effective immunisation programme. All children are offered vaccination at two, three and four months of age.

Tetanus

This serious illness is now relatively rare in England and Wales, largely due to active immunisation of children. The causative organism, *Clostridium tetani*, a gram-positive, anaerobic spore-forming bacillus, is widely distributed in nature and is commonly found in soil. The organism is introduced into the human body by a penetrating injury, for example during gardening. In anaerobic conditions, the spores germinate producing a powerful exotoxin which is neurotoxic. This process takes three to 21 days depending upon the severity of the wound. The average incubation period is about ten days. The patient develops painful muscular contractions initially affecting the facial and neck muscles, but going on to involve the muscles of the trunk. Involvement of the respiratory muscles leads to compromised breathing. In untreated cases, mortality is high (approximately 60%). Treatment of a patient with tetanus involves surgical debridement of the wound, the administration of antitoxin, antibiotics and sedative, and intensive care nursing. People who have injured themselves, for example, by sticking a garden fork into their foot, have probably been exposed to tetanus. The wound should be cleaned and the individuals offered vaccine (depending upon their immunisation history). Long term prevention of tetanus depends upon the childhood immunisation regime.

Mumps

Mumps is a common viral infection of childhood. The mumps virus, a para-myxovirus, is spread by droplets or by direct contact with the saliva of an infected individual. The incubation period is usually about 18 days but may be as short as 12 days or as long as 25 days. The child becomes unwell with a headache, sore throat and a fever, after which the salivary glands, particularly the parotids, become inflamed. The virus persists in the saliva for several days after the onset of parotitis. Subclinical infection occurs in some children, especially youngsters, and is important in perpetuating the spread of the virus.

Mumps infection may be complicated by orchitis in post-pubertal males, oophritis in post-pubertal females, meningitis or encephalitis, and rarely, pancreatitis. Permanent deafness is a rare consequence of mumps meningoencephalitis.

Isolation of cases of mumps does little to halt the spread of this highly infectious disease, although it is prudent to keep children away from school until they have clinically recovered (usually about a fortnight). Routine immunisation in children is the main means of controlling mumps.

CHILDHOOD INFECTIONS FOR WHICH IMMUNISATION IS NOT AVAILABLE

Chickenpox

Chickenpox is caused by the varicella-zoster virus which is a member of the herpes virus family. It is a very common infection worldwide, usually causing a mild illness in children. Chickenpox is one of the most highly infectious diseases occurring in humans and spreads rapidly and readily. It is characterised by the development of fever and a rash which first appears on the trunk. The rash is flat to start with (macular) but swiftly becomes vesicular. The vesicle fluid contains virus particles, although the skin lesions are not as infectious as secretions from the respiratory tract. Transmitted mainly by this means, it is most infectious a couple of days before the onset of the rash up to about five days after the first crop of vesicles appear. The incubation period is usually two to three weeks but can be seven to 26 days.

Usually a mild illness, chickenpox may have a profound effect in immuno-compromised individuals who may suffer a fatal attack. Occasional deaths in otherwise healthy adults occur because of viral pneumonia. Neonates are at risk of a severe generalised infection, and infection in pregnant women in the first trimester might lead to congenital malformations.

Herpes zoster, commonly known as shingles, tends to occur in older adults and is a local manifestation of reactivation of the chickenpox virus. The commonest distribution of the zoster rash is along the skin supplied by the intercostal nerves or over the face in the innervation of the ophthalmic branch of the trigeminal nerve. Severe ophthalmic zoster can permanently damage the cornea.

Herpes simplex infection

Although primary infection with herpes virus can occur at any age, it is most common in young children. Most primary infections are subclinical and it is only when the latent virus is reactivated forming the typical 'cold sores' that it is apparent that the individual is infected. In young children, however, primary infection can be manifest as a very painful acute ulcerative gingivostomatitis. Whether as a result of primary or recurrent infection, the lesions are highly infectious. The virus is usually spread by direct personal contact such as kissing. Health care workers such as dentists may develop lesions on their hands if a patient is excreting virus, the so-called herpetic whitlow.

The incubation period for herpes virus infection is two to 12 days. Halting the spread of infection depends upon avoiding contact with people who have lesions.

In recent years it has been recognised that two forms of herpes virus hominis exist. Type 1 infection leads to the problems described above, whilst Type 2 tends to be sexually transmitted and causes genital herpes.

Cytomegalovirus infection

The importance of this infection, caused by another of the herpes virus group, is in the severe manifestations which can result from congenital infection. As many as 5 to 10% of congenitally infected neonates are estimated to develop significant mental retardation and permanent blindness.

Infants are frequently found to have microcephaly, cerebral calcification and chorioretinitis. In addition the spleen and liver are affected, and sometimes also the kidneys. The virus may be excreted in the child's urine for several months after birth. In view of the serious consequences of this infection it has been suggested that a nationwide screening programme of pregnant women should be adopted in an attempt to identify women who acquire primary infection in pregnancy. This proposal is still the subject of heated debate.

Cytomegalovirus also causes profound problems in immunocompromised patients such as transplant recipients and in individuals infected with human immunodeficiency virus. The incubation period for herpes virus infection is two to 12 days. Halting the spread of infection depends upon avoiding contact with people who have lesions.

INFECTIONS LEADING TO HEPATITIS

Hepatitis A (infectious hepatitis)

Causal agent

Hepatitis virus type A, a human picornavirus.

Frequency and distribution

It occurs in all parts of the world but more often in temperate zones where both sporadic cases and epidemics occur. It is more common in children and young adults. In Britain, epidemics tend to extend over long periods of time and over large geographical areas. Outbreaks are sometimes associated with schools and closed communities for children. There is evidence that the infection is becoming more common in inner city areas of the large urban conurbations.

Identification

Many infections with the type A virus produce no marked symptoms or cause a very mild illness. Other cases have anorexia, abdominal discomfort and pyrexia but no jaundice. Others develop jaundice which may result in a mild illness lasting about a week or a severe illness lasting several months. Recovery is slow in the latter instance but most cases make a complete recovery. Rarely, the disease can involve serious clinical manifestations, including hepatic failure. Hepatitis A is more common in children but also affects adults who usually have a more severe illness. The diagnosis is usually made from the history and clinical features but liver function tests are invariably abnormal. Serological diagnosis is by detection of Hepatitis A specific immunoglobin M (IgM). At the same time Hepatitis B antigen is sought.

Incubation period

Fifteen to 40 days (usually 28–30 days).

Infectivity period

The person is most infectious during the latter half of the incubation period and the early stages of the illness. Most people are not infectious after the first week of jaundice.

Reservoir

Man and some other primates.

Mode of transmission

Person-to-person mainly by faecal-oral route but possibly also by droplet spread. Generally the disease occurs when hygiene is poor; for example, in schools or nurseries where handwashing is not observed and lavatories are kept in a poor state of cleanliness. Sexual transmission has been recorded between male homosexuals. Contaminated water and food act as vehicles and a variety of foods have caused outbreaks notably, shellfish.

Control measures

Strict isolation of the patient is unnecessary because the stools are virus-free shortly after the jaundice appears. However, it is usual to adopt the standard precautions in handling urine, faeces and blood from the patient. Surveillance of close contacts, new cases and undiagnosed cases should be carried out. It is often difficult to trace the source of an outbreak. The long incubation period and the frequency of mild or asymptomatic illness are reasons for this. There is little to be gained from excluding contacts from school but it is wise to remove young people (who are the most susceptible) from food handling for six weeks. A high standard of personal hygiene is especially important when infectious hepatitis is prevalent. Human immunoglobin gives protection for about three months and in special circumstances (such as before travelling to endemic areas or as a prophylactic measure after exposure)may be indicated for some people. The general environmental measures of providing uncontaminated water supply and adequate sewage disposal are important in preventing the spread of infection. A vaccine against Hepatitis A is now available in Britain.

Hepatitis B (serum hepatitis)

Causal agent

Hepatitis virus type B is a hepadnavirus.

Frequency and distribution

The disease occurs throughout the world. The carrier state is of particular importance in this disease. In Britain only 0.2% to 0.5% of the population are carriers but in Southern Europe the carrier rate is up to 5% and in the tropics 10%. In parts of the Far East, some 15–20% of people may have serum which is positive for HBsAg. Most of the carriers in Britain have no previous history of jaundice.

Identification

Patients typically present with gradual onset of 'flu-like symptoms such as malaise, anorexia, nausea, vomiting, abdominal discomfort and aching of muscles and joints. A rash may occur in this early phase of the illness but fever is not usually a prominent feature. Clinical jaundice may then ensue or the patient may remain anicteric, the diagnosis being made by liver function and other tests. The fatality rate and likelihood of permanent liver damage in Hepatitis B is higher than with Hepatitis A infection. In the latter, almost all patients make a full recovery. Three antigenic components of Hepatitis B virus have been identified each with associated antibodies: (i) the surface or capsule antigen (HBsAg) also referred to as the Australia antigen, with the associated antibody (Anti HBs) can be detected by various techniques including radioimmunoassay and electron microscopy; (ii) the core antigen (HBcAg) which is not normally detected because it is neutralised by excess antibody (Anti HBc) which is detectable; and (iii) most recently a third soluble antigen (HBeAg) and antibody (Anti HBe) have been discovered. All are markers of infection. Their presence in the serum of a proportion of the population who have apparently had no clinical infection presents a particular public health problem in the context of blood transfusion and medical instrumentation by medical and non-medical personnel.

Incubation period

Fourteen to 200 days, usually over 40 days.

Infectivity period

The individual is infectious as long as Hepatitis B surface antigen is present in the blood. HBsAg appears several weeks before the onset of symptoms and can be detected for days, weeks or even months after the onset. In about 5–10% of cases, the antigen remains in the serum for a considerable number of years. People who have had hepatitis should not be blood donors, nor should those who give no history of hepatitis but whose serum shows the presence of HBsAg.

Reservoir

Man and possibly other primates.

Mode of transmission

From another human case or more often a carrier, usually by inoculation of blood or blood products. Saliva, semen and vaginal fluids also transmit infection.

Transmission may occur through intravenous drug abuse, tattooing, heterosexual and male homosexual intercourse, acupuncture, ear-piercing and medical and dental instrumentation. It is an occupational risk amongst those involved in handling blood products and dialysis equipment. It can be transmitted from mother to child transplacentally. It has also been suggested that it can be transmitted by insect bites. Blood transfusion is an unlikely method in Britain as strict screening of donor blood is now carried out, but in countries where payment is made to blood donors, the risk of transmission through this means is much greater.

Control measures

Isolation of cases is not necessary but strict precautions are required in the handling and disposal of blood and excreta. Surveillance of contacts is indicated if the source is identified (for example, a tattooist). General preventive measures include adequate precautions as part of the normal routine in all places handling human blood and its products. This includes the correct disposal of used syringes in all settings in which they are used. Specimens must be labelled 'High Risk' and sent in special containers. Special risks apply to patients and staff of renal units where vigilance should be especially high. Patients should be screened before admission to renal dialysis units and those who are positive (HBsAg+) should be nursed at home. The screening of potential blood donors for the carrier state has already been mentioned. Health education is important amongst special and high-risk groups such as drug takers and male homosexuals. Adequate sterilisation of instruments should be undertaken and, wherever possible, disposable needles and instruments should be employed and used once only for each patient. There is a clear need also in this way for closer supervision of tattooing, ear-piercing and acupuncture. Sometimes screening procedures are also carried out on drug addicts and male homosexuals. Patients who are HBsAg positive should be educated about the mode of spread of the disease and counselled as to behaviour to reduce the risk of transmission.

Those in high risk occupations (for example, health care personnel and sewage workers) should be offered the vaccine. Hyperimmunoglobulin can also be given in carefully selected circumstances; for example, after being pricked by a needle from an infected person.

Hepatitis C (Non-A Non-B Hepatitis)

Following the establishment of accurate diagnosis of Hepatitis A and Hepatitis B infection by serological means, it was realised that two or possibly three additional types of viral hepatitis exist. This recognition principally came about because of the persistence of a small number of cases of post-transfusion hepatitis even in circumstances where strict screening of blood donors for Hepatitis B had taken place. The infection is spread by injection of blood, blood products or serum (thus it can be contracted by intravenous drug abusers). There is special significance for the blood transfusion service and particularly with pooled serum. The incubation period is two to 26 weeks. The initial symptoms are usually mild, many patients having no jaundice, but as many as 30% may develop chronic liver damage.

Hepatitis D (Delta hepatitis)

This form of viral hepatitis closely resembles infection with Hepatitis B and the two may co-exist in the same individual. The virus-like infecting particle consists of a Hepatitis B surface antigen in combination with a unique internal antigen: the so called delta antigen. Like Hepatitis B, the infection is spread by injection of infected blood or blood products. The incubation period is probably somewhere between two and 10 weeks.

Hepatitis E

An epidemic form of Non-A, Non-B Hepatitis is spread by the faecal-oral route or by contaminated water. The incubation period is 15 to 64 days and the disease is very similar to Hepatitis A. Hepatitis E is a diagnosis of exclusion and diagnostic tests are still being refined.

INFECTIONS LEADING TO MENINGITIS

Meningococcal infections

Causal agent

Neisseria meningitidis (Meningococcus) is a gram-negative diplococcus. Three main serogroups exist A, B and C. Most infections in Britain are caused by Group B meningococci.

Frequency and distribution

It has a worldwide distribution. In Britain, it is responsible for causing meningitis and septicaemia which occur as sporadic cases and in localised outbreaks, particularly in children and young adults. Overcrowded living conditions facilitate its spread. For example, outbreaks occur in boarding schools and military camps where young people are living and sleeping in close proximity.

During the 1980s, a persistent pocket of high incidence of meningococcal meningitis with fatalities, occurred in Stroud, Gloucestershire. The reason for the higher frequency in this area was not elucidated. It gave rise to great public concern, extensive media coverage and the formation of pressure groups which called for more action and research to combat the disease. Overall, numbers of meningococcal infection increased during the second half of the 1980s. A similar increased incidence was seen in the mid-1970s.

Nasopharyngeal carriage of the organism in asymptomatic individuals can be surprisingly high. The overall prevalence lies somewhere between 2–4% of the population, rising to approximately 20% in epidemic situations and over 50% in outbreaks in closed communities.

Identification

The organism commonly causes a sub-clinical illness. In cases where meningitis does develop, symptoms are fever, headache, neck stiffness and photophobia. Acute septicaemia, which is rapidly fatal if untreated, is accompanied by a purpuric rash. Other symptoms and organs (for example, joints, heart) may be involved. The acute fulminating form of the disease, which occurs especially in children under the age of five years, has a high fatality rate. The laboratory diagnosis is made by observing the organism on direct microscopy of cerebrospinal fluid or by isolating the organism from culture of cerebrospinal fluid or blood. The administration of antibiotics, even before a suspected case is admitted to hospital, is a vital measure in attempting to reduce mortality from this disease. Since the organism can be identified biochemically, administration of antibiotics should not be delayed in order that the organism can be grown in culture.

Incubation period

Between two and ten days, usually three to four days.

Infectivity period

The patient is infective for as long as the organism is present in the naso-pharynx. Penicillin (the antibiotic of choice in the treatment of meningococcal meningitis) suppresses the organism but does not eradicate it. This is important since it means that people who have recovered from meningitis should receive a second antibiotic (usually rifampicin) to eliminate nasopharyngeal carriage of the pathogen.

Reservoir

Man.

Mode of transmission

By droplet spread.

Control measures

A vital measure in saving life is the early administration of antibiotic in suspected cases. Action here rests largely with the general practitioner. Greater awareness amongst general practitioners of the need to take this action would undoubtedly save some lives. Household contacts and other intimate contacts (for example, kissing contacts) should be traced and offered antibiotic prophylaxis as soon as possible after the diagnosis has been made; preferably within twenty-four hours. The use of antibiotic chemoprophylaxis is usually limited to people who came into close contact with the infected person in the five days prior to the onset of the illness. Vaccine is available for Group A and C (and the less common Y and W Groups) and is used on a selective rather than a population basis. The absence of an effective Group B vaccine (research is continuing) is a serious gap in the public health weaponry to combat meningococcal disease. General environmental measures include the avoidance of overcrowding and the maintenance of good ventilation, particularly in sleeping quarters in closed communities containing children and young adults. Here carrier rates may be high.

Haemophilus influenzae

Haemophilus influenzae is a fastidious, gram-negative bacillus. Non-capsulated strains of the organism are not invasive and tend to cause secondary infections of the respiratory tract. They are the commonest cause of otitis media in children. Of greater significance, however, are the six capsulated strains, which produce invasive disease. Most invasive infections are caused by the type B capsulated strain.

Haemophilus influenzae type B infection (also known as Hib) is the commonest bacterial meningitis in children under the age of five years, with a peak incidence at ten to eleven months of age. The disease often has an insidious onset with malaise and a high temperature before the characteristic features of meningitis appear: vomiting, headache, neck stiffness and, in infants, a bulging fontanelle. The incubation period is thought to be short (two to four days). The infection is spread by secretions from the respiratory tract which remain infectious for as long as the organisms are present, but are rendered non-infectious 24 to 48 hours after the commencement of antibiotics. Person-to-person spread, giving rise to secondary cases, does occur. In children under four years of age, being those most at risk, the attack rate is estimated at around 5%. For this reason antibiotic chemoprophylaxis is recommended for all household contacts (including adults) of the index case where there are other under-fours in the family. It should also be considered where two cases occur in children in the same nursery class, but advice on the use of prophylaxis in this specific situation should be sought from the local Consultant in Communicable Disease Control.

In addition to meningitis, *Haemophilus influenzae* type B is also responsible for producing other invasive diseases such as epiglottitis, pneumonia, cellulitis, septic arthritis and osteomyelitis.

A major breakthrough in protecting children against infection by *Haemophilus influenzae* type B has occurred with the successful development of a conjugated vaccine which confers high levels of immunity even in very young children. The vaccine was incorporated into the United Kingdom's childhood immunisation programme in October 1992 and is administered at two, three and four months of age.

Streptococcus pneumoniae (pneumococcus)

Although a less common cause of meningitis than *N. meningitidis* and *H. influenzae* type B, pneumococcal meningitis is important because of its high associated mortality (20 to 40%). It occurs at all ages, but is the commonest bacterial meningitis occurring in the over 50 year old age group. The source of the infection may be an existing respiratory tract infection. Meningitis can also occur as a result of direct extension from chronic otitis media.

Listeriosis

This rare but important cause of neonatal meningitis has been covered in the section on food borne illnesses.

Other organisms

In addition to bacterial meningitis, a variety of other organisms cause the disease. These include viruses (for example, mumps, enteroviruses, herpes simplex), mycobacteria (M tuberculosis and M bovis) and, much more rarely, leptospires and fungi (cryptococcal meningitis usually occurs in immunocompromised people including those with Human Immunodeficiency Virus).

OCCUPATIONAL AND ENVIRONMENTAL HAZARDS

Leptospirosis

Causal agent

Leptospira is a spirochaetal organism which has two species, *Leptospira biflexa* and *Leptospira interrogans* with many different serotypes. Two main serotypes cause most cases of disease in Britain – *Leptospira icterohaemorrhagiae, and Leptospira hardjo.*

Frequency and distribution

The disease is a zoonosis which occurs in all parts of the world. In Britain it was traditionally associated with sewage workers and is usually seen now in farm or abattoir workers or, less commonly, amongst butchers, pest-control workers and veterinary workers. Contact with water contaminated by animal urine causes the disease. Canoeing and other water sports account for a substantial minority of the cases which occur each year. Public Health Laboratory Service reports indicate a relatively stable incidence over recent years with between 40 and 80 cases of leptospiral infection in humans in England and Wales each year. About half of these were due to *Leptospira hardjo* and just less than a third *Leptospira icterohaemorrhagiae*. Imported infections also occur.

Identification

The clinical manifestations are sudden onset of pyrexia, headache, severe muscular pain and sometimes vomiting. Occasionally a petechial rash occurs. More severe cases develop jaundice and haemorrhagic complications. This is classical Weil's disease and up to a fifth of cases can die from it. Spirochaetes can be cultured from patients' blood and sometimes the urine. Antibodies can usually be demonstrated in the serum (a range of tests are available) but not until the end of the first week of illness at the earliest. This means that tests are unhelpful in recognising the disease and initiating treatment in an acutely ill patient. The initial diagnosis should be made on history-taking and physical examination. Early treatment is the most effective especially in reducing fatalities in severe cases.

Incubation period

Usually between seven and 12 days but may extend from four to 19 days.

Infectivity period

Person-to-person transmission is rare.

Reservoir

Many animals carry the different serotypes, including rats and other rodents, dogs, cattle, foxes and squirrels. In Britain the main risks are from rats (*Leptospira icterohaemorrhagiae*), dogs and pigs (*Leptospira canicola*) and cattle (largely *Leptospira hardjo*). Cattle become infected through grazing on fields contaminated by the urine of small rodents. In some surveys over 60 per cent of cattle sera show antibodies to leptospira strains particularly *L hardjo*.

Mode of transmission

Direct contact with water, damp soil or vegetation which has been contaminated by the urine of infected animals or, less commonly, directly from the infected urine of animals. The spirochaete enters via broken skin, via mucous membrane or may be swallowed.

Control measures

Health care professionals should exercise care in handling body excretions, particularly the blood and urine of infected patients. Other people exposed to the primary source should undergo medical surveillance. Protective clothing should be worn by workers in hazardous occupations and wounds and cuts covered. Health education is important. This must be directed both at workers in high risk occupations and at the general public. The latter should be warned about the dangers of infection through swimming in contaminated water such as that in disused canals and through other water sports such as canoeing. The control of the urban rat population is also important. General environmental control measures include extermination of rodents.

Toxoplasma gondii

Causal agent

Toxoplasma gondii, a coccidial protozoan parasite found in the tissues of many animals, including man, but only in the cat is there a stage of development in the intestine. Hence the cat excretes *T. gondii* as oocysts which when ingested by other animals cause the disease. It may also result from the ingestion of contaminated uncooked meat.

Frequency and distribution

It is found in all parts of the world, both in animals and man. In Britain up to 50% of adults have antibodies to toxoplasma indicating previous infection even though the vast majority show no symptoms.

Identification

The primary infection rarely causes symptoms which are severe enough to be reported. In its acute form, the patient has fever and enlarged lymph glands. In immunocompromised individuals, primary infection can cause a much more severe illness affecting the brain, lungs and heart, invariably leading to death. Cerebral toxoplasmosis is recognised as a serious consequence of infection with the Human Immunodeficiency Virus. Congenital infection also occurs and is another important manifestation of this disease.

Incubation period

This is uncertain, but is thought to lie somewhere between 10 and 25 days.

Infectivity period

Infection from person-to-person only occurs in the intrauterine infection. The oocysts excreted by cats become infective one to five days later and can remain viable in moist conditions for up to a year.

Reservoir

The definitive hosts are members of the cat family.

Mode of transmission

The cat becomes infected by eating infected mammals like rodents and birds. The parasite then undergoes a complex process of development in the epithelial cells of the cat's intestine. For a short period of time the cat passes oocysts, a stage of the parasite that can remain potentially infective in the environment for long periods. However, despite the fact that two-thirds of the cat population have been infected, only 1% are likely to be passing oocysts at any one time. It is not known how often people become infested by these oocysts. It is thought that they acquire the infection either directly by injecting oocysts from soil (for example, during gardening) or by eating raw or insufficiently cooked pork, mutton or beef which contains the parasite. Transplacental infection also occurs in humans when the pregnant mother acquires a primary infection. The fetus can be affected at any stage of pregnancy, but is most at risk during the first trimester when infection can lead to foetal death. Congenital infection may also give rise to chorioretinitis, cerebral calcification and hydro-cephalus in up to 60% of survivors. These severe consequences have led to a call for a national screening programme to combat this disease. It is still the subject of debate.

Control measures

The most important are the thorough cooking of meat and advising pregnant women to avoid handling cat litter, especially with bare hands.

Toxocara

Toxocara is a nematode (roundworm) and two species cause concern in the British Isles: *Toxocara canis* (adult form occurs in the small intestine of dogs) and *Toxocara cati* (found in the cat). Each has a complex but different life cycle. It is the minute larvae (about half-a-millimetre long) which invade the tissues of many vertebrates and cause symptoms in humans. Human infestation follows the ingestion of infected eggs from dogs or cat faeces. The transfer may take place directly from hand to mouth (particularly in children) or possibly on salad vegetables. Surveys have shown that 5–25 percent of soil samples in garden, parks and sandpits are contaminated with toxocara eggs. After ingestion the eggs hatch into larvae in the intestine, penetrate the intestinal wall and reach various organs through the bloodstream. The larvae do not develop into adult worms in humans, but the wandering larvae can invade lungs, liver, the brain and eye. In the various tissues larvae produce an immune response and become the centre of an inflammatory reaction with subsequent fibrosis and granuloma formulation. In the great majority of cases, this gives rise to no symptoms but if the lesion is in a vital organ such as the eye it can lead to disturbance of vision or, in the brain, it can result in epilepsy.

It must be remembered that these are rare conditions. There are about 50 cases with ocular involvement reported in Britain each year, mostly children who have been in close contact with dogs. Nevertheless, it is a further reason to ban dogs from beaches, parks and playgrounds. At least 10% of dogs in Britain are infested and up to 35% of cats. Human infection is much more commonly associated with dogs. Between two and five per cent of the adult population in Britain have been found to be infected.

Brucellosis

Causal agent

Brucella abortus, a small aerobic, gram-negative coccobacillus which does not produce spores and induces abortion in cows; the carcases and the milk both become infected. Other serological types are *Brucella melitensis* (which infects goats and sheep), *Brucella suis* (which infects pigs) and *Brucella canis* (which infects dogs), none of which are endemic in Britain.

Frequency and distribution

Worldwide distribution but is more common in Mediterranean areas. By the beginning of the 1990s, following the introduction in Britain in 1971 of a compulsory scheme for eradication of brucella in cattle, the number of laboratory identifications had declined to a small number each year. When the disease does occur it is more often found in rural areas amongst workers (including veterinary surgeons) who are involved with cattle or their untreated milk, and also people who drink unpasteurised milk. Some infections are contracted abroad and imported with the traveller.

Identification

The illness is not sharply defined. Commonly it produces a so-called undulant fever with febrile periods followed by intervals with no increase in temperature. The fever often appears in the afternoons. The diagnosis should be considered in any pyrexia of unknown origin especially in groups with a potential occupational exposure. In about half the cases the organisms may be isolated in blood cultures taken from the patient in the acute stages of the illness. Otherwise the diagnosis is often made by serological tests which are of more value slightly later in the illness.

Incubation period

Usually two to four weeks, but often several months.

Infectivity

Spread person-to-person is virtually unknown.

Reservoir

There are a number of animal reservoirs of the infection, but in Britain the only animal of importance is the cow.

Mode of transmission

Direct contact with infected cattle, particularly the products of conception; and drinking unpasteurised milk from infected cows. The airborne route (inhalation of infected dust) in cattle sheds may occur.

Control measures

Isolation and surveillance of cases is unnecessary. As human immunisation is not available, health education is important. Farmers should be taught how to avoid infection and the public made aware of the dangers of drinking untreated milk. Outbreaks are usually traced to an infected herd if those working with it or drinking its milk become infected. The general measure of raising herds of cattle which are free from *Brucella abortus* infection and the pasteurising of milk would entirely eradicate the disease in humans if carried out meticulously. Whilst the eradication programme in Britain is well advanced with many herds free from brucellosis, each year there are still a small number diagnosed. Close cooperation is required between the health and local authorities, together with the veterinary authorities, when cases or outbreaks occur.

Lyme disease

First described in 1975 in Old Lyme, Connecticut when several children developed acute arthritis, the causal agent, *Borrelia Burgdorferi* (a spirochaete) was not identified until 1982. The organism is transmitted by the bite of the Ixodid group of ticks which live on wild animals (especially deer). It is not transmissible person-to-person. Susceptibility to infection is thought to be universal and the clinical manifestations are divided into two groups. Early symptoms include fever, malaise, headache, lymphadenopathy and a characteristic skin rash called erythema chronicum migrans. Present in about 7% of infected people, the rash develops after about five weeks and spreads slowly during the following months. Late manifestations, which may take years to appear, include arthritis, neurological abnormalities and heart problems.

Although it appears to be uncommon, cases of erythema chronicum migrans have been reported, mostly in the summer months, in Scotland and in the forests of East Anglia and Hampshire. Measures directed at combating this infection include covering exposed areas of skin, particularly legs and ankles, whilst out walking in the forest. If a tick should bite a person it should be removed promptly since transmission of the organism does not seem to occur until the tick has fed for a number of hours.

Orf

This is a common viral disease of sheep and goats and is transmitted to humans by occupational exposure. Farmers, shepherds and vets are usually affected by coming into direct contact with lesions on infected animals. The most common presentation is of a single lesion on the hands which develops into a weeping blister. The lesions, which can measure up to 3 cm in diameter, persist for three to six weeks and then disappear. Occurring mainly in rural communities, this self-limiting illness can be confused with anthrax (see below) or with malignancy.

Anthrax

Causal agent

Bacillus anthracis is a large gram-positive rod which occurs in short chains. The organism grows aerobically and forms heat-resistant spores capable of surviving for many years.

Frequency and distribution

Uncommon in Britain. Nine cases occurred in the ten years up to the beginning of the 1990s. Patients are usually workers dealing with animal products such as carcases, hides, hairs, wool and bonemeal. Sometimes gardeners using unsterilised bonemeal become infected.

Identification

The skin is the organ principally affected in this disease. Although respiratory and intestinal forms are uncommon they may occur and are often fatal. In the cutaneous form, a skin lesion develops usually about two to four days after local infection. It becomes vesicular over a period of several days. After rupture of the vesicle, a deep seated ulcer appears with swollen surrounding skin. It may then become covered by a scab: the characteristic eschar. If left untreated spread to the bloodstream will lead to a septicaemia which is fatal in as many as 20% of cases.

The diagnosis is usually confirmed by microscopy or isolation of the organism in culture of the skin lesion or blood.

Incubation period

Usually two to five days.

Infectivity period

Person-to-person infection has not been reported but, until the patient has received several days of treatment with antibiotics, it is wise to avoid handling the lesion which should be covered with an occlusive bandage.

Reservoir

Spores, often surviving for many years, are shed from the infected animal. Soil may also contain spores from the remains of dead animals.

Mode of transmission

Direct contact of the skin with either contaminated animal material or, less commonly with an animal dying of the disease, leads to the cutaneous form. Even more rarely, inhalation of spores can produce the respiratory form of the disease and the ingestion of undercooked contaminated meat can result in the gastro-intestinal form.

Control measures

Vaccination of workers in conditions where they are exposed to the risk of infection and the education of such workers in personal cleanliness, treatment of minor injuries and the hazards of handling potentially infected material are important control measures for anthrax. Protective clothing, dust reduction and medical supervision of those at risk at work are further preventive steps. Gardeners should take special care when using bonemeal known to be unsterilised. General environmental measures include the sterilisation of hair, wool, hides and bonemeal, particularly of imported products. Early diagnosis of affected animals or people and treatment with appropriate antibiotics is essential, as is the rapid identification of outbreaks in animals. The carcases of animals dying from anthrax should be burnt or deeply buried in quicklime, with any contaminated material and equipment sterilised. Primary contacts (those in contact with the original animal source) should have daily medical surveillance for one week. Contacts of human cases do not require such medical surveillance. Close cooperation between health and local authority together with the veterinary authorities is necessary when cases or outbreaks occur.

INFECTIONS RARELY OCCURRING IN BRITAIN AND INFECTIONS ACQUIRED ABROAD

Malaria

Causal agent

A protozoan, genus (family) name Plasmodium. Four species cause human malaria: two are uncommon (*Plasmodium malariae and Plasmodium ovale*), and two are common (*Plasmodium vivax* the cause of benign tertian malaria and *plasmodium falciparum* which causes malignant tertian malaria, a non-relapsing and serious disease with a high fatality rate).

Frequency and distribution

This is a very common disease in many parts of the tropics and sub-tropics: the vivax form in the Indian subcontinent, Central America and South-East Asia; the falciparum in Africa, South America and South-East Asia. Cases of malaria reported in Britain are almost all imported. They increased steeply during the 1970s, levelled off and started to fall during the late 1980s. However, 1,393 cases were still reported during 1990 and the number of cases of falciparum malaria (the most severe form) continued to rise during the period when overall numbers of reported cases were falling.

Identification

After an initial period of general malaise, pyrexia, shivering and profuse sweating occur in cycles according to the stage of development of the parasite in the human body. These symptoms can vary both in type and severity according to the species of malaria. The diagnosis of malaria should be considered in any patient with a pyrexial illness who has recently been in an endemic area even if the individual has been taking anti-malarial chemoprophylaxis. It is confirmed when the parasite is demonstrated microscopically in blood films.

Incubation period

This depends on the infecting strain. *P. falciparum* approximately 12 days from the infected insect bite, *P. vivax* and *P. ovale* approximately 14 days, and *P. malariae* approximately 30 days.

Infectivity period

The infection is not transmitted within Britain in the usual way by mosquitoes.

Reservoir

Man.

Mode of transmission

Transmitted by the bite of an infected female anopheline mosquito. The mosquito bites the person and ingests human blood containing gametocytes (the sexual stages of the parasite). In the mosquito's stomach, these male and female stages join together to form sporozoites. These concentrate in the salivary glands of the mosquito and are injected into the person when the mosquito next feeds. They pass in the blood stream to the liver where they develop into merozoites (pre-erythrocytic cycle). The clinical attack begins when these are released into the blood stream and invade the red cells, where they can undergo a complete cycle of development (erythrocytic cycle) resulting in further release of merozoites into the blood stream and a further clinical attack. Some also develop into male and female gametocytes which can then be taken up by another mosquito. The life cycle in the mosquito spans eight to 35 days, depending upon the infecting species and the ambient temperature and the pre-erythrocytic cycle in the liver (six to nine days for *P. falciparum, vivax* and *ovale* and 12–16 days for *P. malariae*). The duration of the erythrocytic cycle varies with the species of parasite: 36–48 hours (*P. falciparum*); 48 hours (*P. vivax and P ovale*); and 74 hours (*P. malariae*), which accounts for the different periodicity of clinical attacks in the different forms. A proportion of the merozoites from the pre-erythrocytic cycles continue to develop in the liver (exo-erythrocytic cycle): this provides for the source of infection in relapses which may occur several months after a previous attack. Relapses are particularly common with *P. vivax* infections.

The vast majority of cases of malaria reported in Britain occur amongst people who have sustained a mosquito bite whilst in a part of the world where the disease is endemic and have entered Britain before symptoms have developed. A very small number of cases can occur in more unusual circumstances. Mosquitoes have travelled undetected on aircraft and then left the aeroplane to bite and infect people in the vicinity of the airport; congenital malaria can occur in babies through transplacental spread from an infected mother; and a malaria sufferer who becomes a blood donor (having been undetected on donor screening) can be a rare source of infection of others.

Control measures

Isolation of cases is unnecessary and surveillance of contacts in Britain is only performed to ensure that fellow travellers have not also contracted the disease. However, it is important that a high index of clinical suspicion is maintained and malaria diagnosed and treated early when it does occur. Environmental measures are not required in Britain at the moment, but it is not beyond the bounds of possibility that global warming could allow the insect vector to survive in this country in the future. Travellers going to or passing through endemic areas should take prophylactic anti-malarial drugs and continue taking them for four to six weeks after leaving the endemic area. Drug resistance is a problem and the most up-to-date advice must be given to travellers to particular endemic areas. The World Health Organisation issues information annually about areas where drug-resistance occurs.

The most important groups for health education targeting are members of the ethnic minority populations within Britain, many of whom make relatively frequent trips to their countries of origin and who are not always aware of the risks of malaria and the importance of prophylaxis. Vigilance is also required in ensuring that aircraft do not import the mosquito (or expose passengers travelling between non-endemic areas in aircraft which have previously been used on tropical routes). Maintenance of high standards in screening potential blood donors is another vital control measure.

Rabies

Causal agent
The rabies virus is a rhabdovirus.

Frequency and distribution

Found in many countries throughout the world, it is primarily a disease of animals. The British Isles are at present rabies free with only occasional imported cases. Rabies has been detected in wild life in various parts of Western Europe and progressively closer to ports along the English Channel in recent years, although the introduction of oral rabies vaccine into the animal population has led to a reduction in the number of cases overall. Switzerland, for instance, is now virtually rabies-free. Bat rabies occurs in North America and to a lesser extent within the bat population of parts of Europe.

Identification

It is characterised by an acute encephalitis that is virtually always fatal within a week of first symptoms. The victim is apprehensive, with headache, pyrexia and muscle spasms which progress to paralysis and death. The fear of water (more accurately of swallowing) has led to the name 'hydrophobia'. The laboratory diagnosis of the disease in the brain of a killed infected animal confirms the clinical manifestations in the patient.

Incubation period

Normally this is two to eight weeks. It can be longer but can be as short as five days or as long as two years. It depends on the dose of virus as well as the nerve supply of the area which is wounded and its proximity to the brain. The virus migrates along peripheral nerves from the site of the bite into the central nervous system.

Infectivity period

Dogs and cats are usually infective from between three and 10 days before the onset of clinical illness and remain infectious throughout the course of the illness. Person-to-person transmission has never been demonstrated, although it is a theoretical risk because human saliva does contain the virus in an infected individual.

Reservoir

A variety of wild animals act as a reservoir: including foxes, wolves, dogs, cats and bats. However, for practical purposes the disease is transferred in the majority of cases by a dog bite (or less often a cat bite).

Mode of transmission

By the bite of an infected animal or more rarely by contact between infected animal saliva and the human mucous membrane. The virus cannot penetrate intact skin. A rare mode of transmission is via corneal transplant from an infected person who died of the disease, but in whom it was not diagnosed.

Control measures

Of greatest importance are strict quarantine regulations coupled with legal penalties to prevent the disease being imported by animals. Veterinary surgeons and those who deal with imported animals should be vaccinated with the human diploid cell vaccine. Health education measures should be employed, firstly to encourage travellers to foreign countries to avoid all contact with animals, especially in those countries where rabies is endemic, and secondly, to warn them of the hazards of illegally smuggling animals into this country.

An individual who has been bitten by an animal (for example, a dog, a bat or other wild animal) in which there is a suspicion of rabies or in a foreign country where the disease is endemic should have the wound immediately washed and thoroughly cleansed under medical supervision. Post-exposure treatment with active and passive immunisation (vaccine plus human anti-rabies immunoglobulin) should be considered.

The decision whether to proceed with vaccination depends on the likelihood that the animal is infected. If the animal was not captured and rabies is endemic in the particular country then it is prudent to proceed with post-exposure treatment.

Human diploid cell vaccine is given in a total of six doses intramuscularly: the first immediately, the second on the third day after exposure, the third on the seventh day, the fourth on the fourteenth day, the fifth on the thirtieth day and the last one on the ninetieth day. Human rabies immunoglobulin is injected immediately around the site of the wound, and intramuscularly.

In the context of the British patient, all these measures depend on the quality and availability of medical services in the country which is being visited. An increasingly common occurrence as more people travel abroad, is a history of animal bite in a returning traveller. Medical care may not have been sought or may not have been available in the country concerned. Personal experience indicates that the public health physician often becomes involved in such a situation. For example, a party of schoolchildren returning from a school trip abroad contained two members who gave a history of having been bitten by a dog which had exhibited aggressive behaviour towards them. It was only upon return to this country that parental concern led to the children presenting to the local accident and emergency department some four days after the bite.

Through the Department of Health via its international links the animal was located and found to have remained healthy. Post-exposure treatment was not enforced but would have been commenced immediately if: there was no official record of the incident; the animal had escaped and could not be traced; or the dog had been killed and diagnosed as suffering from rabies.

Because dog bites are such a common and insignificant occurrence in Britain, it is easy to take a casual approach to a stray dog bite sustained by someone returning from abroad (particularly if they appear fit and well). It is important that such cases are taken seriously. Advice can be obtained from the Public Health Laboratory on whether to instigate post exposure rabies treatment in particular circumstances.

If an established case is diagnosed in Britain, rigid rules of isolation usually apply, although the risk of person-to-person transmission is very slight. Attendant medical and nursing staff, and all those potentially exposed to the patient's saliva are offered immunisation. Health care professionals should wear protective gloves and gowns and concurrent and terminal disinfection should be practised.

With the advent of the Channel Tunnel providing easier access to the endemic parts of France, it is possible that rabies will become endemic in the fox population of Britain at some time in the future. The disease will then pose an important public health problem.

Viral haemorrhagic fevers

Some haemorrhagic fevers caused by viruses such as yellow fever have been known from early times. However, since the mid-1950s, new haemorrhagic illnesses have been recognised in humans, although it is likely that they have been acquired from natural animal hosts. The main public health concern is that the viruses, having been transmitted from their natural host to man, are then capable of producing person-to-person transmission. This risk is greatly minimised with strict isolation and meticulous medical and nursing procedures. Cases of this group of diseases are very rare in Britain and are almost exclusively imported by travellers from endemic areas.

Causal agents

Lassa fever – caused by a member of the arena virus family. It was first isolated from an American missionary nurse in the Lassa township in Nigeria during 1969. Since then it has also occurred in Nigeria, Sierra Leone, Liberia and elsewhere in West Africa.

Marburg disease – caused by a virus first described in Marburg in the Federal Republic of Germany in 1967 when 31 cases with seven deaths occurred in Germany and Yugoslavia due to direct contact with the blood, organs and tissues of a batch of African green monkeys originally trapped in Uganda. It is endemic in Central and Southern Africa.

Ebola fever – a very large outbreak of viral haemorrhagic fever with high fatality rates occurred in the Southern Sudan and Zaire in 1976, where it still occurs. The causal virus was found to be morphologically identical to the Marburg virus but serologically distinct and the new strain was named the Ebola virus.

Hantaan virus – produces a haemorrhagic fever with renal syndrome and is a major public health problem in China and Korea, where the case fatality rate reaches about 7%. A milder (but also sometimes fatal) disease occurring in Scandinavia and Eastern Europe is caused by an antigenic subtype: the Puumala virus.

Other haemorrhagic fevers – other infections in this category are endemic in various parts of the World: for example *Dengue fever* (South-East Asia and the Caribbean), *Bolivian haemorrhagic fever* (rural areas of Northern Bolivia), *Omsk haemorrhagic fever* (parts of Siberia).

Frequency and distribution

A very small number of cases of haemorrhagic fever are imported into Britain.

Identification

The disease should be suspected in patients with unexplained pyrexia returning from endemic areas of the world, provided malaria has been excluded as a diagnosis.

Symptoms vary but often there is an insidious onset with a variety of non-specific symptoms including general malaise, pyrexia, sore throat and enlarged lymph glands. Later, the patient's condition worsens with conjunctivitis, chest and abdominal pains, vomiting, and occasionally a mild maculopapular rash. Severe bleeding occurs between the fifth and seventh days most often into the gastro-intestinal tract and lung. Other features vary with the haemorrhagic fever concerned. For example, the severe form of Hantaan fever results in kidney symptoms and in some cases renal failure.

Incubation period

These vary according to the disease, for example:
Lassa fever – usually six to 21 days.
Marburg disease – three to nine days.
Ebola disease – two to 21 days.

The surveillance period for these fevers is usually extended to 21 days as an added precaution.

Infectivity period

Where person-to-person transmission occurs, diseases are infectious as long as blood and body secretions contain the virus, which can be several weeks after clinical recovery.

Reservoir

Lassa fever – a species of wild rodent (*Mastomys natalensis*) in rural West Africa. *Marburg and Ebola disease* – animal reservoir unknown. *Hantaan fever* – field rodents.

Mode of transmission

Lassa fever – Man acquires the infection probably through contact with the rodent's urine. Person-to-person spread may occur via the upper respiratory tract in the acute phase but more often is due to contact with infected blood, urine or secretions of the patient.

Marburg and Ebola diseases – although the original outbreak of Marburg disease occurred as a result of contact with African green monkeys, transmission of the disease from an animal to man has not been demonstrated. Person-to-person spread has usually been due to very close contact with infected individuals. Many outbreaks have been related to hospitals in Africa where unsatisfactory practices have spread the disease amongst patients and staff. In some of these outbreaks the case fatality rate has been over 50%. Such hospitals acted as amplifiers of the infection with secondary cases occurring amongst staff and other patients. However, the introduction of adequate precautionary measures (care in handling a patient's blood, urine and other secretions) quickly brought the disease under control in one outbreak of Ebola fever. In the original outbreak of Marburg fever a number of secondary cases occurred amongst hospital staff who had been exposed to the patient's blood. In Britain, the main risk is to ward and laboratory staff involved in the care of patients with viral haemorrhagic fever.

Control measures

When a suspected case of viral haemorrhagic fever occurs, an infectious diseases specialist must be contacted to exclude malaria as a diagnosis. Where there are good grounds for suspicion the Consultant in Communicable Disease Control is responsible for arranging the patient's admission to a high security isolation unit by a special ambulance crew wearing protective clothing and special respirators. The Department of Health and the Communicable Disease Surveillance Centre must be informed at the earliest opportunity. Close contacts of the patient, either those in the same household or workmates, are kept under strict daily surveillance for 21 days from the last date of exposure. A daily record is kept of temperature and, if a rise occurs or other signs or symptoms are evident, immediate isolation should be effected, and admission to a high security isolation unit considered.

Smallpox

Smallpox is caused by the Variola virus. Until the 1970s smallpox was one of the world's major killing infectious diseases and hence has been the subject of an active vaccination programme world-wide. In 1967 an eradication programme was launched by the World Health Organisation. As a result of this action the last known natural case of smallpox occurred in Somalia on October 26, 1977. However, in 1978, a medical photographer in Birmingham University contracted the disease as a result of an escape of the virus from a laboratory. She died of smallpox but her mother, who was the only other case, survived. Since this accident, rigorous measures have been instituted to reduce the risk of future tragedies of this sort. Global eradication of the diseases was pronounced by the World Health Assembly in 1980.

SEXUALLY TRANSMITTED DISEASES

Gonorrhoea

Gonorrhoea is a sexually transmitted disease which is found in all parts of the world. It is caused by a gram-negative, diplococcus, *Neisseria gonorrhoea*. The initial symptom in the male heterosexual is a urethritis with a purulent discharge. The disease may progress, particularly if treatment is delayed, to cause prostatitis or epididymitis. In women, the shorter female urethra means that symptoms sometimes pass unnoticed. Ascending infection of the female genital tract may cause salpingitis and (in the longer term) infertility. In either sex, rarely, joint inflammation or meningitis can occur. The gonococcus may affect the eyes of a baby born to an infected mother producing ophthalmia neonatorum.

Gonococcal infection is much more common in homosexual than heterosexual men. They present with anorectal and pharyngeal gonorrhoea (both can also occur in heterosexuals but are much less common) as well as urethral infections.

The diagnosis is usually made clinically and confirmed by stained smears of the infective exudate and, subsequently, culture of the organism. Urethral swabs in heterosexual men and women are the usual clinical investigation. In addition, throat swabs and anorectal swabs (during proctoscopy) are important in homosexual men.

The emergence of a penicillin resistant strain, *penicillinase-producing Neisseria gonorrhoeae (PPNG)* has been an important problem in the control of the disease in recent years. So far, resistant strains are those found in other parts of the world (such as the Far East) and penicillin is still effective in cases found in Britain (except for some imported cases).

The incidence of male gonorrhoea declined almost fourfold from nearly 37,000 cases in 1977 to just over 10,000 cases in 1988. Female gonorrhoea reduced threefold over the same time period (over 21,000 cases in 1977 to nearly 8,000 cases in 1988). In both sexes the biggest reduction took place between 1985 and 1988. This was thought to be due, at least in part, to the fear of AIDS and to the increased use of condoms by heterosexuals and by homosexual men. This rapid decline has, however, been shortlived and an upwards trend in the incidence of gonorrhoea was being observed in the early 1990s. Reported gonorrhoea rates are an important marker of unprotected sexual activity, particularly in the high risk groups. This indicator is even more important given the advent of Human Immune Deficiency Virus (HIV) infection.

Non-specific genital infection

In a high proportion of people presenting with symptoms suggesting genital infection, no organism will be isolated. This presentation was originally given the clinical label non-specific genital infection (or non-specific urethritis). Latterly, one organism has been isolated in a substantial proportion of such cases. The organism is called *Chlamydia trachomatis* and there are a number of serotypes which cause diseases. The serotypes concerned cause symptoms similar to gonorrhoea but with much less prominent discharge. It can be complicated by epididymitis, salpingitis and can cause infertility. Treatment is usually with tetracycline. Other serotypes of *Chlamydia trachomatis* cause *lymphogranuloma venereum*.

Trichomoniasis

The protozoan organism *Trichomonas vaginalis* is mainly an infection in women, though their male partners may be infected, remain asymptomatic or have mild symptoms. Women with this infection usually present with a strong smelling vaginal discharge, soreness of the external genitalia and pain during intercourse (dysparunia). A vaginal swab examined by microscopy and culture (and if necessary other more specialised tests) usually confirms the diagnosis. Antimicrobial treatment of both the woman and her partner is necessary to be sure of eradicating the infection.

Syphilis

Syphilis, one of the longest recognised sexually transmitted diseases, is caused by *Treponema pallidum*, a thin spiral organism (spirochaete) which does not stain well and is thus best seen with dark-field illumination microscopy.

It occurs in all parts of the world, and is mainly a disease of young adults. The 1960s and 1970s saw a large increase in the incidence of syphilis in part due to male homosexual spread of infection. The number of new cases is small in comparison with gonorrhoea, but it is more common in sea ports and large cities. A fall in the reported incidence of syphilis in male homosexuals occurred in the late 1980s, believed to be because of fear of AIDS, although heterosexually acquired infection in young adults rose.

Syphilis is invariably acquired by sexual contact. The spirochaete does not survive long outside the human body, hence indirect methods of transmission are not usually important. Congenital syphilis arises from prenatal infection via the placenta.

There are three stages of the acquired disease. The primary lesion (chancre) develops as a painless ulcer on the skin or mucous membrane at the site of entry of the spirochaete usually about three weeks after exposure. Even in untreated cases the primary lesion disappears and is followed within six to eight weeks by a generalised cutaneous rash heralding secondary syphilis. The tertiary stage develops after three to 20 years and can affect various parts of the body including bones, liver, cardiovascular system and the central nervous system, giving rise to classical tabes dorsalis and general paralysis of the insane. Early treatment with antibiotics has greatly reduced the occurrence of the secondary and tertiary stages.

In congenital syphilis, the fetus is frequently aborted or stillborn. If the child survives, handicapping conditions are the usual outcome. The organism may be seen in specimens under dark-field illumination microscopy or using immuno-fluorescent techniques. There are also a number of important serological tests which are used to help make the diagnosis.

The patient is infectious during the primary and secondary stages of the disease and may also be intermittently infectious during latent periods. Effective antibiotic treatment makes the patient non-infectious within one or two days.

Genital herpes

Genital herpes is caused by the *Herpes simplex virus* (usually Type 2) which is transmitted by sexual intercourse. The *Type 1 Herpes simplex virus* is associated with lesions on the mouth and face ('cold sores') but can also cause the genital form of herpes.

Genital herpes is a relapsing condition. The skin heals and then can break down and ulcerate long after the primary infection. Symptoms of the primary infection include pain in the genitals and buttocks, sometimes fever followed by an eruption of vesicles on the skin and mucous membranes of the genital area which gradually break down to produce painful ulcers. Discharge and secondary bacterial infection are common.

Genital herpes occurs in male and female heterosexuals and male homosexuals (in whom it occurs on the penis, in the anorectal area and sometimes in the mouth). Treatment is symptomatic and sometimes antiviral drugs are effective.

The virus becomes latent in the dorsal root ganglia and can then recur at any time although the number and severity of recurrences varies greatly.

Anal and genital warts

Warts in the anal and genital areas are caused by viruses: mainly the *Human Papilloma Virus (HPV)* although another virus also causes a warty-type infection called *Molluscum contagiosum*. Reported cases of anogenital warts have increased in recent years in heterosexuals and homosexual men. It is likely that this represents a true increase in occurrence but greater awareness on the part of patients and disgnosticians has undoubtedly contributed to the increase. An important association is that between HPV and the development of cervical cancer.

Candidiasis

The yeast, *Candida albicans* is a relatively common cause of pruritus, severe vulval discomfort and vaginal discharge. In many cases, the infection is due to spread of the organism from the gastrointestinal tract where it exists as a commensal but, in some instances, it is sexually transmitted. Treatment with antimicrobial pessaries usually resolves the infection.

Other diseases transmitted sexually

A number of other organisms can be transmitted sexually which are not thought of primarily as sexually transmitted diseases. These include *Hepatitis B, Hepatitis A, scabies, cytomegalovirus.*

Control of sexually transmitted diseases

In the 1980s and 1990s the whole field of sexually transmitted diseases has been transformed from a relatively quiet backwater of clinical and public health practice to one of major international importance by the emergence of the Human Immune Deficiency Virus (HIV) which causes the Acquired Immune Deficiency Syndrome (AIDS). This subject is covered in Chapter 3 but many of the control measures which apply to the control of its spread sexually, apply to other sexually transmitted diseases. Thus, HIV directed health promotion and health education programmes aimed at modifying sexual behaviour and encouraging safer sexual practices, particularly in young people, are equally important to the prevention and control of these other diseases.

Traditionally,the focus for the prevention and control of sexually transmitted diseases has been the network of clinics provided around the country within the National Health Service. Prompt diagnosis and investigation of people presenting is vital and, in most diseases, the tracing of contacts of patients is a key control measure. Contact tracing is a skilled exercise requiring considerable diplomacy and is often undertaken by specially trained nurses, health visitors or social workers.

A great deal of effort has been made over recent years to make sexually transmitted disease clinics more welcoming to patients. The premises have been renovated to improve the clinical environment and to rid the service of the old image of the 'pox clinic', which some people shunned even when symptomatic. Similarly, existing codes of confidentiality, operated by staff in sexually transmitted disease clinics, have been reinforced and considerable reassurance given to the public that this has occurred.

Indeed, many of the recent changes in sexually transmitted disease services have been stimulated by experiences of dealing with HIV infection in which it has been important to make sure that risk groups come forward for testing, advice and counselling. The spin-offs for the prevention and control of other sexually transmitted diseases have been important and beneficial.

PARASITIC DISEASES: ECTOPARASITES

Scabies

Causal agent. *Sarcoptes sabiei*, a small mite just visible to the naked eye.

Frequency and distribution. The disease occurs in most parts of the world. In Britain it appears to fluctuate over a 15 year cycle. 'The itch', as it was known, has a long history and it may have been the condition mentioned in the Old Testament for which the treatment advised was bathing in the River Jordan (now known to have a high sulphur content).

Identification. Skin lesions caused by burrowing of the mite are most commonly found between the fingers, on the anterior surfaces of the wrist and the soles of the feet. Symptoms occur when sensitisation develops with a papular rash which may spread to any part of the body except the face. Itching is intense, especially in bed at night. Scratching may result in secondary infection. The diagnosis is confirmed by extracting the female mite from the burrow and identifying it under the microscope.

Incubation period. The initial infestation passes unnoticed until sensitisation occurs about two months later. In people who have been previously infested the time is much shorter (one to four weeks).

Infectivity period. The person is infectious until effective treatment is carried out.

Reservoir. Man. Scabies in animals (such as dogs) does not transfer to man.

Mode of transmission. The parasite is transmitted by close personal contact such as holding hands or sexual intercourse. It has not been possible to demonstrate transfer by indirect means such as bed linen or clothing.

Control measures. There is no need to isolate the patient after treatment but contacts should be examined and treated if necessary. It is helpful to treat all family contacts of the patient simultaneously to avoid reinfection. The maintenance of good personal hygiene standards should also be encouraged.

The common bed bug (*Cimex lectularius*)

This insect is found in temperate climates and man is the preferred host. It lives in the crevices of walls or furniture, particularly in bedrooms and usually seeks out the sleeping host shortly before dawn. Bugs may bite anywhere on the body but hands, arms and head are usually the chosen sites. After feeding on blood, the insect passes liquid urine which leaves a dark brown mark on the sheets and bedding. The bugs are found where standards of hygiene are poor and in old property. They now only rarely occur in most parts of Britain.

Fleas

The association of fleas with man has a long history. For example, the plague which ravaged medieval Britain (the Black Death) was carried by a flea, which although it had the black rat or ship rat (*Rattus rattus*) as its preferred host, would also bite man. In Britain as in most other countries the plague has now been eliminated by controlling the rat population and through it the flea population.

Fleas spend most of their lives in nests or burrows where their eggs hatch and their larvae find food, become pupae and undergo metamorphosis to become adults.

The adult flea then seeks and feeds on the resting host before jumping off again. It could be argued that fleas are not true ectoparasites because they do not actually live on their host. Indeed, many fleas bite other than their preferred host and it is likely that man does not fulfil this role for any type of flea. The so-called 'human' flea (*Pulex irritans*) lives and breeds in association with man usually in bedrooms, in cracks of dirty floors, unwashed bedding and unclean beds where it finds its favourite damp and cool conditions. However, improved standards of housing and hygiene and the widespread use of central heating have resulted in its virtual extinction.

The flea which causes the greatest problem in Britain and other Western countries is the cat flea (*Ctenocephalides felis*). It prefers the warm conditions which are associated with modern centrally heated houses and seeks out the pile of closely fitted carpets and the upholstery of armchairs. It does not usually go under clothing so that bites commonly occur on the exposed parts of the body such as hands, wrists, ankles. The flea bites man when its natural host is absent. It is also often found on dogs. At any time there are twenty times more fleas in the environment than on the cat. The dog flea (*Ctenocephalides canis*), although closely related to the cat flea does not bite man so readily and is relatively uncommon but is the dominant species on racing greyhounds. To control the flea population it is essential to treat the environment as well as the pet.

Lice

General considerations. There are three types of human lice, all are members of the order *Anoplura* (sucking lice) and are parasites exclusively of mammals. All feed on the blood of the host and parasitize only one species, hence they are strongly host-specific. Moreover, many of the 500 known species of lice are so highly specialised that they only colonise one part of the body of their particular host.

Two genera of lice infest man, *Pathirus* and *Pediculus*, although only one species of each is involved. When man began to wear clothes and his hair became restricted to the head, axilla and pubic areas, human lice themselves underwent modifications. The crab louse (*Phthirus pubis*) adapted to live on the hair around the human genitalia, whilst the body louse migrated to clothing, only returning to the host to feed. The head louse became a scalp dweller, and specialised to such a degree that its survival depends on being in almost continual contact with its source of food and warmth. There are two varieties of *Pediculus humanus* – *Pediculus humanus humanus* (the body louse) and *Pediculus humanus capitis* (the head louse).

The body louse *(Pediculus humanus)*

This louse is different from the many species of *Anoplura* in that it lives on the host indirectly (on the clothing), laying its eggs on the seams, near the skin. It visits the body only long enough to obtain meals of human blood. The eggs are laid, attach to the fibres of clothing and, if the temperature is right, hatch within seven days. The young louse matures in about seven days and has an average life-span of 30 days. It is unusual for lice to remain on the body after the clothing has been removed. However, treatment usually consists of topical application of 0.5 per cent malathion lotion or 5 per cent carbaryl dusting talc. A convenient way of delousing clothing is to put it to dry into a tumble-drier for five minutes at the maximum temperature, a manoeuvre which kills both lice and eggs.

Crab louse or pubic louse *(Phthirus pubis)*

This parasite has preference for the coarse widely spaced hair in the pubic area, though occasionally it may be found elsewhere on the hair of legs, beards or eyelashes. The louse tends to feed from the same spot at the base of a hair. It is not easily visible since it blends in with the skin. The eggs are glued onto the hair and hatched in about eight days. The young louse is mature within a week. Spread is nearly always by sexual contact and the treatment of choice is the application of 0.5 per cent malathion or carbaryl lotion to all hairy areas below the neck.

The head louse *(Pediculus humanus capitis)*

This louse is strongly host-specific and for all practical purposes is found in only one place, the hair close to the scalp of human beings.

The eggs (nits) have been found on the hair of an Egyptian mummy and there are numerous references to the louse in literature from the time of the Greek classics. The head louse is about the size of a matchstick head and has a life-span of 30 days, but few survive in the natural state for so long. The eggs are laid in a glue-like medium which attaches them to a hair shaft, very close to the scalp. Usually they hatch within seven days into a nymph which becomes mature within about ten days. The sole food is human blood. The louse moves quickly but does not readily leave the host. The mode of transmission is almost certainly by the louse walking from one person's head to another when they are in close contact. Head louse infestation occurs throughout the world, but it appears to be more common in Western countries. Most infestations are light and the principal symptoms are itching of the scalp with consequent disturbances of sleep. Secondary infection may occur with scratching and, since lice can harbour in their intestines bacteria capable of causing impetigo, wounds may become infected in this way.

If someone, particularly a child or young person presents with an itchy scalp, impetigo or excoriation around the nape of the neck, head infestation must be ruled out. The eggs (nits) are firmly attached to the hair and hence can be distinguished from dandruff. The egg is laid on the hair shaft very close to the scalp and initially is greyish in colour and difficult to see. Later as the hair grows the nit becomes pearl white and easily visible. The eggs are frequently located behind the ears, although they may be found anywhere on the head. Eggs found more than a few centimetres from the scalp can be assumed to be dead. The live lice are difficult to see.

The insecticides of choice for the treatment of head infestation are malathion, benzyl benzoate or carbaryl. Although lotions are the preferred method of applying treatment, shampoos containing these insecticides are effective and of course they are much more acceptable to the patients. The reservoir of infestation is frequently the family so it is important that the whole family is treated at the same time.

PARASITIC DISEASES: ENDOPARASITES

Enterobiasis (*threadworm disease*)

Causal agent. Enterobius vermicularis, a small whitish threadlike nematode (roundworm) 5–12 mm long.

Frequency and distribution. The disease is found in most parts of the world and is the most common helminth infection affecting man. Up to 15 million people infected in the United Kingdom and more often these are children.

Identification. The patient is often symptomless but may notice the threadlike worms on the surface of the stool. The most common symptom is itching around the anus which may lead to scratching and disturbed sleep. The worm may cause appendicitis or, by migration, vaginitis or salpingitis. These complications are however extremely rare and the majority of patients have very mild symptoms. Diagnosis by pressing 'Sellotape' on to perianal skin and then onto a microscope slide. Characteristic eggs are seen under the microscope.

Incubation period. Three to six weeks, though it may take longer before symptoms appear, because the number of worms increases with continuous self-reinfections.

Infectivity period. The patient is infectious for as long as pregnant female worms remain in the gut. An individual worm lives for about two months.

Reservoir. Man. Similar worms in other animals do not infect man.

Mode of transmission. The adult worm lives in the caecum, small and large intestines. The gravid female migrates through the anal orifice and lays small sticky eggs on the skin of the peri-anal region. The eggs are then carried by the fingers to the mouth or indirectly to another individual. They are capable of survival for a few days on clothes, bed-linen or dust if conditions are cool and moist. However, person-to-person transmission is most common. The eggs when swallowed hatch out in the small intestine and the cycle recommences.

Control measures. There is no need to isolate the patient but the family and other close contacts should be screened. Simultaneous treatment of all infected members of the family is essential to prevent reinfection. In addition, there should be education in personal hygiene, frequency washing of the peri-anal region and the need to keep fingernails short and clean. The most important general environmental control measures are frequent washing of personal clothing and bed-linen. The hot cycle of the domestic washing machine is sufficient to destroy the eggs.

In institutions, the eggs may be present in dust so that a general clean up should accompany treatment of patients.

Giardiasis

An increasing number of outbreaks of diarrhoeal disease have been reported due to *Giardia lamblia* (a flagellated protozoan), particularly in travellers from overseas.

Although the incubation period is variable, symptoms usually occur within one to two weeks of the exposure. The main features of the clinical illness are nausea, abdominal pain and profuse watery diarrhoea. Travellers are infected from contaminated drinking water but infection may also be transmitted from person-to-person by the faecal-oral route.

Echinococcus granulosus

This tapeworm is found in all parts of the world. The adult worm is small (usually less than a centimetre in length) and lives in the small intestine of dogs, foxes and wolves, the definitive hosts. In Britain, the main concern is with dogs and there are two well recognised life cycles which almost certainly involve different strains of species. The first has the farm dog as the definitive host and the sheep as the intermediate host. The second involves the fox-hound and the horse. In each case, the intermediate hosts (sheep and horse) acquire the infection by grazing on pastures which are contaminated with dog faeces. The eggs hatch in their intestine and release oncospheres which, via the portal circulation, reach the liver, lungs and occasionally other organs. Over a period of months, a hydatid cyst may develop which is infective and if dogs eat offal containing these cysts, the cycle is completed. Man becomes involved by serving as an alternative intermediate host, acquiring the infection by handling dogs or eating salad vegetables contaminated with eggs from dogs' faeces. In man hydatid cysts are most commonly found in the liver (70% of cases). Cysts grow slowly, taking a year to become one centimetre in diameter and ten years to reach ten centimetres in diameter. Human cases usually involved the dog/sheep cycle and the place of man in the dog/horse cycle is not clear, although the prevalence of echinococcus in horses is around 60%.

Britain lags behind other countries in controlling the disease. In New Zealand and Iceland, for example, the disease in man has been virtually eliminated by breaking the cycle through, more stringent controls of the dog population, the treatment of dogs with antihelminthic drugs and prohibiting the feeding of dogs with infected offal.

HOSPITAL INFECTIONS

Since the end of World War II there has been considerable concern about the frequency of infections acquired by patients whilst they are in hospital (nosocomial infections). This is despite improved methods of sterilisation of equipment and wider adoption of aseptic techniques. The factors involved in this are numerous and include the emergence of resistant strains of organisms (partly due to the increased use of antibiotics); the greater survival of patients with life-threatening illness (for example premature infants) who are more susceptible to infection; the wider use and complexity of surgical techniques; and the advent of modern therapies (such as immuno-suppressive drugs) which lower host-resistance.

Surveys of infection in hospital in-patients in Britain have found around 15–20% had infections, of which almost half had been acquired in hospital. Urinary and wound infections, which are especially likely to develop whilst the patient is in hospital, tend to be endogenous (i.e. a break in the patient's natural body defences causes the patient's own normal bacterial flora to induce infection). Nosocomial infections often lengthen the patient's stay in hospital with attendant economic implications both for the individual and the service as a whole. In the 1960s, the organisms which caused most problems in hospitals were the resistant strains of *Staphylococcus aureus*. This organism is still responsible for a proportion of hospital acquired infections as are some types of streptococcus. The major threat today, however, comes from the gram-negative bacteria including *Escherichia coli, Enterobacter, Klebsiella, Serratia, Pseudomonas* and *Proteus*. Viruses and fungi contribute to a much smaller proportion of such infections.

Although infection is human in origin, coming from other patients, staff or visitors, the source may be either human or the hospital environment (for example, dust, air-conditioning systems or instruments).

Endogenous infection is by far the commonest infection which develops in hospital patients, particularly as a result of surgical procedures or other instrumentation (for example, catheterisation). Cross-infection is classically thought of when hospital-acquired infections are mentioned and this may arise either by contamination of instruments or by transmission of pathogenic organisms on the hands and uniforms of doctors and nurses. Similarly, doctors and nurses who carry organisms in their nasopharynx can induce infection in patients. A classic example of this is the hospital worker who causes an outbreak of staphylococcal infection in a nursery because of nasopharyngeal carriage of staphylococcus aureus. Environmental infection, occurring when organisms can survive and multiply within the hospital environment, is a potential source of problems. Obvious hazards are places like the ward sluice, but more subtle are antiseptic solutions and disinfectants, or even sometimes medication like eye-drops.

It should not be forgotten that some people who develop an infection in hospital might have acquired it at home in the community and have been admitted during the incubation period of illness.

Isolation of cases (and carriers) is advisable. There is no single effective control measure but continuously high standards of hygiene are essential and education of staff is necessary to achieve this. Designers of hospitals should be mindful of the risk of infection at all times. A high standard of building maintenance should be observed. Strict adherence to a routine of cleaning premises is needed. When an outbreak involving a highly infectious agent occurs, it may be necessary to close the ward to interrupt transmission and allow for cleaning and disinfection.

CONCLUSIONS

Communicable disease surveillance and control remains a central component of public health practice. Despite the decline in the relative importance of communicable diseases as causes of death, they remain a major source of morbidity in the population. They can often produce distressing symptoms and complications, and in some cases, they still do cause death. Whilst control of the acute outbreak of illness caused by a micro-organism is vitally important and is the aspect of this field of work which keeps communicable diseases in the public eye, it is only one part of a comprehensive public health approach to communicable disease control. A detailed understanding of the nature, causes, modes of transmission and clinical features of communicable diseases is also essential to an overall strategy of population control of this group of diseases. So too, as in many other fields of public health, is the availability of accurate information and its proper analysis. There is also a need for clear policies for communicable disease control which place strong emphasis on prevention.

10 Environment and health

INTRODUCTION

Environmental issues are a prominent feature of society. They are raised in the classroom, in the media as well as in national and local politics. The relationship between human health and the environment is part of this wider debate. Partly this stems from a growing realisation that the physical environment is far more fragile and susceptible to human destructive influence than was previously believed. Partly it is because of the development of a much broader understanding of the determinants of health and ill-health, which include many environmental factors.

The concept of environment encompasses our physical surroundings, either natural or man-made, the air that we breathe, the pollution we create, the climate and natural life that make up our ecosystem and the social, economic and political infrastructure which regulate and control our lives. It is together that these different facets of a complex environment exert their influence on health. This chapter deals with that relationship.

THE ENVIRONMENT AND HEALTH

Mankind is part inheritor, part creator and part caretaker of the environment. In order both to maintain and promote good health, the environment in which we live must be supportive. It must be a healthy environment. In 1985, as a part of the World Health Organisation's strategy for 'Health for All by the Year 2000', 38 internationally relevant targets were set for the European Region (Table 10.1). Targets 18 to 25 concerned the environment and health. These targets covered specific issues (such as occupational hazards, housing, waste, food contamination, air pollution and water quality) and issues of general importance (such as the need for clear policies for the monitoring, assessment and control of environmental hazards, and the need for multi-disciplinary policies, public awareness, participation and international co-operation).

The ecosystem

The interdependence of people and their environment has been further highlighted by, for example, the World Commission on Environment and Development, the European Charter on Environment and Health and by the British Government's White Paper 'This Common Inheritance'. All of these policy documents for the 1990s and beyond have acknowledged that the earth and its atmosphere is a closed system. If all fossil fuels are allowed to burn, if noxious gases are pumped into the atmosphere, if raw sewage is poured into rivers and oceans and if population growth is allowed to continue unchecked, then it is future generations who will have to live with the consequences. The natural environment does have regenerative qualities but, if in the struggle to develop and survive they are destroyed, the result could be rapid degeneration to the point where the environment is no longer able to support human existence. At current rates of change this future state could possibly be only a few hundred years away.

Table 10.1:   Targets 18–25 of the World Health Organisation "Targets for Health for All by the Year 2000" in the European Region

---

18. By 1990, member states should have multisectoral policies that effectively protect the human environment from health hazards, ensure community awareness and involvement, and effectively support international efforts to curb such hazards affecting more than one country.

19. By 1990, all member states should have adequate machinery for the monitoring, assessment and control of the environmental hazards which pose a threat to human health, including potentially toxic chemicals, radiation, harmful consumer goods and biological agents.

20. By 1990, all people of the Region should have adequate supplies of safe drinking-water, and by the year 1995 pollution of rivers, lakes and seas should no longer pose a threat to human health.

21. By 1995, all people in the Region should be effectively protected against recognised health risks from air pollution.

22. By 1990, all member states should have significantly reduced health risks from food contamination and implemented measures to protect consumers from harmful additives.

23. By 1995, all member states should have eliminated major known health risks associated with the disposal of hazardous wastes.

24. By the year 2000, all people of the Region should have a better opportunity of living in houses and settlements which provide healthy and safe environment.

25. By 1995, people of the Region should be effectively protected against work-related health risks.

Source: World Health Organisation Regional Office for Europe. Targets for Health for All by the Year 2000 in the European Region. Copenhagen: WHO-EURO 1985.

To many this may be too pessimistic a view to be believable. Nevertheless, it is a picture painted by some of the most eminent scientists in the world, based upon current knowledge of the changing environment, population trends and their interrelationship.

The reaction of people in many developed countries such as Britain has been to behave as if they had direct responsibility only for the environment in which they themselves live, effectively treating the environment as an open system. For example, provided that toxic waste is disposed of at sea or in other countries, as long as acid rain does not fall on its creators, as long as enough wealth is generated to obtain the resources needed and as long as population growth is contained, then a wider responsibility for the world's environment does not become a priority. This approach ignores the irrefutable fact that the world's physical environment is one environment (a closed system), albeit a complex one. Pollution of the air and oceans does not recognise national boundaries; destruction of the ozone layer is a global problem; excessive use of natural resources in one part of the world deprives another; and population growth in one part of the world inevitably makes demands on the environment and its resources in other areas.

The realisation of these fundamental principles leads inescapably to the conclusion that people within their own communities must start to look at their local environment as if it were a closed system. This means, for example, recycling waste rather than exporting it; using renewable rather than expendable resources; maintaining an optimum balance between resource use and population growth and maintaining the environment in a supportive state. In addition, the developed world has to start taking an interest in the management of the environment in less developed countries. If it tackles its own environmental problems without helping the developing world, then all that will be achieved is a shift of responsibility for the global environment on to those currently least able to do anything about it. Ultimately the problem will be made worse, not better. What is needed is summed up in the phrase 'sustainable development'.

For most people, environment equates to their immediate home, neighbourhood, village, town or city. Different physical environments surround those who live in a large detached house with a garden compared to those living in a small flat in a high rise block. Similarly, the environment of people living twenty miles from the nearest town is different from those living in the heart of a big city. World population continues to grow rapidly and it is clear that, if nothing else, we have to learn better how to accommodate such growth, live together and share a common future on this planet. The problems associated with such growth and development require a new environmental awareness. Such awareness is a necessary prerequisite to the development of strategies for ensuring mankind's continued survival.

Threats to the environment

The twelve most important problems at an international level, which threaten future wellbeing have been called the Dirty Dozen (Table 10.2). These are all global issues which have major consequences for public health. The responsibility to tackle these issues is also a global one.

It is because people cannot see that addressing these problems will lead to immediate major local health benefits, that many continue to deny the need to act urgently, or indeed, at all. Such attitudes are widespread in society and pose one of the major threats to future human health. Much of the advanced technology required to make industry, agriculture and transport less polluting; to harness renewable energy sources; to stabilise population growth; to provide sufficient food and to ensure global security, already exists. The problem is getting people to change their individual behaviour, policies and organisational practices.

Policies for a healthy environment

Those working within the field of public health and indeed, within the health service as a whole, have an important role to play in keeping these issues constantly in the public mind. They can do this by, for example, focusing attention on those actions which can be taken by individuals and organisations within their localities or region which have a positive environmental impact and similarly, by influencing policy makers.

Table 10.2:   The Dirty Dozen of the ecological
crisis – the 12 most important
problems, at an international level,
which threaten our future well-being

1. Ozone depletion
2. Global Warming
3. The Energy Crisis
4. Air Pollution
5. Soil Erosion and Desertification
6. Deforestation
7. Water Shortages
8. Chemicals
9. Toxic Wastes
10. Arms Spending
11. International Debt
12. Population Growth

Source: Porritt J. *Where on Earth are we Going?* London: BBC
Books 1990.

Local action might begin with all organisations embarking on a process of assessing the impact of their activities on both global and local environments and instituting, where possible, appropriate measures to lessen potentially damaging activities and encourage ones which are protective. Such a programme should be guided by a set of environmental principles. Seven key objectives for environmental policy could be adopted by organisations within a locality or a region both in the public and private sectors (Table 10.3). Actions like these, if taken by a majority of large organisations, will lead to the changes in infrastructure which are necessary to support widespread adoption of more environmentally conscious lifestyles.

The health service itself is a vast organisation. Taken together, its staff, its facilities and the processes of care have a huge environmental impact. The National Health Service is one of the largest users of energy, with expenditure representing 1.6% of the total national consumption. The consumption of fossil fuel is recognised as one of the most important causes of environmental damage, primarily through the generation of carbon dioxide emissions. However, since the first international oil crisis in the 1970s, energy consumption in the National Health Service has been reduced by 30%. During the 1980s, savings of 10% were achieved despite major increases in clinical activity and the rapid growth of new technology (Figure 10.1).

By focusing on the environmental impact of their work, organisations have the potential to produce major change. For example, the use of engineering techniques in the design and maintenance of buildings to increase the efficiency of energy use is of great importance. An illustration of the implication of such techniques in the health service is in the design of low energy hospitals. These have incorporated high levels of insulation and glazing, efficient heat and light control systems and landscaping designed to help reduce heat loss. These features, together with the recycling of waste heat and the use of waste to generate heat and power are all measures which can reduce energy consumption by up to 60%.

Table 10.3:   Seven key objectives for environmental protection

1.   To minimise actions which directly or indirectly cause local or distant pollution of air or water with radiation, biological or chemical sources.

2.   To minimise energy expenditure and maximise energy conservation in all activities.

3.   To minimise the use of non-renewable resources; maximise the use of recycled or renewable resources; and maximise the recycling of all resources used.

4.   To minimise actions which threaten plant or animal life and maximise efforts to conserve and promote wildlife habitats.

5.   To maximise efforts to provide safe, aesthetically pleasing and health promoting indoor and outdoor built environments.

6.   To minimise actions, economic and physical, which are detrimental to sustainable development in the UK or other countries of the world and maximise efforts to promote sustainable development in the same.

7.   To maximise efforts to promote environmental protection through education of the public and professionals, active leadership, community development and collaboration with other organisations in all sectors.

Source: White M. Northumberland Health Authority and the Environment: A Discussion Document. Newcastle: Division of Epidemiology and Public Health, University of Newcastle upon Tyne 1991.

A holistic view is essential to a full consideration of the environment and health. Equally, the promotion of public health requires both a full understanding of these complex issues and a broadly based approach to action programmes to create improvement.

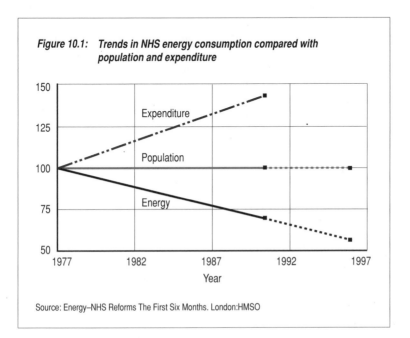

Figure 10.1:   Trends in NHS energy consumption compared with population and expenditure

Source: Energy–NHS Reforms The First Six Months. London:HMSO

In addition, public health is concerned with specific aspects of the physical environment which have the potential to influence health. The remaining sections of this chapter are concerned with some of these specific aspects, the threat which they can pose to human health together with measures required to prevent and protect health.

WATER

Contamination of the water supply in the past has been a major cause of disease and death. It was the provision of a safe water supply, together with proper disposal of sewage, which constituted one of the triumphs of the public health pioneers of the last century.

About 200 litres of water per person per day are used for all domestic purposes. Water can be an important route for the spread of diseases such as cholera, enteric fevers, amoebic and bacillary dysenteries, infective hepatitis and helminthic infections. The main principle in preventing the transmission of water borne diseases is to prevent human and animal excretions from contaminating water intended for human consumption. Similarly, chemical contaminants from industry and agriculture must be prevented from entering a supply which is intended for drinking water. Unfortunately, in most of the water supplies, it is not possible to guarantee that contamination has not occurred. Hence, purification treatment is a routine requirement.

Sources of water

Water is an excellent solvent for most gases and many solids and also for carrying other substances in suspension. Surface water is the main source of public supply in Britain. Water flowing over the ground dissolves minerals and can carry suspended matter, as well as bacteria, algae and various other plants and animals. Upland surface water in natural lakes and man made reservoirs is relatively free from contamination by human and animal life. Rivers, which supply about 70% of drinking water, become more polluted as they flow from their source to the sea. In some parts of Britain, it is necessary to draw on sources from the lower reaches of rivers. Hence, with considerable contamination, a full purification treatment is necessary.

On the other hand, underground water from deep wells and boreholes requires only minimal treatment, being of good quality and almost free from contamination. However, this source contributes only a small proportion to the public water supply. It is hard water because of the dissolved minerals but most people find it palatable. In some areas, water contains significant quantities of dissolved natural radioactivity which requires specialised treatment, except in certain health spas where its 'curative' properties are promoted.

Monitoring the quality of water

Water for human consumption undergoes regular physical, chemical and bacteriological tests.

Physical properties, such as taste, colour and smell are high priorities in determining acceptability, although they may have little bearing on whether the water is safe to drink.

Chemical analysis to determine the type and importance of various chemicals present in water is well established. The presence of nitrogen compounds, either as inorganic ammonium nitrate and nitrites or in its various organic forms, reflects different stages in the decomposition of organic matter in water. High concentrations of chlorides suggest contamination by sewage. Calcium and magnesium salts are an indication of the hardness of the water. The absence of dissolved oxygen is strong evidence of heavy pollution. In addition, chemical analysis may reveal the presence of small quantities of potentially dangerous substances, such as lead.

Bacteriological examination is based mainly on isolating and quantifying coliform organisms. *Escherichia coli* is regarded as an indicator of human or animal faecal pollution.

Purification treatment

The aim of purification is to remove pathogenic bacteria, harmful chemicals, suspended matter and any substance causing colour, odour or undesirable taste.

There are a number of methods of water purification, including filtration, disinfection with chlorine, the use of ozone and activated charcoal. The method most commonly used in Britain is described here. Unlike underground water, which usually only needs the disinfection process, river water requires the full treatment.

Water is first coarse filtered, to remove solid objects and then stored in reservoirs, to allow sedimentation. This storage system has the advantage of allowing the supply from the rivers to be cut off if excessive contamination occurs.

The next step in the purification process is filtration, through either slow or rapid filters. Slow sand filters consist of sand resting on layers of graded gravel. The active part is the slime (algae, worms and suspended substances) which form on the surface, trapping fine suspended matter (including bacteria) and also oxidising organic matter. Rapid sand filters are more widely used and are made of coarser sand which allows the water to flow through more quickly. Salts of aluminium or iron are added to the water to form floccules, which act in a similar, though less efficient, way to the biological layer in the slow sand filters. Bacteria can pass through and their destruction depends on the next phase of purification which is disinfection.

Chlorine is the most widely used disinfectant agent and is automatically delivered, at a concentration of 0.5 ppm (parts per million) by specialised equipment. Before the water is distributed, the level of chlorine is reduced by sulphur dioxide to 0.1–0.3 ppm so that at this residual level disinfection can still be maintained.

After purification, water is held in covered service reservoirs and delivered in main pipes sunk deep enough to avoid frosts.

The process of water supply, purification and distribution is shown diagrammatically in Figure 10.2.

Fluoride and dental health

The presence of fluoride in drinking water at about 1 ppm, has been found to reduce dental decay in the population receiving it by around 60%.

Small amounts of fluoride occur naturally in water that is in contact with the Earth's rocks. In many countries, including parts of Britain, fluoride is also added

Figure 10.2: The process of water supply, purification and distribution

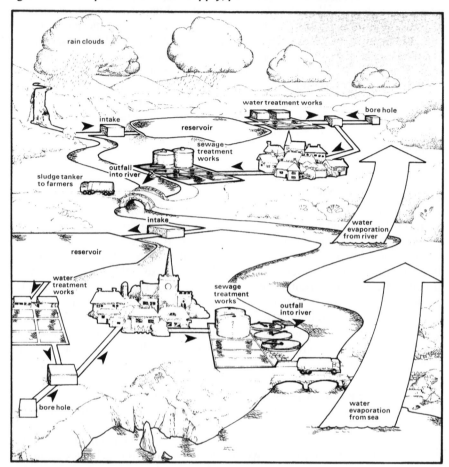

Source: Which? January 1980

to the water supply. Higher levels, which sometimes occur naturally, cause mottling of the dental enamel.

Such measures have been controversial with opponents claiming serious ill effects following the consumption of fluoridated drinking water. However, there is no evidence at all that this is so. Despite this, the influence of a vociferous minority has resulted in Parliament delegating the decision on fluoridation of water supplies for local determination by health authorities and water companies. This is a different approach from that taken in many other countries, which introduced this well-health measure on a national basis. The geographical distribution of fluoridated water is patchy, to the disadvantage of many children's dental health.

Nitrate

Agriculture is the main source of nitrate in the water. Organic nitrogen from the soil and from fertilisers is released into rivers and underground water. The amount which is leached from agricultural land depends on the farming activities as well as the climate. Nitrates in deep underground water may therefore be a reflection of agricultural activities in earlier years.

In parts of Britain the nitrate level in drinking water is higher than the limit set by the European Community (EC) Drinking Water Directive. In order to help overcome this problem the Government has designated nitrate sensitive areas, in which certain agricultural operations are regulated. In addition, farmers may qualify for payments to change their farming operations, such as, switching from arable to grassland cultivation. Another approach is for water companies to install denitrification plants although few have done so in the United Kingdom.

If the nitrate value is 50 mg/litre as nitrous oxide then methaemoglobinaemia can occur in bottle fed babies. This is sometimes called the 'blue baby syndrome' because of cyanosis caused by methaemoglobin preventing the absorption of oxygen by the blood. This tends to occur in rural areas in dry summers. In these circumstances, bottled water is supplied to infants.

Ingestion of nitrates have also been implicated in the causation of cancer in adults, particularly stomach cancer, but the evidence is inconclusive.

Lead

For centuries lead has been recognised as a poison. Lead in tap water is virtually always derived from the domestic plumbing system, particularly where the water is soft and acidic. Installation of lead pipework has been banned in houses since 1964.

In Britain the maximum prescribed level for lead in drinking water is 50 micrograms/litre, which is half the prescribed EC level. There is evidence that lead can cause intellectual impairment in children and therefore levels of lead in drinking water should be even lower. This can be achieved by individuals flushing the pipes before consuming the water and by water undertakings rendering the water more alkaline. The replacement of lead pipes is the most satisfactory but expensive solution.

Aluminium

Water, particularly if it is acidic, can dissolve aluminium from rocks. Large quantities of aluminium are also used in water treatment and careful control is required to prevent it arriving at the tap. The United Kingdom limit is set at the EC Directive Level of 0.2 mg/litre.

Things can go wrong. A load of aluminium sulphate was accidently dumped into a water supply in Cornwall in 1988. The residents of Camelford complained of a variety of symptoms involving the skin and gastro-intestinal system. Whether these symptoms were caused by aluminium or by copper poisoning, as a result of acid water dissolving copper, remains in doubt. However, there was no doubt about the inappropriate manner in which the Water Authority handled the situation by adopting a defensive attitude and by giving confusing and contradictory advice.

A subsequent enquiry attributed the cause of most of the symptoms to anxiety caused by the Water Authority's mishandling of the situation and to alarmist reports in the media.

There is evidence that high aluminium levels in drinking water may contribute to bone disease and there have been widely publicised reports of aluminium being implicated in Alzheimer's Disease. The evidence for this is contradictory but some kidney dialysis patients, using water with high aluminium content, have developed a condition known as 'dialysis dementia'. Investigations are also taking place into the role of aluminium in senile dementia. In this case other factors may be involved, such as, a higher intake of aluminium in the diet and impaired kidney secretion in elderly people.

Sea water

The possible effects on health of bathing in seawater contaminated by sewage is a matter of public concern. In Britain, the Public Health Laboratory Service carried out a retrospective study over a five year period from 1953. This was limited to examining the bathing habits of notified cases of poliomyelitis and enteric fever with a suitable matched control group. For patients with poliomyelitis, it was suggested that sea bathing, three weeks prior to the onset of symptoms, was probably irrelevant as a causal factor. There were four cases of paratyphoid fever in which bathing in sewage contaminated seawater could be implicated.

The general conclusion of this and later studies has been that there is no serious risk of contracting disease through bathing in sewage polluted seawater. Public health requirements would be met by improving grossly insanitary bathing water and preventing the pollution of bathing beaches with undisintegrated faecal matter during the bathing season. This does not address the question of the public's attitude which is likely to reject the idea of any sewage discharges into water used for sea bathing.

EC Directives lay down standards for sea bathing water expressed in total coliform organisms per 100 ml. Sampling is carried out on a regular basis.

WASTE MANAGEMENT AND DISPOSAL

Households in Britain are responsible for some 20 million tonnes of waste each year: about 8 tonnes of waste for each household. Industry generates about 100 million tonnes each year.

About 90% of waste in Britain is disposed of in some 4,000 landfill sites and there are 35 municipal incinerators which burn most of the remaining household waste. In addition, four specialised high temperature incinerators deal with some of the most toxic waste.

Landfill sites require careful design, either in suitable geology (for example, clay) or with impervious linings. To avoid problems with leachate and gas generation, it is necessary to ensure high legislative and enforcement standards, better engineering where necessary and an appropriate programme of monitoring at the site.

Sewage treatment

Domestic sewage contains a large number of intestinal organisms and is, therefore, potentially hazardous. The quantity is roughly equal to the amount of water used. A similar amount of industrial waste, which may contain toxic chemicals, runs into public sewers or directly into rivers as can agricultural waste water. About 90% of domestic refuse and industrial waste (some of it toxic) is disposed of in landfill sites, with the possibility of effluent reaching rivers as surface water or seeping into the underground water table.

From an environmental and public health point of view, therefore, a main concern in controlling disposal of sewage and domestic and industrial waste is to prevent the contamination of the water environment through which, in the end, drinking water is derived.

There is a variety of ways of treating sewage, in addition to the standard and widely used method described here. Sewage is first screened to remove large objects and disperse large solids, before it passes into sedimentation tanks, where further separation occurs. The next stage is biological treatment and the most frequently employed process is known as the *activated sludge* method. Here, in aeration tanks, the sewage is vigorously agitated or air is bubbled through it, to encourage the growth of aerobic organisms. It then passes into settling tanks from which the sludge is removed and the effluent is discharged, usually into rivers.

A variety of methods can be employed to deal with the liquid sludge, which still contains over 90% water. A frequently used, economical method involves putting the sludge into closed tanks to undergo anaerobic fermentation. The gas given off consists of 70% methane and provides the sewage works with an energy source. The resulting digested sludge is then dried, either in lagoons or by mechanical pressure. What remains is then normally free from unpleasant odour and may be used as a fertiliser.

In England and Wales, 96% of domestic properties are connected to the sewage system, the highest proportion in Europe. About 6,500 inland treatment works receive 83% of all sewage and most of the effluent is discharged into rivers. Unfortunately, by 1990, nearly one in five sewage works were failing to meet their discharge consent conditions, set by the National Rivers Authority. Failure to comply was often because the plant was inadequate to deal with an increased load. The water industry now has in place a very large investment programme which is designed to improve the situation over a period of years.

An even more unsatisfactory situation pertains with the proportion of sewage (17%) which is discharged into the sea. Much of this has had little or no treatment. Even when outfall pipes are laid far out from the shore (and a few are not even past the low tide mark) wind and tide wash sewage ashore. A large investment programme is required to address this situation.

Industrial waste

Most chemicals in rivers are by-products of industrial processes but some, like pesticides, also come from agricultural activities. The Government has compiled a 'Red List', which is drawn from a European Community Directive of Dangerous Substances in Water. These substances are persistent, toxic and liable to accumulate in living tissues. They include heavy metals, pesticides, chlorinated industrial chemicals and solvents. Renewed efforts are being made to reduce levels by applying environmental quality standards, by reviewing discharge consents and through government controls on the production and use of harmful substances.

Agricultural waste

Farm slurry, because of the amount of organic matter it contains, is a hundred times more polluting than raw sewage. Silage effluent is even more polluting. Farm waste contains a wide variety of micro-organisms, some of them pathogenic to man. In addition, it contains chemicals, particularly nitrates and phosphates. Some waste flows directly into streams and rivers. Much of it is returned to the land where it may be carried by erosion to ponds, lakes, streams and rivers. In lakes and ponds a problem known as eutrophication may occur. This is a process in which the water becomes richer and richer in nutrients, particularly phosphates and nitrates. There is then an accelerated growth of aquatic plants and algae, resulting in deoxygenation of the water, which becomes lifeless and foul smelling. These nutrients also come from industrial and domestic waste. Detergents contribute up to half the phosphate content of domestic sewage.

The National Rivers Authority has carried out surveys in several regions, which indicate a scale of agricultural pollution more widespread than the number of reported incidents suggest. In the late 1980s, the British Government introduced 50% grants to provide, replace or improve facilities for storage, treatment and disposal of agricultural waste and silage effluent. Other measures, such as a free advisory service, were also put in place.

PESTICIDES

The extensive use of pesticides makes it almost impossible for an individual to avoid some exposure.

Pesticides can enter the human body by inhalation, ingestion or through the skin. In the case of the general public, however, pesticide exposure is primarily through eating food or drinking water. The potential risks to health from diet are a frequent cause of fear and alarm in the public, often enhanced by somewhat sensationalised reports in the media. Nevertheless, the public have a right to expect no harmful effects from food and water consumption.

The Ministry of Agriculture, Fisheries and Food (MAFF) is responsible for co-ordinating the monitoring of pesticides. Maximum Recommended Levels (MRLs) are set for pesticide residues in the main fruit and vegetable components of diet. The levels of residue both in home produced and imported food are monitored. In addition, surveys are carried out of residues in humans, wild life and in the environment.

Modern analytical methods allow detection of very small amounts of pesticides in water. Samples containing pesticide residues at levels higher than those recommended as safe have been reported from various places, particularly supplies drawing water from agricultural areas.

Effects on health

The health effects of acute exposure and acute poisoning by pesticides are well documented. Illnesses usually follow, either accidental or deliberate ingestion or skin contamination following careless handling. The symptoms occur shortly afterwards and, in the majority of cases, there is complete recovery without long-term complications.

The main interest to public health is the effect of small doses over a long period of time. Here the evidence is much less clear. One way of attempting to identify the long-term health effects of exposure to low level or intermediate doses of pesticides, is to study groups of people who have been exposed. Possible outcomes of pesticide exposure which have been considered are cancer, the effect on the fetus, damage to the nervous system, as well as mutagenicity and allergies. However, in most studies, the link between these conditions and pesticides has been tenuous.

LOCAL ENVIRONMENT QUALITY

The importance which people attach to their immediate environment is emphasised by a population survey carried out in one of Britain's larger cities. When people on Tyneside were asked 'Do you have any ideas about how we could work towards making Newcastle a healthier city?', the most common comments related to improvement in the environment (Figure 10.3). The general public was making a clear and explicit link between their environment and health. Some of the issues raised related to making the environment more pleasant, with less litter, more green spaces and less traffic noise and pollution. Others were about making it safer, with less risk of ill-health from vermin, city centre traffic and unsafe play facilities.

This study provided a fascinating glimpse into people's perceptions of health. Aside from traditional notions of freedom from disease and positive lifestyles, experiencing a healthy environment was seen to be part of being healthy. It also places in a somewhat different light traditional environmental improvement activities at local level (control of dogs, litter, noise, and nuisances) which some have considered as unfashionable and having no place in a modern conceptualisation of public health. This section reviews the public health approach to a number of issues which are of importance to the quality of the local environment.

Nuisance

The term 'nuisance' has been used in legislation since the last century. Nuisances were thought to be responsible for ill health at a time when it was believed that odours were the cause of disease. Nuisances are currently concerned with physical and psychological discomfort (for example, smoke, odours, noise). Local authorities have a legal obligation placed on them, by various Acts, to take action to abate 'statutory' nuisances.

Noise

Noise is an unwanted sound which causes discomfort to the listener. Sound is a form of energy which is transmitted through the air by rapid cyclic pressure changes. Noise in excess is regarded as a pollutant in the environment.

There is a wide range of literature on the effects of noise on hearing, sleep, communication, work and leisure, as well as other general physiological and psychological parameters. The evidence is not always convincing, with examples which are contradictory and inconclusive. On the other hand, there is ample indication of very high degrees of annoyance caused by noise to sections of the

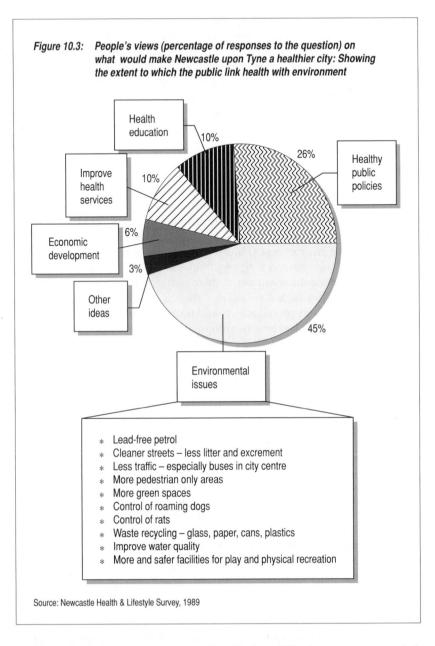

Figure 10.3: **People's views (percentage of responses to the question) on what would make Newcastle upon Tyne a healthier city: Showing the extent to which the public link health with environment**

Health education — 10%

Improve health services — 10%

Economic development — 6%

Other ideas — 3%

Healthy public policies — 26%

Environmental issues — 45%

* Lead-free petrol
* Cleaner streets – less litter and excrement
* Less traffic – especially buses in city centre
* More pedestrian only areas
* More green spaces
* Control of roaming dogs
* Control of rats
* Waste recycling – glass, paper, cans, plastics
* Improve water quality
* More and safer facilities for play and physical recreation

Source: Newcastle Health & Lifestyle Survey, 1989

population. Such factors are easy to identify but difficult to measure and thus, ultimately also difficult to control.

Workers have a high risk of noise induced deafness if their environment has noise levels equivalent to a continuous level of 90 dBA or more. However, occupational deafness is the result of fairly lengthy exposure. Permanent deafness may also result from a single, loud explosive sound. Transient deafness (temporary threshold shift) may also be the sequel of exposure to a sudden loud noise or to prolonged intense noise. It is unlikely that environmental noise will cause hearing loss, except in special situations like discotheques. Studies suggest that sleep is disturbed above 35 L_{eq} (see below for an explanation of this term). Although the noise may not be sufficient to cause wakening, the quality of sleep may be impaired, resulting in poor task performance.

In the experimental situation, noise affects people physically in many ways. In laboratory work changes are induced in the circulatory system including raised blood pressure, elevated skin conductive levels and increased secretion of hormones indicative of sympathetic nervous system activity and generalised stress reaction. Environmental noise, which produces a high degree of annoyance in a section of the population, can interfere with periods of rest and relaxation and produce stress. Many studies in Britain and other countries, concerning noise, relate to the effect of aircraft noise on health.

The main causes of complaints about noise relate to domestic premises (60%) and industrial and commercial sources (20%). Aircraft noise causes considerable annoyance but tends to be localised near airports.

Level, frequency, loudness and time are four characteristics of sound which are important when assessing noise.

Level

Sound is transmitted through the air in waves giving rise to positive and negative fluctuations in pressure. The greater the fluctuations, the greater is the intensity of sound. The difference between positive and negative pressure is known as amplitude. Sound level meters measure pressure on a logarithmic scale which is expressed in decibels (dB).

Frequency

Frequency is dependent on the length of the sound waves, hence, their rate of repetition. The higher the frequency, the higher the pitch of the sound. Very low frequencies and very high frequencies are not audible to the human ear. It is measured in the number of cycles per second or hertz (Hz).

Loudness

Loudness is the listener's impression of sound and it is not a measurable quantity, although it is closely related to sound pressure and changes in frequency. An increase of 10 dB will seem twice as loud, while a change of less than 3 dB is hard for the human ear to detect, although sound energy will, in fact, have doubled.

Sound level meters incorporate filters and electronic circuits which simulate the function of the human ear. In practice, the so called 'A scale' is most used (dBA) and has been found to correlate well with responses of the human ear to various sound sources.

Time

Most environmental noise sources fluctuate over time. A number of measurements have been devised to take account of the level of fluctuations. One commonly used unit is the 'continuous equivalent sound level' (L_{eq}). This is the level of sound energy delivered over a defined period of time, which would be the same as the fluctuating source. Aircraft noise is assessed by a 'noise and number index' (NNI), which takes account of the sound level of each aircraft and the number of movements in a given time.

Housing

Living accommodation is designed to provide shelter, security, privacy and comfort. Whether it be in the form of a house, a flat, a bed-sitting room, a caravan, a houseboat or a residential institution, all are covered by legislation.

The Industrial Revolution led to small houses and large tenements, crowding the centres of the new towns and cities, in narrow streets with little open space. Those dwellings were poorly ventilated, ill lit, lacking in sanitary facilities and the practice of burning coal on open fires created a smoke polluted environment.

The recognition of the association between poor housing and poor health was a main focus of the sanitary reformers of the last century. In the first half of this century, with the great improvements in sanitary conditions, emphasis changed to the link between inadequate housing and communicable diseases, particularly tuberculosis. Stress was placed on the design of houses to provide good ventilation, natural lighting, heating and the eradication of overcrowding. There is general acceptance that these measures contributed to the decline in tuberculosis and in other infectious diseases, prior to the advent of vaccination and effective therapeutic measures. By the 1950s, the great decline in communicable diseases lessened the emphasis on housing as a factor in ill health. There has been a paucity of research into the relationship between housing and health. Much of what has been carried out, has flaws in its methodology. It is now well established that there is a significant association between damp dwellings and respiratory symptoms in children. There is less convincing evidence for this as a cause of adults developing an excess of respiratory symptoms or for links between poor housing and other diseases. In studying this problem, it is difficult to eliminate the effect of confounding variables such as social deprivation which themselves increase the likelihood of respiratory and other illnesses. Moreover, in studies based upon individuals' reports of symptoms there is a further source of bias. For example, people in damp houses are more likely to report symptoms.

In the past, the main process for dealing with unfit housing was slum clearance. This started in 1930 and continued, with a break for World War II, until the mid-1970s. The emphasis then changed to renovation of existing houses with demolition of properties being an exceptional action. In 1979, there were 24,000 dwellings demolished in slum clearance areas but by the end of the 1980s this had fallen to 3,500. On the other hand, the number of major renovations of dwellings doubled over the same time period.

The Local Government and Housing Act 1989 encouraged local housing authorities to assess the need for clearance and renovation on a systematic and area basis.

A new statutory concept of 'renewal areas' was introduced to allow a comprehensive approach covering renovation and development of housing alongside action on social, economic and environmental problems. It is envisaged that this activity would be spread over ten years. Thus, the authorities would have real scope to improve the housing, general amenities and environmental problems in an area.

Before declaring a renewal area authorities must carry out an assessment and consider various options. The assessment team will include, environmental health officers together with other officials, such as planners, valuers and accountants.

Standards for housing are set through local and national legislation and enforced by local authorities. The statutory standards for fitness for human habitation include, structural stability, freedom from dampness and serious disrepair, adequate lighting, heating and ventilation, satisfactory facilities for cooking food, piped supply of wholesome water, fixed bath or shower with hot and cold water, a toilet and effective drainage system.

Virtually all housing authorities take account of any medical problems when considering an application for housing. Many operate a points system to which certain priority factors contribute. Time on the waiting list, family size, over-crowding and poor social circumstances, are some examples. When the required number of points are achieved, the family is rehoused. There is a wide variation between authorities in the number of points allowed for medical priority. Little has been reported on the improvement in health brought about by rehousing.

Pest and vermin control

Various insects, birds and mammals can be pests in certain environments, such as households, institutions and hospitals. Control of pests is important to ensure the quality of local environments.

Insects

The common house fly (*Musca domestica*) and other flies, like bluebottles, feed on human and animal excreta, as well as on food. They can transfer pathogenic organisms to food, either mechanically on their feet, via their faeces or by regurgitation as part of the feeding process. In that they are readily visible, action can be taken to deal with the problem by observing strict rules of cleanliness, adequate disposal of waste food and other matter and the use of fly screens and insecticides.

Of the 4,000 different species of cockroaches, the German cockroach (*Blattella germanica*) and the oriental cockroach (*Blatta orientalis*) or 'steam fly' are commonly found in hospitals, hotels and similar establishments. Cockroaches are nocturnal insects so that occupants of premises may be unaware of their presence until heavy infestation has occurred. They are omnivorous and regurgitate their food leaving characteristic vomit marks or 'spotting'. During the day they hide in safe harbourages, for example, under floors, behind panels, in cupboards, refrigerator insulation and lagging on hot water pipes. Pathogenic bacteria have been isolated from the hind gut and external surfaces of cockroaches. The organisms found tend to reflect those that are present in the environment. Cockroaches in hospitals have been found to carry a wide range of bacteria and viruses with the potential to cause food poisoning and other diseases. Information from surveys suggests that over 50% of hospitals have cockroaches, making them the most common pest.

Of even greater concern is the Pharaoh's ant (*Monomorium pharaonis* (L)). This ant is of tropical origin and is found in permanently heated premises, particularly hospitals but also in other similar institutions and private property. They nest within the building fabric and the worker ants forage along well defined trails. They are omnivorous and have been found, like cockroaches, to carry a range of pathogenic organisms which reflect those found in their environment. Surveys suggest that about 10% of hospitals are infested. They are a major problem because they have been found under wound dressings, in premature baby incubators, in sterile supplies and with their ability to chew through plastic, in sets for giving intravenous fluid.

Mammals

The main mammal pests are rats and mice, which can spoil animal and human food stocks and spread disease. The brown rat (*Rattus norvegicus*), is most commonly encountered in Britain. Less common is the black rat (*Rattus rattus*) which is well known for its historical association with bubonic plague.

Although mice present a less serious problem, they also have a destructive effect on food and spread gastro-intestinal disease.

Feral cats are regarded as pests in hospitals and similar institutions where they can colonise the underground ducting systems.

Birds, such as pigeons and sparrows, can cause considerable trouble by infesting a hospital's kitchens and wards. Many of these birds have been demonstrated to be carriers of food poisoning organisms, which have been implicated in outbreaks of gastro-enteritis. Birds not only cause problems by the fouling of areas with their droppings, they also cause annoyance from their noise.

Control of pests

There are three main approaches to controlling pests. The first is exclusion, incorporating structural features to ensure the building prevents access to various types of pests, and by devices, such as fly screens. The second is good hygiene, which denies pests food and harbourage. Thirdly, and only after the preventive measures have been taken, is elimination. This involves the use of appropriate pesticides which should be handled by experts.

Most hospitals have their pest control undertaken by the private sector and failures often relate to poorly specified contracts. Model contracts for pest control are available from the Department of Health.

ATMOSPHERIC POLLUTION

In the eighteenth and nineteenth centuries, the Industrial Revolution brought increasing problems of atmospheric pollution from the chimneys of factories and houses in the new industrial towns. Legislation to control pollution at that time was directed mainly at industry. The zeal of the sanitary reformers, more than 100 years ago, in achieving safe drinking water and proper disposal of sewage, was not matched by an attack on the other environmental evil, air pollution, which had effectively turned the atmosphere over the large towns into an air sewer. Over the years, the public showed little interest. Indeed, a major contributor to air pollution, the domestic open coal fire, was stoutly defended.

A dramatic turning point in attitudes to atmospheric pollution occurred in December, 1952. A London 'smog' (the word 'smog' was coined to describe fog filled with smoke) coincided with a steep rise in the number of deaths. Although excess deaths had been noted in other smog episodes, nothing quite as striking had occurred before. The matter received wide media coverage and a curious occurrence made the story even more sensational. A number of prime young cattle, at a show in London, also succumbed from the effects of pollution. Some cynical observers attributed the swift action that followed as a testament to the British love of animals.

Legislation

The results of the events in the early 1950s in London, led to the first Clean Air Act of 1956 and subsequent legislation. This set a framework for action and was enhanced by other factors, such as the trend towards central heating and the switch in the 1960s to natural gas, which is smoke free and virtually sulphur free.

A major feature of the legislation was to create smoke control areas. In general in these areas it is an offence to emit smoke from a chimney. They are not 'smokeless zones' because controlled amounts of smoke from specific buildings are permitted, for example, as the result of lighting up a furnace. The main thrust of the scheme was to reduce smoke from the domestic fire, which had been identified as contributing to 80% of pollution.

The result was a dramatic improvement. The average visibility on a winter's day in London increased from one to four miles. The concept in the legislation has been adopted by other countries and it formed the basis for the quality standards in European Community Directives. By 1980, the perceived success of the reduction of atmospheric pollution led to the demise of the very bodies which helped to solve the problem: the Clean Air Council and the Medical Research Council's Air Pollution Unit. Furthermore, much of the monitoring network for air quality was dismantled. The consequence of these measures has been that the high quality of research into the effects of atmospheric pollution, which started at the time of the London smog, ceased in the 1980s in Britain.

Yet there are gaps in knowledge about the association between current pollutants in the air and diseases of the lung. Comprehensive monitoring and high quality research is needed to assess the affects of atmospheric pollution on the population, especially the more vulnerable members.

Types of pollutants

There are three main statutory Air Quality Standards in Britain which are the subject of EC Directives. Smoke and sulphur dioxide; lead in the air and nitrogen dioxide.

Smoke and sulphur dioxide

As already described, smoke in the atmosphere is greatly reduced from domestic sources (householders can receive grants for conversion to smoke free heating).

Other sources of smoke, such as diesel engines and the burning of straw stubble (to be banned in the United Kingdom) are set for tighter controls by the EC Directives. There is concern about the carcinogenic effect of smaller particles from diesel exhaust fumes.

In Britain, over 70% of emissions of sulphur dioxide are from power stations. Although emissions have decreased by 40% from 1970 levels, proposals are in place under the EC Large Combustion Plants Directive to make further substantial reductions in the 1990s. This can be done by installing equipment to remove sulphur from flue gases or to switch fuels from coal to gas.

Lead in the air

Lead is a particularly dangerous heavy metal. During the 1980s, concern was expressed that the average blood-lead concentration of the population was high. A major contributor to lead in the atmosphere is the petrol engine. As a result, measures were taken, combined with tax incentives, to introduce unleaded petrol. By 1990, one third of all petrol sold was unleaded.

Certain industrial processes also emit lead into the air. However, only at one site was the level above that allowed by the EC Directive.

Nitrogen dioxide

Whereas sulphur dioxide gas is only produced when sulphur is present in the fuel being burnt, oxides of nitrogen are formed when any material is burned. The main sources of oxides of nitrogen are from power stations, large industrial plants and, in particular, motor vehicles, which contribute 80% of the nitrogen dioxide in urban environments.

During the latter part of the 1980s, with growing vehicle emission, levels of nitrogen dioxide were increasing, especially in urban centres. This is now being tackled in the European Community through Vehicle Emission Standards.

Ozone is formed by the action of sunlight on nitrogen oxides and occurs in increased concentrations when hydrocarbons are present. The climate in Britain is less likely to produce this photochemical chain reaction, unlike the well publicised situation in Los Angeles.

Nitrogen oxides and sulphur dioxide contribute to the formation of acid rain. The gases which are involved can be carried long distances by the wind and can cross national boundaries to affect neighbouring countries. Consequently, acidic air pollution can have a widespread effect on buildings, fish, wild life and vegetation.

Other pollutants

Carbon monoxide, which is produced by incomplete combustion of fuel, has increased in the same way and for the same reasons as the oxides of nitrogen. In Britain 85% of carbon monoxide emissions come from car exhausts. The application of EC standards should reduce this. Some radioactive gases, such as argon-41, are routinely released from nuclear power stations and reprocessing plants. Such discharges are subject to site specific authorisations in the United Kingdom and represent a minor component of radiation exposure of the general public.

Incineration of waste has introduced the risk of dangerous pollutants, such as polychlorinated biphenyls and dioxins. EC Standards are set to control such pollutants.

Monitoring

Monitoring is carried out at Government stations at key sites for the three EC Statutory Standards.

Key sites are connected directly to the Department of Environment so that information can be immediately available. This can be made public by weather bulletins to help people who might be affected by air pollution to take necessary steps.

Pollution from industry is the responsibility of HM Inspectorate of Pollution and of local authorities. They have responsibilities for ensuring air and water quality standards and that solid waste is properly disposed of. They also have enforcement powers to ensure that standards are met. The Department of Transport has the responsibility to control pollution from vehicles. This is done by testing emissions from vehicles, through MOT tests and road side checks.

The effects of atmospheric pollution on health

There is wide agreement that patients with established respiratory or cardiac disease, particularly the elderly, suffer adverse effects of atmospheric pollution when it reaches peak level. Prior to the implementation of the Clean Air Act 1956, it was estimated that 4,000 extra deaths per annum could be attributed to atmospheric pollution. Studies showed, from 1952 until 1963, the daily death rate and hospital admission rate increased during periods of fog. Since then, this relationship has not re-appeared.

There is relatively little systematic evidence on the effects of the long term exposure to atmospheric pollutants and more research is urgently needed. Sulphur dioxide, the oxides of nitrogen and ozone, in relatively low concentrations, have an adverse effect on lung function of healthy individuals. There is also evidence of them increasing the hypersensitivity of asthmatics. The acute effects of carbon monoxide are well known.

Indoor air quality

The population spends, on average, 90% of their time indoors and of that time 70% is in their own homes. Thus, air is breathed primarily in a closed environment and more attention is now directed at the micro climate.

Indoor pollution can arise from the activities of individuals (such as cigarette smoking), from combustion of fossil fuels, the growth of moulds in damp conditions from materials of which the building is constructed and emissions from the ground, such as radon, a naturally occurring radioactive gas. The increasingly recognised dangers from radon are discussed in the section on radiation.

Production of carbon monoxide can result through improper installation of gas or solid fuel fires, where there is an inadequate supply of air. Lethal concentrations cause up to 100 deaths every year and at lower levels, the well documented symptoms of chronic carbon monoxide poisoning occur.

Smoking tobacco can give rise to a variety of pollutants in the indoor climate. There is an increased incidence of respiratory illness in children and of lung cancer for non-smokers. It is estimated that several hundred lung cancer deaths a year in Britain can be attributed to passive smoking. In addition, smoking enhances the risk posed by radon, which is estimated to be ten times greater for the smoker than the non-smoker.

A number of volatile chemicals found in products such as paint strippers and glues, can be dangerous if used in poorly ventilated spaces.

Sick building syndrome

Reports of higher incidence of symptoms amongst people who work in certain buildings have given rise to the label 'sick building syndrome'. The type of symptoms reported relate to the eye, headaches, respiratory tract infections and sore throats. A variety of causes have been suggested, including poor air quality and the design of buildings. Research is continuing but has not yet established a specific link between any of the suggested causative factors and illness. However, improved ventilation seems to be helpful in reducing symptoms.

RADIATION

Concern and attention in environmental and public health has centred primarily on ionising, nuclear radiation, though reference will be made later to non-ionising radiation whose effects are of increasing importance.

Most elements have stable forms, their nuclei comprising configurations of *protons* (positively charged particles) and neutrons (particles of similar mass having no charge) effectively in equilibrium. However, some natural elements such as radium and uranium, have no stable form and are said to be *radioactive* emitting *radiation* from their nuclei in moving towards a more stable configuration. Radioactive forms of stable elements (widely used in medicine and industry) can be produced artificially, for example by bombardment with neutrons.

Three types of radiation are emitted principally. *Alpha particles* are essentially identical to the helium nucleus, comprising two protons and two neutrons and consequently having a double positive charge and relatively large mass. *Beta* particles are identical to electrons but emitted from the nucleus after the internal transformation of a neutron into a proton and an electron. *Gamma rays* are electro-magnetic radiation, like x-rays and similar to light but of much higher frequency, and they may be regarded as quanta (or packets) of photons emitted usually during de-excitation of the nucleus, commonly after emission of a beta particle.

In passing through matter, including tissue, each form of radiation loses energy by *ionisation,* removing electrons from the orbital shells of atoms or molecules in the matter and leaving behind ions or free radicals as chemically active species.

However, the alpha particle by its nature is densely ionising, depositing more energy per unit track length, having a high *linear energy transfer* (LET). Consequently, alpha particles have a relatively short range and greater propensity within the body for damaging cells. In contrast to alpha particles, which outside of the body are completely absorbed by a thin sheet of paper or the dead layers of skin, beta and gamma radiation have a lower LET and are more penetrating. Up to

1 cm of aluminium is required to absorb beta radiation and about 4 cm of lead to reduce the gamma ray intensity from, for example, a radium source by a factor of ten. Clearly, beta and gamma radiation can pose a potential risk outside of as well as inside the body.

Concepts of radiation dose to individuals and populations

The *absorbed dose* corresponds to the energy deposited per unit mass. Its unit is the gray (symbol Gy), named after a British scientist, and is equivalent to 1 joule per kilogram.

As might be expected, because of its high LET, 1 Gy of alpha radiation in tissue will cause more harm than 1 Gy of beta or gamma radiation. To provide a common measurement of potential harmfulness the *equivalent dose* is used which is equal to the absorbed dose multiplied by a factor to take account of the LET for that type of radiation. The unit of equivalent dose is called the sievert (symbol Sv), named after a Swedish scientist. For beta and gamma radiation the factor is 1 so that the absorbed dose and equivalent dose are numerically identical. In the case of alpha particles emitted within the body from inhaled or ingested material, the factor is 20 and an absorbed dose of 1 Gy corresponds to an equivalent dose of 20 Sv. Finally, it is necessary to recognise that the susceptibility of different tissues to the induction of malignancy is not the same. For example, the risk of fatal malignancy per Sv is greater for lung than the thyroid. To take account of these differences and the risk of serious hereditary effects, the equivalent dose is multiplied by a risk weighting factor for the different tissues, which can then be summed to give the *effective dose* (commonly abbreviated to 'dose'). A benefit of using the measure effective dose is that the risk to health for non-uniform distribution of equivalent dose in the body can be broadly expressed as a single number.

As the sievert is a relatively large dose of radiation, sub-multiples are commonly used. The microsievert is one-millionth of a sievert and the millisievert is one-thousandth of a sievert. The gray and sievert are Standard International (S.I.) units and earlier literature used the previous terminology of the rad (100 rad = 1 gray) for absorbed dose and the rem (100 rem = 1 sievert) for the equivalent dose.

Although radiation doses to individuals are generally of greatest interest, it is sometimes appropriate to have a measure of the total dose from a particular source to groups of people or a whole population. This total dose is expressed as the *collective effective dose* (commonly abbreviated to 'collective dose'). By analogy with man-hours, the collective dose is expressed in man sieverts (symbol man Sv) and is obtained by summing the average effective dose to each group multiplied by the number of people in that group. For illustration, as will be seen shortly, the average annual effective dose from natural background radiation to inhabitants of the United Kingdom is 2200 microsieverts. As the population of the United Kingdom is about 56 million, the collective dose for the population is the product of these numbers and is thus about 123,000 man Sv. However, it is important to recognise that, although the collective dose would be the same for a population half this size and receiving twice the average dose, the personal risk to these individuals would obviously be doubled.

Effects of ionising radiation on health

Soon after the discovery of X-rays by Roentgen in 1895 and of radioactivity by Becquerel in the following year, the harmful effects of radiation were noticed. The effects are dependent on the dose, dose-rate and tissues exposed, as summarised in Table 10.4.

Table 10.4:   *Principal harmful radiation effects: conditions for occurrence and sources of information*

Effect	Condition	Information
Early	Very high dose and dose rate:	Human data from various sources
Death	to much of body	
Erythema	to area of skin	
Sterility	to testes and ovaries	
Late Malignant diseases	Any dose or dose rate. Probability depends on dose. Manifested years later.	Risk data for humans by linear extrapolation from high doses and dose rates. Various sensitivities of organs
Hereditary defects	Any dose or dose rate. Probability depends on dose. Manifested in descendants.	Risk data for humans by inference from mouse data.
Non-malignant changes	Very high dose. Various times to manifestation.	Human data from various sources
Developmental changes	Irradiation of embryo. Manifested after birth.	Limited human data

Source: Living with Radiation. The National Radiological Protection Board, 1989 edition.

Early effects

Early effects are associated with exposure to high dose and dose-rates. At the extreme, an absorbed dose of 5 Gy or more to the whole-body delivered almost instantaneously is liable to be fatal because of acute damage to the gastro-intestinal, erythropoietic and central nervous systems. Brief exposure of a limited area of the body to a very large dose may be sub-lethal but some early effects may be generated. Whole-body doses of about 1 to 3 Gy may create the symptoms of acute radiation sickness, including vomiting, diarrhoea and epilation but with a substantial probability of survival. Exposure of the skin to an almost instantaneous absorbed dose of 5 Gy would probably produce erythema within about a week and more serious damage would result with higher doses. Such doses to the testes or ovaries would be liable to cause sterility.

However, with whole-body doses rather less than 1 Gy or larger total doses received more protractedly, no early signs of injury may be apparent but may be manifested much later as malignancy or hereditary effects in offspring.

Late effects

The two most important late effects of radiation are the induction of malignant disease and hereditary effects.

In studies of groups of people, such as the Japanese survivors of atomic bombing and others, a greater incidence of various malignant disease was recorded in those exposed to relatively high doses of radiation some years previously. From these data, risk factors have been derived by UNSCEAR and the International Commission on Radiological Protection (ICRP), relating the excess of fatal cancers to the radiation dose received. Importantly, it is further assumed that there is no threshold below which fatal cancer might not be induced by radiation. The number of cancers increase with increasing radiation dose.

Clearly, these risk factors are based on relatively high doses received in a short period of time. Whereas, in the normal course of events, relatively small doses are received over longer periods. It would seem reasonable to expect reduced risks in the latter circumstances and indeed there is substantial evidence, at least for beta, X and gamma radiation that the risk is less at low doses and low dose rates. The risk factors, recently revised by ICRP, are expressed as a mathematical probability, for example 1 in 20 per Sv (or 5×10^{-2} Sv^{-1}) incorporate a dose and dose rate effectiveness factor of 2 to make some allowance for this effect.

Similar considerations apply to hereditary effects. However, in human offspring there has been no conclusive evidence for hereditary defects attributable to exposure from natural or artificial radiation. The Japanese data failed to show statistically significant increases in hereditary defects but these negative findings, representing an upper estimate, together with animal data, were used by ICRP to estimate a risk factor for serious hereditary damage in humans. When all generations subsequent to a radiation exposure during reproductive life are taken into account, the value of the risk factor for severe hereditary effects is about 1 in 100 per Sv (or $1 \times 10^{-2}\,Sv^{-1}$).

To maintain proper perspectives it is important to recognise corollaries arising from the basic assumption of a proportional relationship between dose and risk, without a threshold. It implies that exposure to any dose of radiation, no matter how small, carries some risk. Consequently, even the smallest additional risks to a population will inevitably lead to a prediction of some associated deaths or hereditary effects which can be alarming. For example, a very small increase (of 20 microsieverts, about 1 per cent of the average annual dose from natural background radiation) in the average dose to a population would give a calculated additional risk of only 1 in a million, but for the United Kingdom (population of 56 million) would lead to a prediction of 56 attributable cancer deaths and in other European countries (population 650 million) 650 attributable cancer deaths. It is sometimes necessary to remember that even for a fatal risk of 1 in 10,000, there is a probability of 99.99 per cent that death will occur from some other cause.

Radiation doses to the general public in perspective

The principal sources of radiation exposure to the general public include natural background radiation, medical exposures and discharges from the nuclear industry.

Natural background radiation arises from extra-terrestrial cosmic rays and through naturally radioactive elements in the earth's crust, notably uranium, thorium and potassium-40. Uranium occurs in soil and rock in concentrations varying from a few parts per million (ppm) to more than 1000 ppm. Uranium-238 is the parent of a long chain of radioactive daughters of several elements. The decay products include the alpha-emitting radioactive gas radon (radon-222), some of which escapes to the atmosphere continuing decay to radioactive daughters. Polonium-210 is another natural alpha-emitting decay product and has a radiotoxicity similar to that of plutonium-239. Thorium is similarly distributed in the earth and radon-220 (called thoron) is akin to radon-222, being a daughter product of thorium-232. Potassium comprises 2.4 per cent by weight of the earth's crust and naturally radioactive potassium-40 in turn constitutes 120 ppm of the stable element. Consequently, the public is exposed to *external radiation* from cosmic rays and gamma rays from radioactivity in the earth and to *internal radiation* through inhalation of radon, thoron and their daughter products and also through ingestion of foodstuffs and water incorporating natural radioactivity.

The primary source of medical exposures for the public as a whole is through diagnostic X-ray examinations, being much more common than radiotherapy procedures and outweighing the greater individual dose of the latter.

Discharges of radioactive waste from the nuclear industry occur at various stages of the fuel cycle; fuel preparation, reactor operation and fuel processing. However, fuel processing at Sellafield, Cumbria, England is the principal contributor to the population dose from waste discharges, particularly discharges of caesium-137, plutonium-239 and americium-241. However, the routes of exposure are essentially identical to those associated with natural background radiation.

Experience suggests that the public (and the media) has little if any concern about natural background and, indeed, medical exposures but other man-made exposures attract such epithets as 'deadly'. It is important to establish if these perceptions and the priorities given to protection of the public from these sources are correct.

Average exposures

Figure 10.4, published by the National Radiological Protection Board (NRPB) shows that, for the general public, about 87% of the annual radiation dose is attributable to natural sources (primarily radon and its daughter products), about 12% is due to medical exposures and less than 0.1% is associated with nuclear discharges. This situation is clearly at variance with public perception. Expressed differently, the average annual dose due to natural background is about 2200 units (a unit being one micro-sievert), the corresponding dose from medical exposures is about 300 units and that from nuclear waste discharges less than 1 unit, giving a total of some 2501 units. If discharges from the nuclear industry disappeared overnight, the average annual dose would only decrease from 2501 units to 2500 units, which is scarcely a major reduction. However, these are average exposures and it is also necessary to consider the range of exposures of the general public from each of these sources.

Range of exposures

The range of annual doses to the public from natural background and radioactive waste discharges is illustrated in the bar chart Figure 10.5 together with the average for medical exposures.

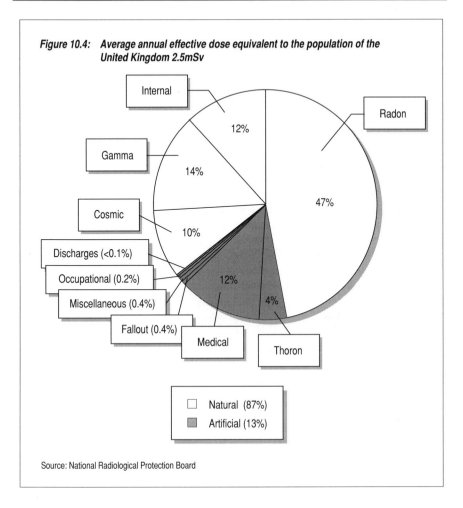

Figure 10.4: Average annual effective dose equivalent to the population of the United Kingdom 2.5mSv

Internal — 12%

Radon — 47%

Gamma — 14%

Cosmic — 10%

Discharges (<0.1%)

Occupational (0.2%)

Miscellaneous (0.4%) — 12%

Fallout (0.4%)

Medical

Thoron — 4%

☐ Natural (87%)
▨ Artificial (13%)

Source: National Radiological Protection Board

Again, by far the largest exposures are attributable to natural background with doses ranging from 1000 units (1 mSv) up to 100,000 units (100 mSv), and again, primarily attributable to radon and its daughters. About 6,000 members of the public are exposed to more than the current annual dose limit for occupational workers of 50,000 units (50 mSv) compared to less than 50 occupational workers (primarily non-coal miners) in that situation. Similarly, only about 9000 workers receive occupational annual doses exceeding 5000 units (5 mSv) compared with about 600,000 members of the public due to natural background. The average annual dose in Cornwall is about three times greater than that for Britain as a whole. However, only some £200,000 per annum is spent in studying radon exposures. Discretionary grants of up to about £1,000 are available for remedial work on a dwelling to reduce radon levels but only if the exposure of its occupants is likely to exceed an 'action limit' of 20,000 units (20 mSv) per year (now being reduced to 10,000 units (10 mSv) per year).

As indicated earlier, the routes of exposure for the general public due to the nuclear industry are directly analogous to those from natural background; external

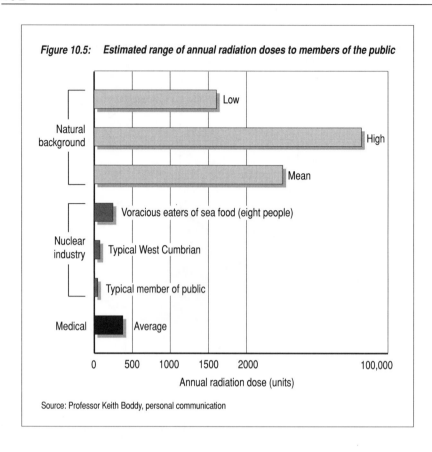

Figure 10.5:   Estimated range of annual radiation doses to members of the public

Source: Professor Keith Boddy, personal communication

radiation, inhalation and ingestion. However, as Figure 10.5 shows, both the range and magnitude of exposures are much smaller. For one 'critical group' near Sellafield, Cumbria, which comprises a group of about eight voracious consumers of seafood (particularly winkles), the associated annual dose would be equivalent to about 190 units (microsieverts). For other residents of the locality working in the fishing industry, the corresponding annual dose would be about 30 units whilst for a typical resident of West Cumbria it would be about 3 units per year. Background radiation is not above average and the annual dose attributable to discharges for such an individual would be similar to that from spending only a couple of hours in areas of Devon and Cornwall at the Action Limit. The monitoring programme carried out by British Nuclear Fuels Limited (BNFL) costs in the region of £2.5 million per year and probably about the same for other nuclear establishments and authorising departments taken together. Discharges of alpha and beta emitters from Sellafield have been reduced dramatically from the unnecessarily high levels of the 1970s with an associated reduction in exposures to the critical groups. Currently, levels of naturally radioactive potassium in fish exceed those of caesium-137 and doses from natural polonium-210 in winkles exceed those from plutonium and americium. Coincidentally, the additional dose for a regular air traveller, in this case as a result of increased exposure to cosmic rays, is practically identical to that of the heavy consumers of seafood in West Cumbria referred to earlier. In this context, a regular air traveller is someone who travels once per week between Newcastle upon Tyne and London, England and back or equivalent.

Of course, accidental releases represent a further potential source of radiation exposure for the general public. The unforgivable accident at Chernobyl in 1986 had major health consequences for those workers who were involved in the incident itself and in the subsequent clearing up operations. There were also major social consequences for many members of the public who were evacuated from their homes; to which some will probably never return. Nevertheless, and despite considerable uncertainty, some perspectives on the radiation doses to the public can be derived. The villagers in Pripyat, closest to the site and evacuated first, received effective doses on average estimated at about 28 per cent of their lifetime dose due to natural background but obviously over a much shorter period. In the 30 km zone, where the population was evacuated rather later, the average dose was greater, about the same as their lifetime dose from background. Some members of the public received almost ten times the average dose, the effect of which would have been to increase their cancer risk from about 22% to 22.1%. In the Western Soviet Union, about 4% of the background dose was received by 75 million people but, as pointed out earlier, this small additional individual risk leads to a prediction of 3000 attributable cancer deaths in such a large population (of which about 16 million will die naturally from cancer). In the United Kingdom, it has been estimated that, over the fifty years following the accident, the average individual dose will amount to 46 microsieverts which is about 2 per cent of the average dose received from natural background every year. The effect of the additional exposure to the United Kingdom population would be a small increase in the cancer risk from 22% to 22.00005%. To provide a further perspective, for the 90,000 people near Pripyat who received double the background dose, there are about 60,000 people in Devon and Cornwall who receive six times that dose annually.

However, it must be recognised that these perspectives apply to the reported effective doses and are dependent on their accuracy. For more local populations, the intake of released radioiodine resulted in greater doses to the thyroid gland with an increased incidence of thyroid cancer already having been observed. In any case, the perspectives presented here are no excuse whatsoever why such a disgraceful accident ever happened.

Figure 10.4 illustrates that by far the greatest source of exposure to man-made radiation for the general public as a whole, arises from medical diagnostic procedures. However, in contrast to the nuclear industry, monitoring is far less extensive and costs only about £200,000 per year. Although the number of examinations per thousand of the population per year is less in Britain than in most comparable countries, there is an increasing number of radiographs undertaken per year. The best dose reduction measure is to eliminate all unnecessary radiographs, including repeats. Relatively low cost improvements can produce dose savings of 15% using a carbon fibre couch top (£800), savings of 7% using a carbon fibre cassette (from £67) and savings of 25% using a carbon fibre grid cover (£55). Selective replacement of medical equipment, at a total cost of £150 million over 15 years, would reduce exposure of the public by 3400 population dose units (man-sieverts). In contrast, BNFL is currently spending £500 million to reduce doses further. Yet, stopping discharges entirely would reduce the population dose by only

30 population dose units (man-sieverts). It will be self-evident which of these measures is cost-effective and which is not.

Non-ionising radiation

Non-ionising radiation is radiation that does not produce ionisation in matter. Non-ionising radiation is of two types: optical (ultra violet, visible and infrared) and electromagnetic fields (microwave, radio frequency and extremely low frequency). Radiations are described in terms of their wavelengths or frequency. For convenience, optical and microwave radiations can be considered as packets of energy (photons) travelling through space. Radio frequency and extremely low frequency fields can be considered as time varying electric and magnetic fields moving through space in wave like patterns.

Harmful effects

The harmful effects of non-ionizing radiations are of three main types: photochemical, thermal and electrical effects. Examples of adverse photochemical effects are ultraviolet induced sunburn and snow blindness. There is good evidence that ultraviolet radiation especially can cause non-malignant skin cancer. Cutaneous malignant melanoma is much less common but of considerable public health concern, because of its serious nature and its rapid increase during the last few decades. Although direct evidence of a link with ultraviolet radiation is absent, there is epidemiological evidence that short term, intermittent exposure to high levels of solar ultraviolet radiation, especially at an early age may be a contributory factor in the causation of cutaneous malignant melanoma. Risks are likely to be increased through the effects of depletion of the ozone layer.

The longer wavelengths in infrared and microwave regions of the non-ionizing spectrum produce thermal injury. Intense sources of optical and infrared radiations, such as lasers, also produce thermal burning. The lens of the eye lacks a direct blood supply and is therefore more susceptible to injury from heat. Hence, infrared and microwave radiation can produce cataracts. Exposure to intense electro magnetic fields can result in shock and burns. Epidemiological studies of occupational and population exposures to various electrical and magnetic sources have suggested associations with a variety of health effects. These include various cancers, miscarriages and fetal abnormalities. The evidence is still inconclusive but warrants further investiation.

ENVIRONMENTAL PROTECTION

Measures to protect and improve the quality of the environment are contained in the Environmental Protection Act 1990 and in a number of other pieces of legislation, relating particularly to the role and responsibilities of the local authority.

The Department of the Environment is the Government department with overall responsibility for coordinating and implementing environmental protection. There are a number of inspectorial and standards enforcement bodies (in particular Her Majesty's Inspectorate of Pollution, the National Rivers Authority, the Health and Safety Executive and local authorities).

The Government is also advised by a separate body on the impact of natural and man-made radiation on human health. The Committee on Medical Aspects of Radiation in the Environment (COMARE) was established following an enquiry into the incidence of childhood leukaemia in the mid 1980s near to Sellafield. It produces regular publications and technical reports. In addition, there are many other advisory groups and working parties which advise Government on radioactivity in relation to the environment.

Her Majesty's Inspectorate of Pollution (HMIP) has overall responsibility for control of the most polluting industrial processes which may contaminate any aspect of the physical environment. It runs a control system known as integrated pollution control (IPC). Now also included in the HMIP role is the Radiochemical Inspectorate.

The National Rivers Authority (NRA) has powers and responsibility for managing water resources. It monitors water quality and assesses the extent to which water quality standards are being achieved, taking enforcement action where necessary.

Local authorities have wide-ranging powers and responsibilities concerning environmental protection. These relate to air quality, pollution control, toxic substances, waste, noise, nuisances, pests and vermin, dog control and litter. At a day to day level much of this work is carried out by environmental health officers who also have responsibilities in relation to communicable disease control and food hygiene.

Britain is now subject to a great deal of environmental protection legislation produced by the European Commission (EC). For example, Directives cover drinking water, bathing water, air quality, larger combustion plants and hazardous waste.

CONCLUSIONS

The importance of the relationship between the quality of the physical environment and people's health has long been recognised. Moreover, in recent years, there have been a number of major incidents around the world which have all too dramatically highlighted some of the contemporary threats and hazards both to the well being of individuals and to the planet itself. With the current growth in interest and rapidly rising concerns about wider environmental issues, the future will see the current focus on environment and health evolving to the point when they become inextricably linked. One of the important roles of public health will be to promote this wider view of health as well as establishing measures to protect populations from the adverse impact of specific environmental hazards.

References

CHAPTER 1

1. Hunt S M, McKenna S P, McEwan J, Backett E M, Williams J, Papp E. A quantitative approach to perceived health status: a validation study. Journal of Epidemiology and Community Health, 1990; 34: 281.

CHAPTER 3

1. Vallery Radot R. The life of Pasteur, London: Constable, 1902.
2. Lalonde M. A new perspective on the health of Canadians. A working document. Ottawa: Information Canada, 1974.
3. U.S. Surgeon General. Healthy People: The Surgeon General's report on health promotion and disease prevention. Washington DC: Department of Health, Education and Welfare (PHS 79: 55071), 1979.
4. World Health Organisation. Targets for health for all: targets in support of the European regional strategy for health for all. Copenhagen: World Health Organisation, Regional Office for Europe, 1985.
5. Secretary of State for Health. The Health of the Nation: a strategy for health in England. HMSO, 1992 (Cm 1986).
6. Wilson J M G, Jungner G. The principles and practice of screening for disease. Public Health Papers, 34. Geneva: World Health Organisation, 1968.
7. Shapiro S. Evidence of screening for breast cancer from a randomised trial. Cancer 1977; 39: 2772–82.
8. Breast Cancer Screening. Report to the Health Ministers of England, Wales, Scotland and Northern Ireland by a working group chaired by Sir Patrick Forrest. London: HMSO, 1987.
9. Department of Health and Social Security. Inequalities in health: report of a research working group (The Black Report). London: HMSO, 1980.
10. Townsend P, Phillimore P, Beattie A. Deprivation and health: inequality and the north. Beckenham: Croom Helm, 1987.

CHAPTER 4

1. Donabedian A. Explorations in quality assessment and monitoring. Vol 1. The definition of quality and approaches to its assessment. Ann Arbor, MI: Health Administration Press, 1980.
2. Department of Health and Social Security. Medical audit. Working paper 6. London: HMSO, 1989.
3. Buck N, Devlin H B, Lunn J N. The report of a confidential enquiry into perioperative deaths. London: Nuffield Provincial Hospitals Trust, Kings Fund, 1988.
4. Deming W E. Out of the crisis. Cambridge: Cambridge University Press, 1986.
5. Juran J M. Managerial breakthrough. New York: McGraw-Hill, 1964.
6. Berwick D. Continuous improvement as an ideal in health care. New England Journal of Medicine 1989: 320: 53–56
7. Department of Health. The Patient's Charter. London: HMSO, 1991.

CHAPTER 5

1. World Health Organisation. International Classification of Impairments, Disabilities and Handicaps. Geneva: World Health Organisation, 1980.

CHAPTER 6

1. Health for all children: a programme for child health surveillance. The report of a joint working party on child health surveillance. Hall DMB (Ed). Oxford: Oxford University Press, 1989.

CHAPTER 7

1. Faris R E L, Dunham H W. Mental disorders in urban areas: an ecological study of schizophrenia and other psychoses. Chicago: University of Chicago Press, 1939.
2. Hollingshead A B, Redlich F C. Social class and mental illness. New York: John Wiley, 1958.

Index